Level Set Method in Medical Imaging Segmentation

Level Set Method in Medical Imaging Segmentation

Authored by

AYMAN EL-BAZ AND JASJIT S. SURI

CRC Press
Taylor & Francis Group
Boca Raton London New York

CRC Press is an imprint of the
Taylor & Francis Group, an informa business

CRC Press
Taylor & Francis Group
6000 Broken Sound Parkway NW, Suite 300
Boca Raton, FL 33487-2742

First issued in paperback 2023

ISBN 13: 978-1-03-265306-8 (pbk)
ISBN 13: 978-1-138-55345-3 (hbk)
ISBN 13: 978-1-315-14859-5 (ebk)

DOI: 10.1201/b22435

Library of Congress Cataloging-in-Publication Data

Names: El-Baz, Ayman S., editor. | Suri, Jasjit S. editor.
Title: Level set method in medical imaging segmentation / [edited by] Ayman El-Baz and Jasjit S. Suri.
Description: Boca Raton : Taylor & Francis, 2019. | Includes bibliographical references.
Identifiers: LCCN 2019005809 | ISBN 9781138553453 (hardback : alk. paper) | ISBN 9781315148595 (ebook)
Subjects: | MESH: Image Interpretation, Computer-Assisted—methods | Image Processing, Computer-Assisted—methods | Mathematical Computing
Classification: LCC RC78.7.D53 | NLM WN 182 | DDC 616.07/54—dc23
LC record available at https://lccn.loc.gov/2019005809

Visit the Taylor & Francis Web site at
http://www.taylorandfrancis.com

and the CRC Press Web site at
http://www.crcpress.com

With love and affection to my mother and father,
whose loving spirit sustains me still

Ayman El-Baz

To my late loving parents, my wife, and loving children

Jasjit S. Suri

Contents

Preface

In the medical imaging field, accurate segmentation of structures is crucial in many applications; for example, in detecting lesions and abnormalities. However, segmentation is highly challenging due to such factors as the low contrast between different tissues types that makes it difficult to even segment the desired object manually, and the motion artifacts associated with the scans which adds noise to images. This book covers the state-of-the-art approaches for medical imaging segmentation based on the level set technique that was implemented by Osher and Sethian. The level set technique mainly relies on the theory of curve and surface evolution, in addition to the link between front propagation and hyperbolic conservation laws. This makes it easy to follow shapes that change topology.

Among numerical techniques, level sets are significantly powerful at interpreting interface motion. Level set methods have provided great advances to clinicians in assessing abnormalities through computer-aided diagnostic (CAD) systems that can analyze images from these different modalities; for example computed tomography (CT), magnetic resonance imaging (MRI), and optical coherence tomography (OCT). Different modalities will be discussed in this book for different applications.

In summary, the main aim of this book is to survey an illustrative subset of past and current applications of level set technique in medical imaging segmentation. It focuses on major trends and challenges in this area, identifies new techniques and presents their use in biomedical image analysis.

Ayman El-Baz
Jasjit S. Suri

Biographies

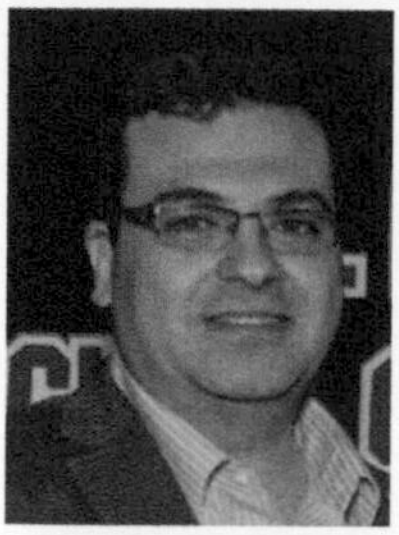

Ayman El-Baz is a professor, university scholar, and Chair of the Bioengineering Department at the University of Louisville, Kentucky. Dr. El-Baz earned his B.Sc. and M.Sc. degrees in electrical engineering in 1997 and 2001, respectively. He earned his Ph.D. in electrical engineering from the University of Louisville in 2006. In 2009, Dr. El-Baz was named a Coulter Fellow for his contributions to the field of biomedical translational research. Dr. El-Baz has 17 years of hands-on experience in the fields of bio-imaging modeling and non-invasive computer-assisted diagnosis systems. He has authored or coauthored more than 500 technical articles (133 journals, 25 books, 57 book chapters, 212 refereed-conference papers, 143 abstracts, and 27 US patents and disclosures).

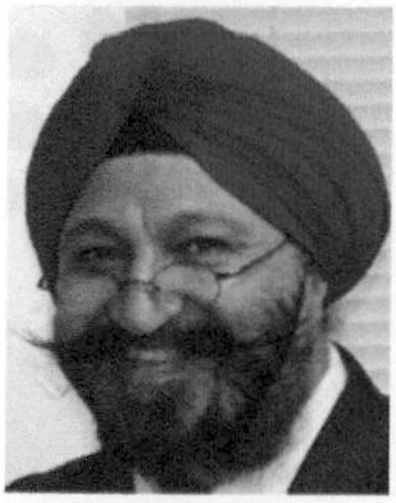

Jasjit S. Suri is an innovator, scientist, visionary, industrialist and an internationally known world leader in biomedical engineering. Dr. Suri has spent over 25 years in the field of biomedical engineering/devices and its management. He received his Ph.D. from the University of Washington, Seattle and his Business Management Sciences degree from Weatherhead, Case Western Reserve University, Cleveland, Ohio. Dr. Suri was awarded the President's Gold medal in 1980 and made Fellow of the American Institute of Medical and Biological Engineering for his outstanding contributions. In 2018, he was awarded the Marquis Life Time Achievement Award for his outstanding contributions and dedication to medical imaging and its management.

Acknowledgements

The completion of this book could not have been possible without the participation and assistance of many people; all of whose names may not be enumerated. Their contributions are sincerely appreciated and gratefully acknowledged. However, the editors would like to express their deep appreciation and indebtedness particularly to Dr. Ali H. Mahmoud and Ahmed ElTanboly for their endless support.

Ayman El-Baz
Jasjit S. Suri

Contributors

Sebastian Bautista
Computer Science Department
Engineering School, Universidad de Cuenca
Cuenca, Ecuador

Tien D. Bui
Department of Computer Science and Software Engineering
Concordia University
Montréal, Quebec

Elisabetta Carlini
Mathematics Department, "Sapienza"
University of Rome
Rome, Italy

Yuncheng Du
Department of Chemical and Biomolecular Engineering
Clarkson University
Potsdam, New York

Dongping Du
Department of Industrial, Manufacturing, and System Engineering
Texas Tech University
Lubbock, Texas

Ahmed ElTanboly
Bioimaging Laboratory, University of Louisville
Louisville, Kentucky

Magdi El-Azab
Department of Engineering Mathematics
Mansoura University
Mansoura, Egypt

Ayman El-Baz
Department of Bioengineering
University of Louisville
Louisville, Kentucky

Maurizio Falcone
Mathematics Department, "Sapienza"
University of Rome
Rome, Italy

Bin Fang
Department of Computer Science
Chongqing University
Chongqing, China

Jiangxiong Fang
Department of Measure and Control
East China University of Technology
Nanchang, China

Aly A. Farag
Electrical and Computer Engineering Department
University of Louisville
Louisville, Kentucky

Roberto Ferretti
Mathematics Department "Sapienza"
University of Rome
Rome, Italy

Thomas Fevens
Department of Computer Science and Software Engineering
Concordia University
Montréal, Quebec

Mohammed Ghazal
Department of Electrical and Computer Engineering
Abu Dhabi University
Abu Dhabi, UAE
and
Bioengineering Department
University of Louisville
Louisville, Kentucky

Deepak K. Ghodgaonkar
RF Lab, DA-IICT
Gandhinagar, Gujarat
India

Hassan Hajjdiab
Department of Electrical and Computer Engineering
Abu Dhabi University
Abu Dhabi, UAE

Robert Keynton
Bioengineering Department
University of Louisville
Louisville, Kentucky

Alexandra La Cruz
GBBA
Universidad Simón Bolívar
Caracas, Venezuela

Laquan Li
School of Automation
Huazhong University of Science and Technology
Wuhan, China

Ali Mahmoud
Bioengineering Department
University of Louisville
Louisville, Kentucky

Ruben Medina
Biomedical Engineering Group (GIBULA)
Electronics and Communications Department
Universidad de Los Andes
Merida, Venezuela

Villie Morocho
Computer Science Department
Engineering School, Universidad de Cuenca
Cuenca, Ecuador

Hossam Abd El Munim
Computer and Systems Engineering Department
Ain Shams University
Cairo, Egypt

Padmasini N
Department of Biomedical Engineering
Rajalakshmi Engineering College
Chennai, India

Hardik N. Patel
RF Lab, DA-IICT
Gandhinagar, Gujarat
India

Françoise Peyrin
Creatis Laboratory
INSA-Lyon
University of Lyon
Lyon, France

Ahmed Shalaby
Bioengineering Department
University of Louisville
Louisville, Kentucky

Mohamed Yacin Sikkandar
Department of Medical Equipment Technology
CAMS
Majmaah University
Kingdom of Saudi Arabia

Manavi D Sindal
Senior Consultant
Vitreo-Retina Services
Aravind Eye Hospital
Pondicherry, India

Bruno Sixou
Creatis Laboratory
INSA-Lyon
University of Lyon
Lyon, France

Jasjit S. Suri
Global Biomedical Technologies, Inc.
Roseville, California
and
AtheroPoint LLC
Roseville, California
and
Department of Electrical Engineering
Idaho State University
Pocatello, Idaho

Shaghayegh Taheri
Department of Computer Science and Software Engineering
Concordia University
Montréal, Quebec

Umamaheswari R
Department of Electrical and Electronics Engineering
Velammal Engineering College
Chennai, India

Lin Wang
Creatis Laboratory
INSA-Lyon
University of Lyon
Lyon, France

Shenhai Zheng
Department of Computer Science
Chongqing University
Chongqing, China

1

Tomography Reconstructions With Stochastic Level-Set Methods

Bruno Sixou, Lin Wang, and Françoise Peyrin

CONTENTS

1.1 Introduction

The level-set methods are now a well-known tool for the computation of evolving boundaries since their introduction by Osher and Sethian [1]. They have been designed newly to reconstruct solutions of inverse problems with non-smooth and piecewise constant solutions [2–4]. The numerical results indicate their sucess. Yet, inverse problems with piecewise constant solution are non-convex and the reconstructed solution is a local minimum of the regularization functional. It may be interesting to escape this local minimum with global optimization methods. Stochastic algorithms based on stochastic differential equations have been proposed for the global optimization of non-convex functions [5–9]. Let $(\Omega, \mathcal{F}, P)$ be a probability space, in order to obtain the global minimum of a function $g : \mathbb{R}^m \rightarrow \mathbb{R}^m$, a random trajectory $X(t)$ governed by the following diffusion process is often used [5–9]:

$$dX(t) = -\nabla g(X(t))dt + \mu(t)dW(t) \tag{1.1}$$

where $W = (W_1(t), \ldots, W_m(t))$ is the standard m-dimensional Brownian motion and $\mu(t)$ the noise strength. For an appropriate annealing schedule $\mu(t)$ and under appropriate condition on g, the probability law of $X(t)$ converges weakly to a probability law which has its support on the set of the global minimizers of g [5–9]. In the field of image processing, stochastic partial differential equations applied to level-set functions have been used for segmentation tasks [10]. The right way to study stochastic evolutions in the level-set framework is through the Stratonovich integral so that evolution of the boundary curve is independent of the level-set function used for its representation [10]. The aim of this chapter is to show that this type of approach can be generalized to inverse problems with piecewise constant solutions.

In the first section, we summarize some results about stochastic calculus and the level-set regularization of inverse problems. Then, the stochastic level-set approach is applied to the binary tomography and to the phase contrast tomography inverse problem.

1.2 Preliminaries

In this first section, we present the level-set regularization approach of inverse problems and some aspects of stochastic calculus.

1.2.1 Level-Set Regularization of Inverse Problems

In this section, we detail the level-set regularization approach of inverse problems. Let $R : H_1 \to H_2$, a linear operator mapping two Hilbert spaces H_1 and H_2, and $g \in H_2$. Our aim is to find a piecewise constant solution f of the inverse problem:

$$Rf = g \tag{1.2}$$

For Ω a bounded Lipschitz open subset in $\mathbb{R}^2$, we assume that the function to be reconstructed f is the characteristic function of a regular set $\Omega_1 \subset \Omega$, $f = \chi_{\Omega_1}$. It can be represented with the Heaviside distribution and with a level-set function $\theta \in H_1(\Omega)$ as $f = H(\theta)$, where $H_1(\Omega)$ is the first-order Sobolev space and with $H(\theta) = 1$ if $\theta > 0$ and 0 otherwise.

Assuming that the noisy data are such that $\|g^\delta - g\| \leq \delta$, where δ is the noise level, the reconstruction problem becomes nonlinear and consists in determining the level-set function θ minimizing the regularization functional:

$$E(\theta) = \frac{\|RH(\theta) - g^\delta\|_2^2}{2} + F(\theta) \tag{1.3}$$

where F is a regularization term for the level-set function. We have considered here a Total Variation-H_1 regularization functional [2,3]:

$$F(\theta) = \beta_1 |H(\theta)|_{TV} + \beta_2 \|\theta\|_{H_1}^2 \tag{1.4}$$

where $|.|_{TV}$ is the Total Variation semi-norm. The regularization parameters β_1, β_2 determine the relative weights of the stabilizing terms.

Since H is discontinuous, it is necessary to consider generalized minimizers of the regularization functional [2, 3]. These minimizers can be approximated by minimizers of smoothed regularization functional with an approximation H_ϵ. The following smooth approximations of the Heaviside function H has been used $H_\epsilon(x) = \frac{1+2\epsilon}{2}(erf(x/\epsilon) + 1) - \epsilon$ where ϵ is a real positive constant. The smoothed regularization functional is given by:

$$E_\epsilon(\theta) = \frac{\|RH_\epsilon(\theta) - g^\delta\|_2^2}{2} + \beta_1 |H_\epsilon(\theta)|_{TV} + \beta_2 \|\theta\|_{H_1}^2 \tag{1.5}$$

The minimizers of the Tikhonov functionals are found with a first-order optimality condition for the smoothed functionals, $E'_\epsilon(\theta) = 0$, with:

$$E'_\epsilon(\theta) = H'_\epsilon R^* \left(RH_\epsilon(\theta) - g^\delta\right) + \beta_2 (I - \Delta)(\theta) + \beta_1 \frac{\partial |H_\epsilon(\theta)|_{TV}}{\partial \theta} \tag{1.6}$$

where R^* denotes the adjoint of the forward operator. From the current estimate θ_k, the update $\theta_{k+1} = \theta_k + \delta\theta$ is obtained with a classical Gauss-Newton method with a linearization of the condition $G(\theta_k + \delta\theta) = 0$ [22].

This method can be generalized to nonlinear operators and R must be replaced by the Fréchet derivative of the direct operator. For high noise levels, the solution θ may be trapped in a local minima. In that case, the data term

$\|RH_\epsilon(\theta) - g^\delta\|$ at the end of the optimization is largely higher than the noise level δ and the many reconstruction errors are still present. In order to escape from these stationary points, we propose stochastic global optimization methods.

1.2.2 Some Notions of Stochastic Calculus

The stochastic evolution of the level-set function is based on the Stratonovich integral. In this first section, we summarize some useful notions of stochastic calculus [11,12]. We explain the difference between the Itô and Stratonovich stochastic integrals. Let $(\Omega, \mathcal{F}, \mathcal{F}_t, P)$ represent a probability space and $W_{t\geq 0}$ a one-dimensional Brownian motion. The paths of the Brownian motion are only $\frac{1}{2}$-Hölder continous and nowhere differentiable, and in order to define $dW(t)$, it is usual to start with the stochastic integral. Given a square integrable process $(\phi(s,\omega))_{s\geq 0}$ and a subdivision $\Delta = \{0 = t_1 < \dots . < t_n = t\}$, the stochastic Itô integral $\int_0^t \phi(s,\omega)dW(s)$ with respect to the Brownian motion is defined as the limit of the Riemann sum:

$$\sum_{1\leq i\leq n} \phi(t_i,\omega)(W(t_{i+1}) - W(t_i)) \tag{1.7}$$

when $|\Delta| = min|t_{i+1} - t_i| \to 0$. The limit obtained $\{I(\phi)\}_{t\geq 0}$ is a square integrable martingale. This definition can be extended to an arbitrary dimension.

Considering a process $X = (X_t)_{t\geq 0}$ and a smooth function α of class C^2, the process $Y_t = (\alpha(X_t))$ satisfies the Itô formula:

$$dY(t) = \alpha'(X(t))dt + \frac{1}{2}\alpha'' d < X, X > (t) \tag{1.8}$$

The drift term involves the quadratic variation $< X, X >$ of the process X which depends on the stochastic part of the dynamics. For a stochastic process, $X(t) = \int_0^t f(s)dW(s) + A(t)$, where f is a continuous square integrable function and $A(t)$ is continuous and increasing, the quadratic variation can be calculated as:

$$< X, X > (t) = \int_0^t f(s)^2 ds \tag{1.9}$$

It is possible to give another definition of the stochastic integral so that the classical chain rule is satisfied. Considering two processes $X(t) = M(t) + B(t)$, $Y(t) = N(t) + C(t)$ where M, N are local continuous martingales and B, C are increasing processes, the Stratonovich integral of Y with respect to X is given by the formula

$$\int_0^t Y(s) o dX(s) = \int_0^t Y(s)dX(s) + \frac{1}{2} < M, N > (t) \tag{1.10}$$

Then, it can be shown that the classical chain rule formula is satisfied [11,12]:

$$\alpha(X_t) = \alpha(X_0) + \int_0^t \alpha'(X(s)) o dX(s) \tag{1.11}$$

The principle of the stochastic level-set evolution framework is to transfer the contour evolution to the level-set function. The dynamics of the level-set contour should not be modified by a change of the level-set function. This invariance property is not guaranted by the Itô rule. If the Itô integral is replaced by the Stratonovich for the stochastic evolution, the additional drift term disappears and the invariance property is verified.

The Stratonovich evolution equation can be implemented with an implicit scheme. The Stratonovich integral with respect to the Brownian motion W can be approximated as:

$$\int_0^T Y(s) o dW(s) = \lim_{|\Delta|\to 0} \sum_{1\leq i\leq n} Y\left(\frac{t_i + t_{i+1}}{2}\right)(W(t_{i+1}) - W(t_i)) \tag{1.12}$$

with $W(t_{i+1}) - W(t_i) \sim \sqrt{(t_{i+1} + t_i)}\mathcal{N}(0,1)$, where $\mathcal{N}(0,1)$ is a Gaussian of standard deviation 1.

In [10], it was proposed to simulate the Stratonovich evolution with the Itô formalism and an additional drift term. Using the formula Eq. 1.10, it can be shown that, for a level-function θ:

$$\begin{aligned}|\nabla\theta(x,t)| o dW(t) &= |\nabla\theta(x,t)| dW(t)\\ &+ \frac{1}{2}(\Delta\theta(x,t) - |\nabla\theta(x,t)| div\left(\frac{\nabla\theta(x,t)}{|\nabla\theta(x,t)|}\right)\end{aligned} \tag{1.13}$$

This evolution equation has been used for image segmentation tasks leading to stochastic active contours [10]. It is the basis of the approaches presented in the following. Some proper type of solutions can be defined for these equations with stochastic viscosity solutions [10].

1.3 Binary Tomography Reconstructions of Bone Microstructure from Few Projections with Stochastic Level-Set Methods

1.3.1 The Binary Tomography Problem

The tomographic reconstruction from few projections is a very ill-posed problems with many applications in medical imaging or material science. The binary tomography methods can be used to set a simpler inverse problem [13]. The binary tomography problem can be formulated as an under-determined linear system of equations with the linear Radon projection operator R and binary constraints:

$$Rf = p^{\delta} \quad f = (f_1, \ldots\ldots f_n) \in \{0,1\}^n \tag{1.14}$$

relating the pixel values $(f_i)_{1\leq i\leq n}$ of the image and the noisy projection data p^{δ}. Very often it is assumed that the non-noisy projections p are corrupted by an additive Gaussian noise.

Various approaches have been investigated to solve this reconstruction problem [14, 15, 19, 20]. The minimization of a functional with a data term and a binary constraint may be performed with stochastic techniques [16] or convex analysis optimization [17, 18]. A variational method based on Total Variation regularization can also be used for this reconstruction problem [21–23].

Yet, the discrete tomography problem is non-convex and the reconstructed solution may be trapped in local minima of the regularization functional. The reconstruction errors are very often localized on the boundaries [22]. We use here stochastic level-set methods for the discrete tomography problem to improve the reconstruction obtained with a deterministic level-set scheme [22, 23]. The reconstruction results obtained with this new approach are compared with the ones obtained with the classical simulated annealing method [24–26] in terms of reconstruction quality and convergence speed.

1.3.2 Global Optimization with Stochastic Level-Set Evolution and Simulated Annealing

1.3.2.1 Stochastic Level-Set Evolution

We use here the level-set regularization and represent the function f with a level-set function θ, $f = H(\theta)$. Let Ω be the domain of the image to be reconstructed, we propose to improve the reconstruction image with the following stochastic partial differential equation for the level-set function θ, for $x \in \Omega$, given by:

$$d\theta(x,t) = \delta\theta(x,t) + \mu(t)|\nabla\theta(x,t)| o dW(t) \tag{1.15}$$

where o denotes the Stratanovich convention [12] and $\delta\theta$ is the gradient calculated as explained in Section II.A, Eq. 1.6.

As explained in Section II.B, using the definition of the Stratonovich integral, the equation can be transformed to get the following Itô stochastic differential equation:

$$d\theta(x,t) = \delta\theta + |\nabla\theta(x,t)| dW(t) + \frac{1}{2}\left(\Delta\theta(x,t) - |\nabla\theta(x,t)| div\left(\frac{\nabla\theta(x,t)}{|\nabla\theta(x,t)|}\right)\right) \tag{1.16}$$

The level-set and stochastic level-set schemes are applied successively on random time intervals. In the framework of the intermittent diffusion algorithm, the coefficient for the intermittent diffusion is defined as:

$$\mu(t) = \sum_j \mu_j I_{[S_j,T_j]}(t) \tag{1.17}$$

where $I_{[S_j,T_j]}$ is the characteristic function of the interval $[S_j, T_j]$. The time intervals length and the diffusion strengths μ_j are chosen at random in the range $[0, T]$ and $[0, \mu_{max}]$ where $\mu_{\max}$ is the scale for the diffusion strength and T is the scale for the diffusion time [8]. With probability arbitrarily close to 1, the intermittent diffusion method can find the global minimum of the regularization functional in a finite simulation time.

1.3.2.2 Classical Simulated Annealing

Simulated annealing methods are reviewed extensively in [24–26]. Let f_b be the binary reconstructed image, and U the data term $U = \|Rf_b - p^\delta\|$, our aim is to minimize the objective function U on a finite configuration space E which is the set of binary images:

$$E = \{f_b = (f_k)_{1\le k\le N} \quad f_k \in \{0,1\} \quad \forall k \in [1,N]\} \tag{1.18}$$

The classical simulated annealing algorithm is based on the definition of a Markov chain, $(f^n)_{n\in\mathbb{N}}$ on the finite state space E. Each point f^n in the state space is defined by the set $(f_k^n)_{0\le k\le N}$ of the pixel values. A stochastic search is performed on E with a "cooling down" algorithm. The boundary between the 0 and the 1 regions is first calculated with a Sobel filter. Then one pixel is selected at random on the boundary and is changed and this rule defines the neighborhood system $N(f_b)$ of a point $f_b \in E$:

$$g_b \in N(f_b) \iff \exists! k, f_k \neq g_k \tag{1.19}$$

It is thus possible to define a communication kernel $q_0(f, g)$, in which all the new states in the neighbourhood of f are equiprobable:

$$q_0(f_b, g_b) = \begin{cases} \frac{1}{|N(f_b)|} & \text{if} \quad g_b \in N(f_b) \\ 0 & \text{otherwise} \end{cases} \tag{1.20}$$

The classical simulated annealing algorithm defines an inhomogeneous Markov chain, with transitions constructed recursively as follows: $P(f^{n+1} = g|f^n = f) = q(f, g)$ with

$$q(f,g) = \begin{cases} q_0(f,g)exp(-\beta_n(U(g) - U(f))^+ & \text{if } g \neq f \\ 1 - \sum_{h\neq f} q(f,h) & \text{if } g = f \end{cases} \tag{1.21}$$

where [a]+=max(a,0), $(\beta_n)_{n\in\mathbb{N}}$ the cooling schedule, f^0 an arbitrary initial point.

From the current state f^n, a test image f_{test} is sampled randomly according to Eqs. 1.20 and 1.21. If $U(f_{test}) > U(f^n)$ the proposal f_{test} may be accepted. In the beginning of the simulation, the temperature is high and the state space is explored freely. As β increases, the images distribution is more and more concentrated around the minima of U [24–26]. Under some restricting conditions on the cooling schedule, the convergence towards the global minimum is obtained by the convergence rate may be very slow. Several techniques have been used to speed up the simulated annealing method but the modifications are rather empirical [27, 28] and the results obtained seems to be very dependent on the complexity of the objective function. They will not be considered here.

1.3.3 Comparison of the Algorithms: Results and Discussion

1.3.3.1 Simulation Details

The simulated annealing algorithm and stochastic level-set methods have applied to simulated projections of an experimental bone cross-section acquired with synchrotron micro-CT (voxel size:15 μm) [29]. Figure 1.1 displays the 256×256 bone cross-section f^* reconstructed from 400 projections with 400 rays per projections with Filtered Back Projection (FBP). The discrete approximation of the Radon transform is the operator implemented in the Matlab Toolbox.

First, the deterministic level-set scheme regularization is applied. To obtain a good accuracy, the ϵ was set to $\epsilon = 0.03$. The initial level-set function chosen is $\theta_0 = 0$. The regularization parameters were chosen to obtain the best decrease of the regularization functional. The iterations are stopped when the iterates stagnate, $\| f_{k+1} - f_k \|_2 < 0.01$. At the end of this first optimization step,

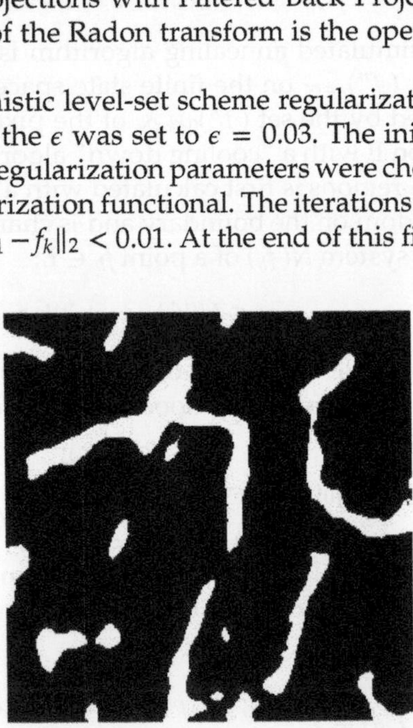

FIGURE 1.1
Reconstruction of the bone cross-section from 400 projections with the FBP algorithm. The bone fraction is 14.20%.

the Morozov discrepancy principle [30] is not satisfied. The discrepancy term is much higher than the noise level, $||p^\delta - Rf|| >> \delta$. This image is the initial image used for the application of the stochastic algorithms. For the simulated annealing algorithm, the initial temperature value is chosen so that most transitions are accepted, with an acceptance ratio around 0.8.

For the simulation of Eq. 1.16, we use an explicit scheme with finite differences, the WENO scheme with $\Delta x = 0.5$ and $\Delta t = 0.1$. The noise strength μ and the number of iterations T are chosen randomly with a uniform distribution in $[0.01, 0.1]$ and $[1, 100]$. A binary image is then obtained by thresholding and a signed distance is then used for reinitializations before the stochastic level-set step. The optimization method was applied for M equally spaced noisy projections, with $M = 10$ and $M = 15$, with $N = 367$ rays per projections and with a Gaussian noise added to the projections with a standard deviation $\sigma_p = 3$ (PSNR=20 dB) and $\sigma_p = 6.5$ (PSNR=7 dB). The noise level δ can estimated by $\delta = \sqrt{MN}\sigma_p$.

1.3.3.2 Numerical Results

The reconstructed cross-sections obtained with 10 projections and 367 rays per projection, for the standard deviation $\sigma_p = 3$ after the level-set algorithm and after the stochastic level-set algorithm are displayed in Figure 1.2a and Figure 1.3a respectively. The difference maps are displayed in Figure 1.2b and Figure 1.3b. The reconstruction errors on the boundaries of the homogeneous regions are reduced.

At the end of the deterministic optimization, the discrepancy term $||Rf - p^\delta||$ is well-above the noise level for different number of projections. A local minimum is obtained and the level-set algorithm can not escape this

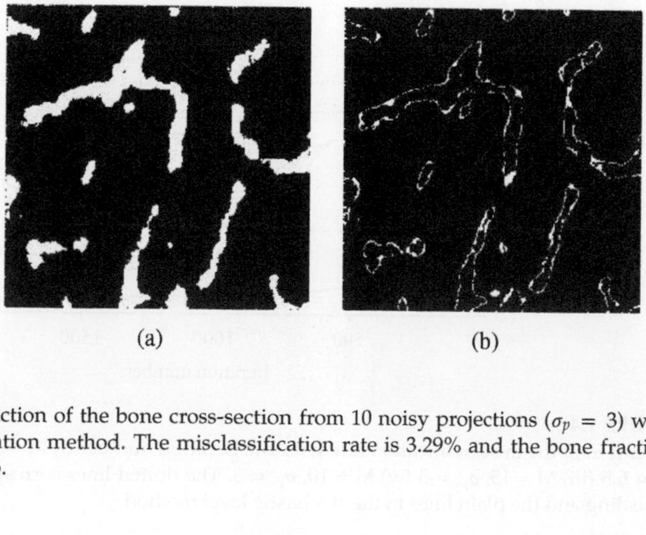

(a) (b)

FIGURE 1.2
(a) Reconstruction of the bone cross-section from 10 noisy projections ($\sigma_p = 3$) with the level-set regularization method. The misclassification rate is 3.29% and the bone fraction is 12.27% (b) Error map.

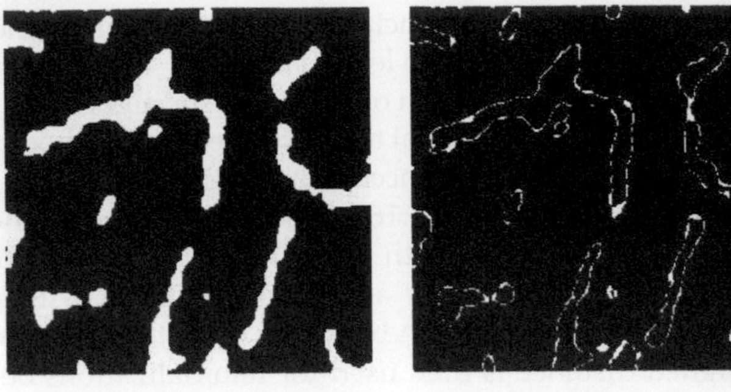

FIGURE 1.3
(a) Reconstruction of the bone cross-section from 10 noisy projections ($\sigma_p = 3$) with the stochastic level-set regularization method. The misclassification rate is 2.56% and the bone fraction is 14.14% (b) Error map.

local minimum. With the iterations, a significant decrease of the data term is obtained towards these noise levels for both stochastic methods.

The decrease of the misclassification rate as a function of the number of iterations is displayed in Figure 1.4 for the same number of projections and noise levels. The misclassification rates obtained at the end of the simulations are summarized in Table 1.1. Better reconstruction results are obtained with

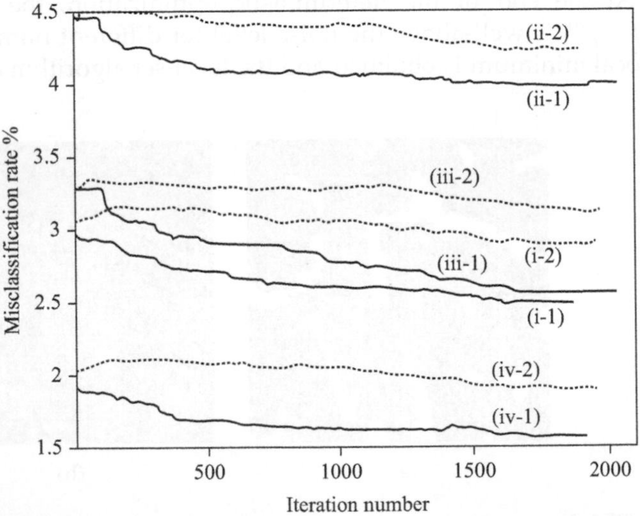

FIGURE 1.4
Evolution of the misclassification rate with the iteration number (i) M = 15, $\sigma_p = 6.5$ (ii) M = 10 $\sigma_p = 6.5$ (iii) M = 15, $\sigma_p = 3$ (iv) M = 10, $\sigma_p = 3$. The dotted lines corresponds to the simulated annealing and the plain lines to the stochastic level method.

TABLE 1.1

Misclassification Rates Obtained with the Stochastic Algorithms

	Simulated Annealing	Stochastic Level-Set
$\sigma_P = 3$, M = 15	1.89	1.56
$\sigma_P = 3$, M = 10	3.12	2.55
$\sigma_P = 6.5$, M = 15	2.9	2.48
$\sigma_P = 6.5$, M = 10	4.23	3.97

the stochastic level-set algorithm than with the simulated annealing minimization, for all noise levels and numbers of projections. At the end of the simulations, the errors on the boundary of the images are much lower.

1.4 Stochastic Level-Set Reconstruction in Nonlinear Phase Contrast Tomography

In this section, we detail the results obtained with stochastic level-set methods for phase contrast tomography. The inverse problem considered is nonlinear but the optimization methodology is very similar to the one applied to the binary tomography problem.

1.4.1 Nonlinear Phase Contrast Tomography

X-ray in-line phase contrast tomography is a very sensitive technique for soft tissues within dense materials. This imaging technique is based on a coupling of tomography and phase retrieval [31, 32] and it aims at reconstructing the complex refractive index [33]. For coherent X-rays obtained with synchrotrons, the Fresnel intensity is recorded for one or several propagation distances and for several projection angles after interaction of the X-rays with the object [34,35]. The inverse problem set by the reconstruction of the refractive index is nonlinear.

For volumes with several homogeneous materials, the imaginary and real part of the index are piecewise constant [33], and the level-set regularization can account for this a priori on the index map. Assuming that the discrete real and imaginary parts of the index are known, the inverse problem is then formulated as a shape optimization problem. Yet, the nonlinear phase contrast tomography problem is non-convex and the reconstructed solution obtained with the deterministic level-set regularization is a local minimum. We investigate here stochastic perturbations of the boundaries performed with tools similar to the ones used for binary tomography in [36] to improve the reconstruction and escape the critical point of the cost functional obtained with the deterministic method.

1.4.2 Level-Set Regularization in In-Line Phase Contrast Tomography

The real and imaginary parts of the complex refractive index to reconstruct from the Fresnel intensity measurements, denoted as δ and β are defined on a 3D bounded domain (Σ) with spatial coordinates (x, y, z). We denote (x_θ, y_θ, z) be the rotated spatial coordinate system for an angle θ around the z-axis (Figure 1.5). The sample is irradiated with a monochromatic, coherent, parallel X-ray beam propagating in the y_θ direction with the wavelength λ. The complex refractive index is given by [37,38]:

$$n(x, y, z) = 1 - \delta(x, y, z) + i\beta(x, y, z) \tag{1.22}$$

where δ is the refractive index decrement and β is the absorption index. Let $X_\theta = (x_\theta, z)$, the intensity detected at a distance D after the sample is given by the squared modulus of the following convolution product [33]:

$$I_{D,\theta}(X_\theta) = |T_\theta(X_\theta) * P_D(X_\theta)|^2 \tag{1.23}$$

where the Fresnel propagator is written:

$$P_D(X_\theta) = \frac{1}{i\lambda D} exp\left(i\frac{\pi}{\lambda D}|X_\theta|^2\right). \tag{1.24}$$

The transmittance function T_θ is given by:

$$T_\theta(X_\theta) = \exp[-B_\theta(X_\theta) + i\varphi_\theta(X_\theta)] \tag{1.25}$$

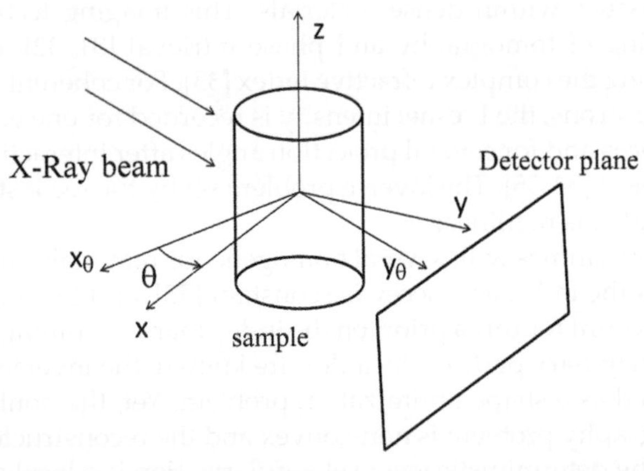

FIGURE 1.5
Experimental set-up in propagation based phase contrast tomography with a single propagation-distance showing the X-ray beam, the rotated coordinate system (x_θ, y_θ, z) for a rotation angle θ, the sample, and the detector.

with

$$B_\theta(X_\theta) = \frac{2\pi}{\lambda}\int \beta(y_\theta, X_\theta)dy_\theta \tag{1.26}$$

and

$$\varphi_\theta(X_\theta) = \frac{2\pi}{\lambda}\int (1 - \delta(y_\theta, X_\theta))dy_\theta \tag{1.27}$$

Let $L(\theta, x_\theta)$ the line defined by $L(\theta, x_\theta) = \{y_\theta\bar{\theta}^* + x_\theta\bar{\theta} : \tau \in \mathbb{R}\}$, with $\bar{\theta} = (cos(\theta), sin(\theta))$ and $\bar{\theta}^* = (-sin(\theta), cos(\theta))$, for parallel beam projection, with a beam parallel to the $X = (x, y)$ plane and $f \in L^1(\Sigma)$, the Radon transform of f is defined as:

$$Rf(\theta, x_\theta, z) = R_\theta f(x_\theta) = \int_{t\in L(\theta,x_\theta,z)\cap\Sigma} f(t)dt \tag{1.28}$$

where $L(\theta, x_\theta, z)$ is the $L(\theta, x_\theta)$ line for the coordinate z. The intensity $I_{D,\theta}$ can be reformulated with the Radon transform R.

For simplicity, we assume that δ and β are piecewise constant and that they can take two values δ_1, δ_2 and β_1, β_2 on disjoint subsets Σ_1, Σ_2 such that $\Sigma = \Sigma_1 \cup \Sigma_2$. In order to represent the unknown functions δ and β, we have used a level-set function of the first order Sobolev space $\eta \in H_1(\Sigma)$:

$$\beta = \beta_1 + H(\eta)(\beta_2 - \beta_1) \tag{1.29}$$

$$\delta = \delta_1 + H(\eta)(\delta_2 - \delta_1) \tag{1.30}$$

A variational approach is considered with the following regularization functional:

$$F[\eta] = \|I_{D,\theta}[\eta] - I_{\delta_n}\|_2^2 + \alpha_1\left(\|\eta\|_{L_2}^2 + \||\nabla\eta|\|_{L_2}^2\right) \tag{1.31}$$

where I_{δ_n} are the noisy intensity data and α_1 a regularization parameter.

The minimizers of the regularization are found numerically with first order optimality conditions for the smoothed functional where the Heaviside function is replaced by its approximation:

$$I'^*_{D,\theta}[\eta][I_{D,\theta}[\eta] - I_{\delta_n}] + \alpha_1(I - \Delta)[\eta] = 0 \tag{1.32}$$

where I'^*_D denotes the adjoint of the Fréchet derivative of the intensity operator with respect to L_2 spaces. I represent identity and Δ the Laplacian operator. The solutions of the optimality system are obtained with a Gauss-Newton method. The update is given by $\eta_{k+1} = \eta_k + \delta\eta$ and $\delta\eta$ is obtained with the linear system:

$$\left([I'^*_{D,\theta}[\eta^k]I'_{D,\theta}[\eta^k]\right)\delta\eta + \alpha_1(I - \Delta)\delta\eta = -F'[\eta^k] \tag{1.33}$$

An explicit formula can be derived for the Fréchet derivative of the intensity $I_D[\delta, \beta]$ and its adjoint are given in [39].

1.4.3 Stochastic Level-Set Methods for Phase Contrast Tomography

Stochastic level-set evolution The deterministic optimization of the level-set function is often stopped in local minima. We propose to improve the reconstruction image obtained with the deterministic level-set evolution with the following stochastic partial differential equation for the level-set function η, for $\vec{r} \in \Sigma$ by:

$$d\eta(\vec{r},t) = \delta\eta(\vec{r},t) + \rho(t)|\nabla\eta(\vec{r},t)|o dW(t) \tag{1.34}$$

where o denotes the Stratanovitch convention and $\delta\eta$ is the deterministic change calculated with the Gauss-Newton method of Eqs. 1.32, 1.33 as explained in the former section. We obtain the following Itô stochastic differential equation with the definition of the Stratonovich integral:

$$\begin{aligned} d\eta(\vec{r},t) &= \delta\eta + \rho(t)|\nabla\eta(\vec{r},t)|dW(t) + \frac{1}{2}\rho(t)(\Delta\eta(\vec{r},t) \\ &\quad - |\nabla\eta(\vec{r},t)|div\left(\frac{\nabla\eta(\vec{r},t)}{|\nabla\eta(\vec{r},t)|}\right) \end{aligned} \tag{1.35}$$

The deterministic level-set and stochastic level-set schemes are applied successively on random time intervals with an intermittent diffusion similar to the one proposed for the binary tomography. For the stochastic evolution, the time interval lengths and the diffusion strengths ρ are chosen at random with a uniform distribution in the range $[0, T_{max}]$ and $[0, \rho_{max}]$ where $\rho_{\max}$ is the scale for the diffusion strength and T_{max} is the scale for the diffusion time.

The minimization scheme is summarized in Algorithm 1:

Algorithm 1

Let Δt be the time step of the discretization of Eq. 1.35,
For k=1 to Maxiter:

Step 1: chose a projection angle θ at random with a uniform distribution chose at random $t \in [0, T_{max}]$, and $\rho \in [0, \rho_{max}]$, for the iteration number $N_{iter,sto} = t/\Delta t$, use the discrete version of Eq. 1.35.

Step 2: calculate $\delta\eta$ with Eqs. 1.32, 1.33, for $N_{iter,deterministic} = 100$ iterations.

Step 3: reinitialize the level-set function η with the signed distance function.

end

The derivative in Eq. 1.32 and Eq. 1.33 describes the sensitivity of the regularization functional with respect to deterministic changes of shape of the boundary between the regions of constant values of the index. The equation Eq. 1.35 corresponds to stochastic perturbations of the geometry. Topology changes like splitting and merging of domains can be obtained with the level-set approach [40]. It has also been proposed to add some new component or small holes far from the boundaries to modify the topology of the reconstructed images [39].

1.4.4 Numerical Results and Discussion

In the following, we compare the deterministic level-set algorithm with the modified algorithms with the stochastic evolution.

1.4.4.1 Simulation Details

The deterministic and intermittent stochastic level-set algorithms and the deterministic algorithm are compared in this section on one multi-material object made up of two homogeneous materials. It is possible to extend these results to objects with more than two materials with multi-level regularization.

The simulated test object (O_1) consists of an Al cylinder of 20 μm in diameter and 110 μm in height embedded in PMMA. Some horizontal sections of the β and δ maps of the simulated object (O_1) are displayed in Figure 1.6.

Let $\mu = \frac{4\pi\beta}{\lambda}$, the δ and μ values used for PMMA and Al for 24 keV X-rays are summarized in Table 1.2. The β and δ values were discretized on a regular grid with a pixel size of 1.5 μm. The cylinder is included in a rectangular volume of size $N_1 \times N_1 \times N_2$ pixels with $N_1 = 74$ and $N_2 = 109$ used for the simulations. The number of projection angles N_θ used for the simulation are $N_\theta = 75, 125$ and 180. A single sample-to-detector distance D = 100 mm is considered. The Radon transform is the projection operator implemented in the Mablab Toolbox. The intensity data were corrupted with additive Gaussian white noise. This noise distribution corresponds to the noise measured experimentally. The signal to noise ratio was measured with the peak-to-peak signal to noise ratio (PPSNR). To obtain a good accuracy, the ϵ parameter of the smooth approximation of the Heaviside function was fixed to $\epsilon = 0.03$.

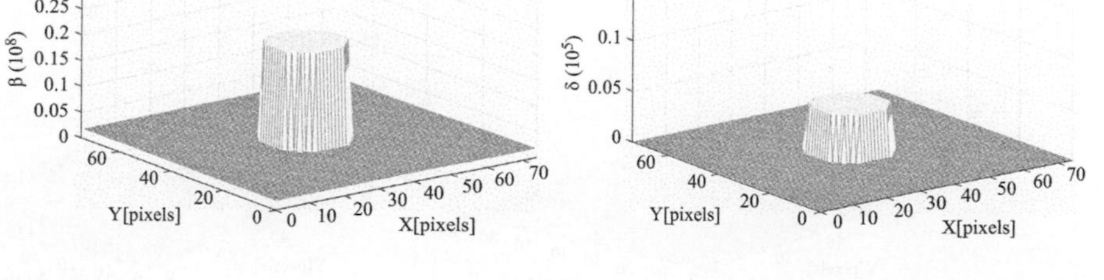

FIGURE 1.6
Ground truth β and δ maps for the object (O_1).

TABLE 1.2
Values of the δ and μ Values for the Materials in the Object, at 24 keV X-rays from http://henke.lbl.gov/optical_constants

Material	$\delta(10^{-7})$	$\mu(m^{-1})$
PMMA	4.628	41.2
Al	9.396	502.6

In order to evaluate the efficiency of the reconstruction, the relative mean square errors (RMSE) using the $L_2(\Sigma)$ norm, $\|\delta^* - \delta\|_2/\|\delta^*\|_2$ and $\|\beta^* - \beta\|_2/\|\beta^*\|_2$ have been studied. Let $D_k = \frac{\|I_{D,\theta}[\eta_k]-I_{\delta_\eta}\|}{\|I_{\delta_\eta}\|}$ the value of the data term for the projection angle θ and the value η_k. The iterations are stopped when the average value of the variation of the data term $D_{k+1} - D_k$ evaluated on 10 iterations is below 0.05.

1.4.4.2 Numerical Results for Deterministic Level-Set Method

For piecewise constant δ and β maps, the reconstruction results are improved with the level-set regularization with respect to Tikhonov regularization because some a priori information on the possible values of δ and β is included. Some simulations have been performed to reconstruct the object (O_1) with an initial diameter of the central Al cylinder equal to 40 μm, twice the diameter of the cylinder to be reconstructed and noise levels of 30 and 48 dB. With this starting map for the refractive index, the inverse problem is an easier shape optimization problem in which only the possible discrete values of the real and imaginary parts of the refractive index are known but not the shape of the regions where the refractive index takes constant values.

Figure 1.7 displays the horizontal section of the initial β and δ maps. Figure 1.8 presents some horizontal sections of the errors for the real and imaginary part of the reconstructed index map for a PPSNR of 48 dB after 500 iterations. These figures show that the reconstruction errors have been significantly reduced. Some errors are still present on the boundaries between the

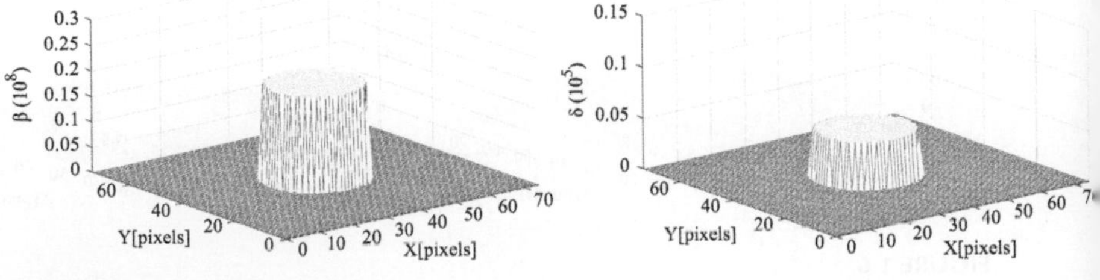

FIGURE 1.7
Horizontal section of the initial β and δ maps for the object (0_1).

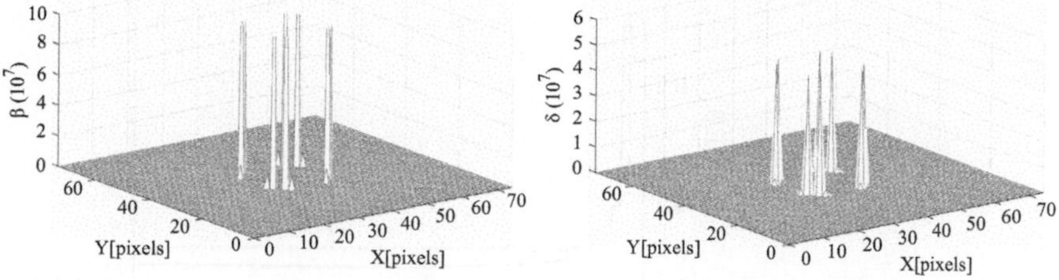

FIGURE 1.8
Horizontal section of the final error map for β and δ for a PPSNR of 48 dB.

two materials. Similar results are obtained for the other sections and the noise level of 30 dB with reconstruction errors at the interface between the different regions.

In order to have more quantitative information about the convergence of the method, the evolution of the relative mean square errors (RMSE) $\|\delta^* - \delta\|_2/\|\delta^*\|_2$ and $\|\beta^* - \beta\|_2/\|\beta^*\|_2$, are displayed as a function of the number of iterations for a PPSNR of 30 dB and 48 dB in Figures 1.9 and 1.10. The relative mean square errors on the two components β and δ of the refractive index are much decreased.

1.4.4.3 Deterministic Level-Set versus Stochastic Level-Set Algorithm

For higher noise levels and initializations maps with very different shape from the ground truth, the level-set regularization algorithm may be stuck in local optima. The stochastic level-set algorithm improves the reconstruction results. In order to perform a comparison of the deterministic and stochastic level-set algorithm, a first reconstruction is performed on the simulated

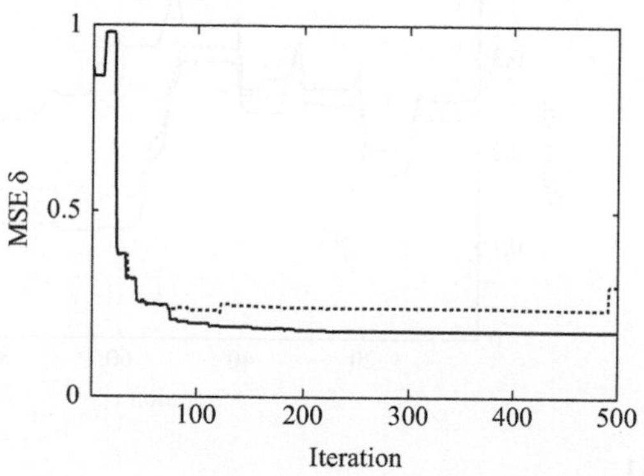

FIGURE 1.9
Evolution of the RMSE on δ with the iterations for the noise levels 30 dB (dotted line) and 48 dB (plain line).

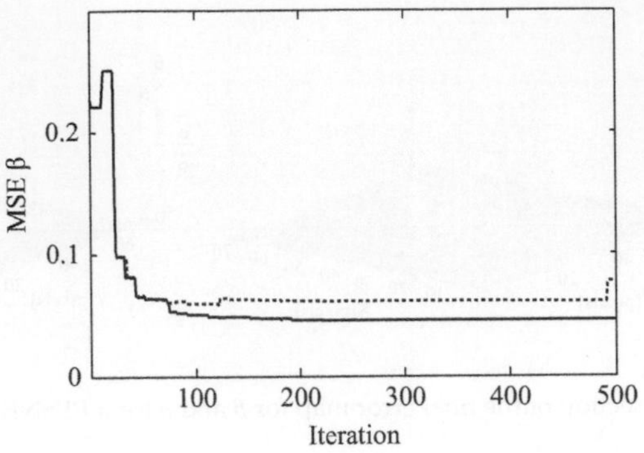

FIGURE 1.10
Evolution of the RMSE on β with the iterations for the noise levels 30 dB (dotted line) and 48 dB (plain line).

object (O_1). The initial guess is a large cylinder with a diameter twice the diameter of the object (0_1). Then algorithm 1 is applied to this initial reconstruction for PPSNR of 24 and 18 dB. Following algorithm 1, the numbers of stochatic iterations are chosen randomly with a uniform distribution between 1 and 50 and the noise strength in the range $[1, 10^{-3}]$. For the simulation of Eq. 1.35, we use an explicit scheme with finite differences, the WENO scheme [41] with $\Delta x = 0.1$ and $\Delta t = 0.01$. An iterated deterministic minimization is performed for comparison with periodic reinitialization of the level-set function and projection angles chosen at random.

The evolutions of the data term, $\|I_{D,\theta}[\eta] - I_{\delta_n}\| / \|I_{\delta_n}\|$ are displayed in Figure 1.11 for the deterministic and intermittent stochastic algorithms

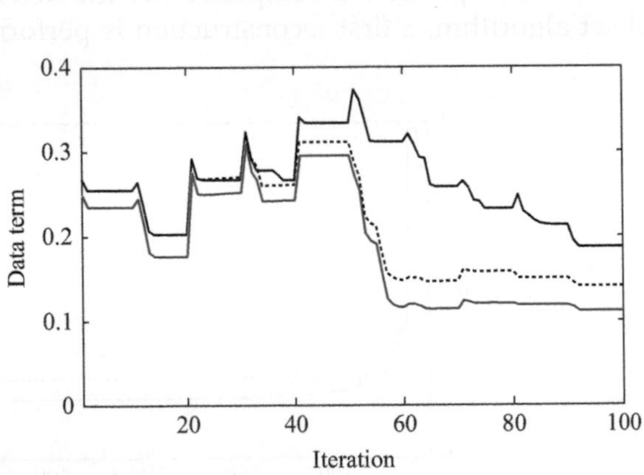

FIGURE 1.11
Evolution of the data term for the deterministic level-set algorithm for 24 dB (black line), for the intermittent stochastic level-set algorithm for 24 dB (blue line) and for the intermittent stochastic level-set algorithm for 18 dB (dotted line).

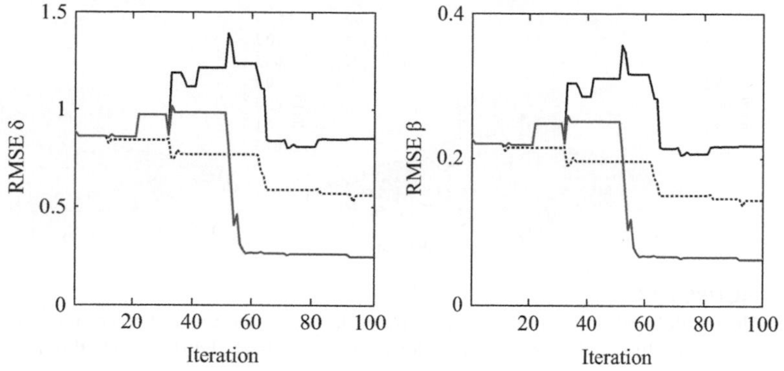

FIGURE 1.12
Evolution of the RMSE for β and δ for the deterministic level-set algorithm for 24 dB (black line), for the intermittent stochastic level-set algorithm for 24 dB (blue line) and for the intermittent stochastic level-set algorithm for 18 dB (dotted line).

starting from the initial reconstruction for the noise levels 18 dB and 24 dB. The deterministic algorithm is not efficient to achieve lower reconstruction errors. Different behaviours are obtained depending on the random projection angles θ for similar noise levels. Yet, after hundred iterations, only small fluctuations are observed on the real and imaginary parts of the refractive index, β and δ, and the uncertainty on the RMSE given in the Tables is below 5% for a given noise level.

The evolution of the normalized mean square error, $\|\delta^* - \delta\|_2/\|\delta^*\|_2$ and $\|\beta^* - \beta\|_2/\|\beta^*\|_2$, are displayed as a function of the number of iterations for the deterministic and stochastic algorithms in Figure 1.12. The iterated deterministic minimization can not escape the local minimum corresponding to the initial reconstructed δ and β volumes. A larger decrease is obtained with the stochastic scheme. Table 1.3 presents the reconstuction quality results for different noise levels and the different algorithms. The results correspond to an average over three trials. This table shows the efficiency of the stochastic optimization.

Some horizontal sections of the difference image between the ground truth image and the reconstructed real index map obtained for the minimum of the discrepancy term for 24 dB with the stochastic or the deterministic methods are displayed in Figure 1.13. These figures show that the

TABLE 1.3
RMSE for β and δ for Deterministic Level-Set and Stochastic Level-Set

	RMSE β, LS	RMSE δ,LS	RMSE β, Stochastic LS	RMSE δ, Stochastic LS
PPSNR=18 dB	0.28	0.85	0.15	0.55
PPSNR=24 dB	0.22	0.80	0.06	0.26

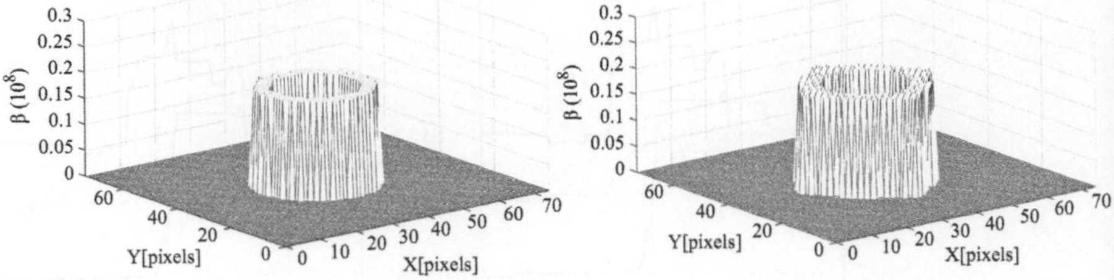

FIGURE 1.13
Horizontal section of the difference image between the ground truth and the reconstructed β maps with the stochastic and the deterministic level-set algorithms for the noise level 24 dB.

reconstruction errors have been significantly reduced. Similar results are obtained for the imaginary part of the refractive index.

1.4.5 Conclusion

We have studied some aspects of the nonlinear inverse problem associated with the reconstruction of the real and imaginary parts of the refractive index in phase contrast tomography and with the binary tomographic reconstruction problem. Both are regularized with level-set functions and with Total-Sobolev penalty term. The deterministic optimization of the regularization functional leads to local minima with large reconstruction errors. The reconstruction results are improved with a stochastic perturbation of the shape of the reconstructed regions with a stochastic level-set evolution. The evolution is based on a stochastic partial differential equation with the Stratonovich formulation. The stochastic algorithm leads to a decreased reconstruction errors localized on the boundaries for different noise levels. The method gives better reconstruction results than the classical simulated annealing method.

References

1. J. A. Sethian, "Level Set Methods and Fast Marching Methods", Cambridge Monograph on Applied and Computational Mathematics, Cambridge University Press, 1999.
2. A. Egger and L. Leitao, "Nonlinear regularization for ill-posed problems with piecewise constant or strongly varying solutions", *Inverse Problems*, vol. 25, pp. 115014, 2009.
3. A. DeCezaro, A. Leitao and X. C. Tai, "On multiple level-set regularization methods for inverse problems", *Inverse Problems*, vol. 25, pp. 035004, 2009.
4. M. Burger, "A level set method for inverse problems", *Inverse Problems*, vol. 17, pp. 1327–1355, 2001.

5. S. Geman and C. R. Hwang, "Diffusion for global optimization", *J. Control Optim.*, vol. 24, pp. 1031–1043, 1986.
6. B. Gidas, "Metropolis-type Monte Carlo simulation algorithm and simulated annealing", *Topics in Contemporary Probability and Its Applications*, Probability Stochastics Series, CRC, Boca Raton, FL. pp. 159–232, 1995.
7. P. Parpas, B. Rustem, "Convergence analysis a a global optimization algorithm using stochastic differential equations", *J. Control Optim.*, vol. 45, pp. 95–110, 2009.
8. S. Chow, T. Yang and H. Zhou, "Global optimization by intermittent diffusion", National Science Council Tunghai University Endowment Fund for Academic Advancement Mathematics Research Promotion Center vol. 121, 2009.
9. T. S. Chiang, C. R. Hwang and S. J. Sheu, "Diffusion for global optimization in $\mathbb{R}^n$" *SIAM J. Control Optim.*, vol. 25, pp. 737–753, 1987.
10. O. Juan, R. Keriven and G. Postelnicu, "Stochastic Motion and the Level-Set Method in Computer Vision: Stochastic Active Contours", *International Journal of Computer Vision*, vol. 69, pp. 7–25, 2006.
11. I. Karatzas and S. Shreve, *Brownian motion and stochastic calculus*, Springer Verlag, New York, 1991.
12. G. Da Prato and J. Zabczyk, "Stochastic equations in infinite dimensions", *Encyclopedia of Mathematics and Its Applications*, Cambridge:Cambridge University Press, 1992.
13. G. T. Herman and A. Kuba, "Advances in discrete tomography and its applications", Birkhauser Boston, 2007.
14. K. J. Batenburg and J. Sijbers, "Generic iterative subset algorithm for discrete tomography", *Discrete Applied Mathematics*, vol. 157, pp. 438–451, 2009.
15. W. Cai and L. Ma, "Comparison of approaches based on optimization and algebraic iteration for binary tomography", *Computer Physics Communications*, vol. 181, pp. 1974–1981, 2010.
16. L. Rusko and A. Kuba, "Multi-resolution methods for binary tomography", *Electonics Notes in Discrete Mathematics*, vol. 20, pp. 299–311, 2005.
17. T. D. Capricelli and P. L. Combettes, "A convex programing algorithm for noisy discrete tomography", *Advances in discrete tomography and its applications*, Boston, MA, pp. 207–226, 2007.
18. T. Schule, C. Schnorr, S. Weber and J. Hornegger, "Discrete tomogrphy by convex-concave regularization and D. C programming", *Discrete Applied Mathematics*, vol. 151, pp. 229–243, 2005.
19. H. Y. Liao and G. T. Herman, "Automated estimation of the parameters of the Gibbs priors to be uses in binary tomography", *Discrete Applied Mathematics*, pp. 149–170, 2004.
20. E. Gouillart, F. Krzakala, M. Mezard and L. Zdebrova, "Belief propagation reconstruction for discrete tomography", *Inverse Problems*, vol. 29, pp. 035003, 2013.
21. L. I. Rudin, S. Osher, E. Fatemi, "Nonlinear total variation based noise removal algorithms", *Phys. D*, vol. 60, pp. 259–268, 1992.
22. B. Sixou, L. Wang and F. Peyrin, "Binary tomographic reconstruction of bone microstructure from few projections with level-set regularization", *IEEE Symposium on Biomedical Imaging*, San Francisco, 2013.
23. Sixou B. "Binary tomography reconstruction with stochastic level-set methods" *IEEE Signal Processing Letters* vol. 22, pp. 920–924, 2015.

24. R. Azencott, "Sequential simulated annealing: speed of convergence and acceleration techniques", *Simulated annealing:parallelization techniques* Wiley, New York, pp. 1–10, 1992.
25. O. Catoni, "Rough large deviation estimates for simulated annealing algorithms", *Annals of Probability*, vol. 20, pp. 1109–1146, 1992.
26. C. Cot and O. Catoni, "Piecewise constant triangular cooling schedule for generalized annealing algorithms", *Annals of Applied probability*, vol. 8, pp. 375–396, 1998.
27. R. Szu and R. Hartley, "Fast simulated annealing", *Physics Letters A*, vol. 122, pp. 157–162, 1987.
28. L. Ingber, "Very fast simulated annealing", *Journal of Mathematical Computer Modelling*, vol. 12, pp. 967–973, 1989.
29. L. Apostol, V. Boudousq, O. Basset, C. Odet, S. Yot, J. Tabary, J. M. Dinten, E. Boller, P. O. Kotzki and F. Peyrin, "Relevance of 2D radiographic texture analysis for the assessment of 3D bone microarchitecture", *Medical Physics*, vol. 33, pp. 3546–3556, 2006.
30. H. W. Engl, M. Hanke and A. Neubauer, "Regularization of Inverse Problems", Dordrecht: Kluwer Academic, 1996.
31. A. Momose, T. Takeda, Y. Tai, Y. Yoneyama and K. Hirano, "Phase-contrast tomographic imaging using an X-ray interferometer", *J. Synchrotron. Rad.* vol. 5, pp. 309–314, 1998.
32. P. Cloetens, M. Pateyron-Salome, J. Y. Buffiere, G. Peix, J. Baruchel, F. Peyrin and M. Schlenker, "Observation of microstructure and damage in materials by phase sensitive radiography and tomography" *J. Appl. Phys.* vol. 81, pp. 5878–5886, 1997.
33. M. Langer, P. Cloetens, A. Pacureanu and F. Peyrin, "X-ray in-line phase tomography of multimaterial objects" *Optics Letters* vol. 37, pp. 2151–2154, 2102.
34. B. Sixou, V. Davidoiu, M. Langer, F. Peyrin, "Absorption and phase retrieval in phase contrast imaging with nonlinear Tikhonov regularization and joint sparsity constraint regularization" *Inverse Problems and Imaging* vol. 7, pp. 267–282, 2013.
35. K. A. Nugent, "Coherent methods in the X-rays science" *Advances in Physics* vol. 59, pp. 1–99, 2010.
36. L. Wang, B. Sixou and F. Peyrin, "Binary tomography reconstruction with stochastic level-set method" *Signal Processing Letters* vol. 22, pp. 922–924, 2015.
37. M. Born and E. Wolf "Principles of Optics". Cambridge University Press; 1997.
38. J. W. Goodman "Intoduction fo Fourier Optics" Roberts, Greenwood Village, CO 2005.
39. B. Sixou, "Deterministic versus stochastic level-set regularization in nonlinear phase contrast tomography" *Inverse Problems in Science and Engineering* 2016.
40. S. Osher and R. P. Fedkiw, "The Level-Set method and Dynamic Implic Surfaces" Springer, New York; 1988.
41. G. S. Jiang and D. Peng, "Weigthed ENO schemes for Hamilton-Jacobi equations" *SIAM J. Control Optim.* vol. 21, pp. 2126–2143, 2000.

2

Application of 3D Level Set Based Optimization in Microwave Breast Imaging for Cancer Detection

Hardik N. Patel and Deepak K. Ghodgaonkar

CONTENTS

2.1 Introduction

The incidence of breast cancer is increasing rapidly with high levels of mortality, according to Globocan [1]. However, early breast cancer detection can reduce the rate of mortality. At present, mammography, which uses ionizing X-rays for breast imaging, is the 'gold standard' technique for breast screening. However, there are a number of limitations. It uses ionizing X-rays for breasts imaging. High radiation doses of X-rays or frequent mammography screenings increases the risk of cancer. In mammography, false negative and

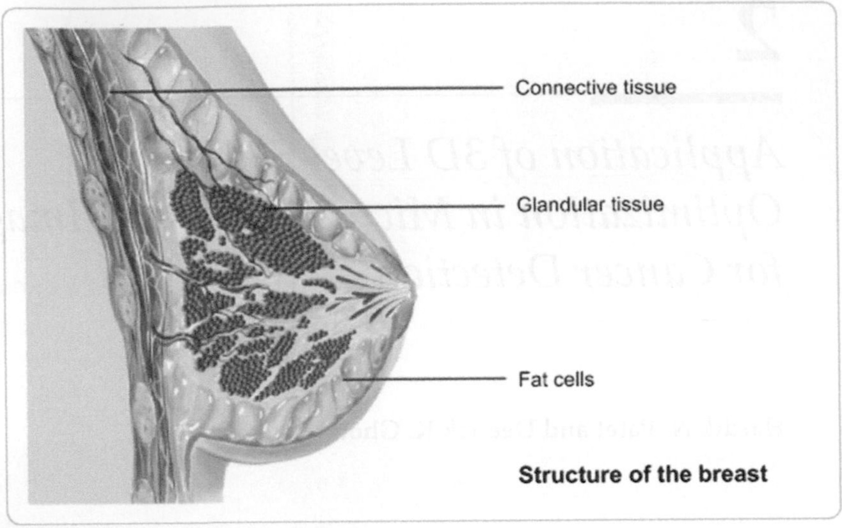

FIGURE 2.1
Breast anatomy.
Image courtesy: www.aboutbrachytherapy.com

false positive rates are about 15% and 13% respectively, which lead to additional imaging and biopsies [2]. As well, in mammography, breasts are pressed between two plates for better contrast, which makes it painful and uncomfortable for patients. An alternative technique is required to overcome the disadvantages of mammography. In the last decade, microwave imaging for breast screening has emerged as a new diagnostic option [2]. Advantages of microwave imaging are described below. Significant contrast exists between the dielectric properties of healthy and malignant breast tissues over microwave frequencies [3–5]. The non-ionizing nature of microwave radiation constitutes a key advantage over X-ray based mammography. The use of a low power microwave signal for breast screening does not harm the patient. It is extremely important to understand breast anatomy and tumour cell properties. Breast anatomy provides a clear picture of different tissues and their locations. (See Figure 2.1.) Breasts mainly contain fatty and fibro-glandular tissues as shown in Figure 2.1 [6]. General properties of tumour cells are quite intuitive. In tumour detection, it is extremely important to know tumour cell properties, as outlined below [7].

- Dielectric properties of tumour tissues are different from healthy tissues in their microwave frequency range.
- Cell reproduction rate is higher than in healthy cells.
- Glucose and blood consumption are high due to abnormal reproduction rate.

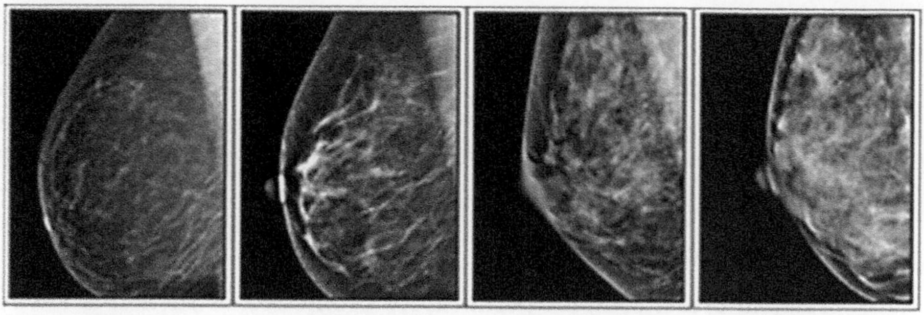

FIGURE 2.2
Classification of breast according to density. Class I, Class II, Class III, and Class IV breasts. (Left to right)
Image Courtesy: www.acsh.org

- Temperature is high due to the abnormal reproduction rate.
- Shape and size are abnormal.
- Electrical properties are also different.
- Tumour cells neither become mature nor commit suicide.
- Tumour cells don't follow commands of surrounding healthy cells.

Microwave imaging is based on the first property of tumour cells. Positron emission tomography (PET) is based on the third property of tumour cells. Thermography is based on the fourth property of tumour cells. Electrical impedance tomography (EIT) is based on the sixth property of tumour cells. Of these techniques, microwave imaging is the most promising [2].

There are four classes of breasts according to the Breast Imaging Reporting and Data System (BI-RADS). Mammography based images of four breast classes are shown in Figure 2.2 [8]. Class I breasts have only 25% glandular tissues which make them almost entirely fatty. Class II breasts have 25% to 50% scattered glandular tissues. Class III breasts are heterogeneously dense due to 51% to 75% glandular tissues. Class IV breasts are known as extremely dense due to more than 75% glandular tissues. Women with class III and class IV breasts have a high risk of breast cancer [9–12]. The colour of a breast tumour is white in mammography images. Accordingly, it is very difficult to detect tumours in class III and class IV breasts because of glandular tissues are also white. If a tumour is hidden inside glandular tissues then it results in false negative detection. On the other hand, if the higher density of glandular tissues is detected as tumour, then it results in false positive detection. Thus, false positive and false negative rates are higher in class III and class IV breasts [13]. In microwave breast imaging, low power microwave signals are transmitted on the breast using antennas. Now, these incident signals are scattered according to dielectric properties of breast tissues. The scattered waves are then received by antennas. This process is known as forward problem solution. Then, noise is added to known scattered fields. A dielectric (complex permittivity) profile of the breast is reconstructed from noisy scattered fields data. This process is known as an inverse scattering problem solution.

2.1.1 Motivation

Human breast complex permittivity profile reconstruction is always challenging in three dimensions. Both shape and value reconstructions are important in three dimensions. Shape reconstruction is not involved in most of the current optimization techniques. This is considered a major drawback in 3D reconstruction. However, this limitation is avoided using 3D level set functions. Novel 3D level set based optimization is used to reconstruct values as well as the shape of complex permittivity profile. Debye parameter values and 3D level set functions are updated to minimize cost function. Ill-posed system matrix and noisy scattered field data make 3D reconstruction very challenging. Therefore, regularization is used in 3D level set based optimization to overcome these challenges. The performance of 3D level set based optimization is evaluated using Tikhonov and total variation regularization schemes. 3D FDTD is used in this optimization to calculate the total electric field at each voxel.

2.2 Multiple Frequency Inverse Scattering Problem Formulation

The multiple frequency inverse scattering problem is solved to reconstruct a microwave image of the breast. Simulation is done using a class 3 numerical breast phantom developed in [14]. Y-Z, X-Z, and X-Y views are shown in Figure 2.3. Fibro-glandular tissues are represented by white (bright) colour and adipose tissues are represented by black or gray (dark) colour. MRI

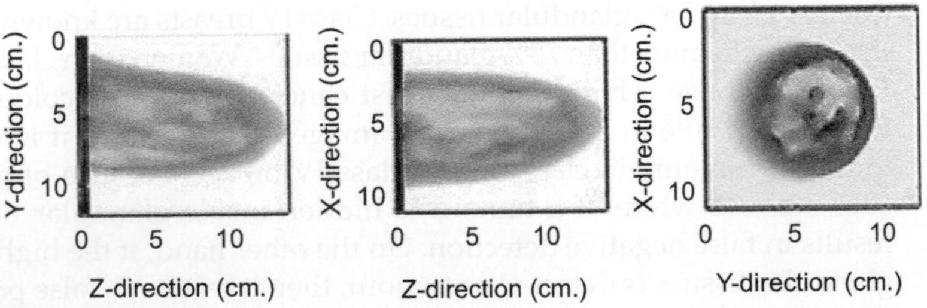

FIGURE 2.3
Y-Z, X-Z and X-Y view of a class 3 MRI derived numerical breast phantom.

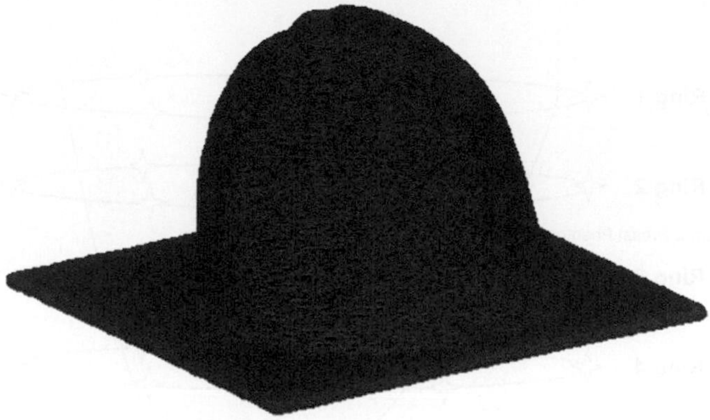

FIGURE 2.4
3D view of numerical breast phantom.

derived numerical breast phantom is used to make the simulation more realistic. A 3D view of a class III numerical breast phantom is shown in Figure 2.4. Relative permittivity of human breast tissues is a function of temperature and frequency. Temperature is assumed to be constant. The dispersion and polarization effect of human breast tissues are incorporated in FDTD by using the single pole Debye model [15]. The single pole Debye model is given by equation 2.1.

$$\epsilon(\omega) = \epsilon_{\infty} + \frac{\Delta\epsilon}{1 + j\omega\tau} + \frac{\sigma_s}{j\omega\epsilon_0} \tag{2.1}$$

In equation 2.1, ϵ_{∞} is infinite frequency permittivity, $\Delta\epsilon$ is difference between static permittivity (ϵ_s) and infinite frequency permittivity (ϵ_{∞}), and σ_s is static conductivity. τ is relaxation time constant which is 15ps for all breast tissues. Relaxation time constant is assumed to be spatially invariant.

Consider antenna placement surrounding numerical breast phantom for inverse scattering problem formulation. (See Figure 2.5.) There are five rings of antennas around numerical breast phantom [17,21,22]. Each ring has eight infinitesimal dipole of area 2cm×2cm, which lead to 40 antennas in the system [17]. Scattered fields at antenna locations are calculated using equation 2.2.

$$\vec{E}^s(\vec{r}) = \iiint G(\vec{r}, \vec{r}') \cdot \vec{J}(\vec{r}')dv' \tag{2.2}$$

In equation 2.2, $\vec{E}^s(\vec{r})$ is scattered electric field at antenna locations $\vec{r}$, $G(\vec{r}, \vec{r}')$ is Green's function for homogeneous background medium, and $\vec{J}(\vec{r}')$ is polarization current density. Equation 2.3 is obtained by substituting polarization current density into 2.2.

$$\vec{E}^s(\vec{r}) = \omega^2\mu \iiint G(\vec{r}, \vec{r}') \cdot \vec{E}_t(\vec{r}')[\epsilon(\vec{r}') - \epsilon^b(\vec{r})]dr' \tag{2.3}$$

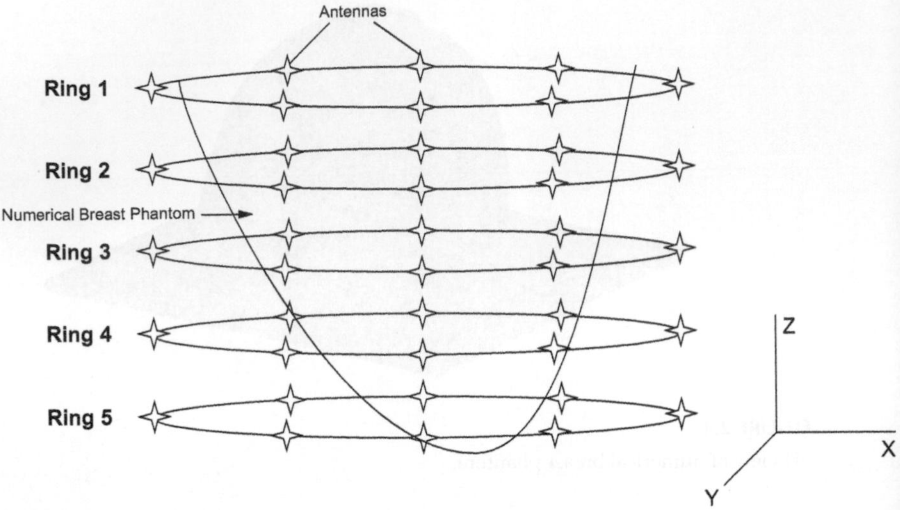

FIGURE 2.5
Antenna placement surrounding the numerical breast phantom.

In equation 2.3, $\epsilon(\vec{r}') - \epsilon^b(\vec{r})$ is contrast in permittivity with respect to homogeneous background medium, $\vec{E}_t(\vec{r}')$ is total electric field intensity at location $\vec{r}'$. Linear approximation of equation 2.3 is obtained using [16,17]. Numerical breast phantom is represented by K voxels after discretization. There are 40 antennas surrounding the breast, as shown in Figure 2.5. Each antenna works as a transceiver. One antenna transmits microwave signal on the breast while the other antennas receive scattered signals due to breast tissues. This process is repeated for each antenna present in the system. Let us consider that there are N antennas in the system. There is F number of frequencies. Ideally there are N^2F measurements possible. There are only $M = (N(N-1)/2)F$ measurements possible after removing redundancy. There are N-1 receivers when first antenna transmits. There are N-2 receivers when the second antenna transmits. In this way, there are channels among transmitters and receivers. By considering N antennas, M number of channels, F number of frequencies, and K voxels equation 2.4 is obtained from equation 2.3.

$$\begin{bmatrix} Re(A_1^{\infty}) & Re(A_1^{\Delta}) & Re(A_1^{\sigma}) \\ Im(A_1^{\infty}) & Im(A_1^{\Delta}) & Im(A_1^{\sigma}) \\ & \cdot & \\ & \cdot & \\ Re(A_M^{\infty}) & Re(A_M^{\Delta}) & Re(A_M^{\sigma}) \\ Im(A_M^{\infty}) & Im(A_M^{\Delta}) & Im(A_M^{\sigma}) \end{bmatrix} \begin{bmatrix} \delta(\epsilon_{\infty}) \\ \delta(\Delta\epsilon) \\ \delta(\sigma_s) \end{bmatrix} = \begin{bmatrix} Re(E_1^s) \\ Im(E_1^s) \\ \cdot \\ \cdot \\ \cdot \\ Re(E_M^s) \\ Im(E_M^s) \end{bmatrix} \quad (2.4)$$

In equation (2.4), $\delta(\epsilon_\infty) = (\epsilon_\infty)_k - (\epsilon_\infty)_b$, is the difference between kth voxel's infinite frequency permittivity and background medium's infinite frequency permittivity, $\delta(\Delta\epsilon) = (\Delta\epsilon)_k - (\Delta\epsilon)_b$ and $\delta(\sigma_s) = (\sigma_s)_k - (\sigma_s)_b$ are defined same as above. Re(.) and Im(.) represent real part and imaginary part, respectively. By comparing equation (2.4) with $A\epsilon = b$, Sizes of A, ϵ and b are $2MF \times 3K$, $3K \times 1$ and $2MF \times 1$, respectively. There are total 2MF equations, and 3K unknowns. Let's consider an example with 40 antennas, 18 frequencies, and 64000 voxels. There are 28,080 equations and 192000 unknowns in our system. It means that this approximated linear system of equation (2.4) is under-determined. In equation (2.4), each element of matrix A is represented by equation (2.5) and scattered fields column vector of the right hand side is given by equation (2.6).

$$A_p^e = \begin{bmatrix} C_e(\omega_1)\left[a_1^p(\omega_1) \ldots\ldots a_k^p(\omega_1)\right] \\ \vdots \\ C_e(\omega_F)\left[a_1^p(\omega_F) \ldots\ldots a_k^p(\omega_F)\right] \end{bmatrix} \tag{2.5}$$

$$E_p^s = \begin{bmatrix} E_y^t(\vec{r}_n|\vec{r}_m, \omega_1) - E_y^i(\vec{r}_n|\vec{r}_m, \omega_1) \\ \vdots \\ E_y^t(\vec{r}_n|\vec{r}_m, \omega_F) - E_y^i(\vec{r}_n|\vec{r}_m, \omega_F) \end{bmatrix} \tag{2.6}$$

Where, $a_k^p(\omega_1) = \omega_1^2\mu\epsilon_0 \cdot E_y^t(\vec{r}_j|\vec{r}_m, \omega_1) \cdot IG_y(\vec{r}_n|\vec{r}_j, \omega_1)$ and $C_\infty(\omega) = 1$, $C_\Delta(\omega) = (1 + j\omega\tau)^{-1}$, $C_\sigma(\omega) = (j\omega\epsilon_0)^{-1}$. $E_y^t(\vec{r}_j|\vec{r}_m, \omega_l)$ is y direction electric field present at j^{th} voxel location due to a transmitter at location $\vec{r}_m$ for angular frequency ω_l, $IG_y(\vec{r}_n|\vec{r}_j, \omega_l)$ is y direction component of the integration of the Green's function at angular frequency ω_l. Where, $\vec{r}_n$, p and k represent receiver location, particular channel number and total number of voxels, respectively. Incident electric field of [3, 4, 7] is replaced by total electric field in this formulation. Scattered electric field matrix of equation (2.4) is known due to forward simulation. Left hand side matrix A of equation (2.4) is also known. Permittivity contrast profile column matrix is only unknown in equation (2.4).

$$C(\epsilon) = \frac{1}{2}\sum_{f=1}^{F}\sum_{n=1}^{M} |E_m^s(\vec{r}_n, \omega_f) - E_r^s(\vec{r}_n, \omega_f, \epsilon(\vec{r}'))|^2 \tag{2.7}$$

$$C(\epsilon) = \frac{1}{2}\sum_{i=1}^{FM} |R_i|^2 \tag{2.8}$$

In equation (2.7), $C(\epsilon)$ is cost function, $E_m^s(\vec{r}_n, \omega_f)$ is known scattered field (measured) at location $\vec{r}_n$ for frequency ω_f, $E_r^s(\vec{r}_n, \omega_f, \epsilon(\vec{r}'))$ is reconstructed scattered field at location $\vec{r}_n$ for frequency ω_f and dielectric profile $\epsilon(\vec{r}')$, F is the number of frequencies, M is the number of measurements (channels), $\vec{r}_n$ is receiver location, ω_f is angular frequency. Now, Cost function is represented in residual form using equation (2.8).

2.3 3D Level Set Based Optimization Approach

The level set method was proposed by Osher and Sethian in 1988 [18]. There are many applications of level set methods in different areas of science and technology. Image segmentation, topology reconstruction, and inverse scattering problem solution are some of the most popular applications of the level set method. The Hamilton-Jacobi equation is solved by using moving fronts with curvature dependent speed [18]. This article forms the base for level set methods. The algorithm proposed in [18] handles topology merging and breaking naturally which makes it attractive for shape reconstruction. Level sets with the fast marching method and extension velocity are described with great detail in [19]. Level set based evolution and optimization approaches are described in great detail for inverse problems involving obstacles [20]. Deconvolution and reconstruction of diffraction screen examples are also covered. Results are very promising for the above two examples. The problem of instability and regularization are left as a future work in reference [20]. Electromagnetic tomography using adjoint fields and level set is given in [21], which requires heavy computations. Level set based solutions are given for inverse problems with considerable mathematical detail. The level set based novel frequency hopping technique is given in [23], which can avoid local minima. A classical survey on level set methods for inverse scattering problems is described with great detail in [22, 24, 25]. Inverse scattering problem of two dimensional microwave breast imaging is solved using the level set based steepest descent method in [26,27,32]. The generalized parametric level set method is given for inverse problems and reconstruction in [28, 29]. Computationally efficient 3D level set method is implemented for microwave breast imaging in [30], which requires only one FDTD simulation per iteration (inverse scattering problem is solved iteratively). The level set based adjoint method requires two FDTD simulations per iteration so method of [30] is quite efficient. A modified level set method is given for microwave imaging and parameter reconstruction in [31]. The method shown in [31] can reconstruct values and shape of dielectric profile simultaneously. Level set functions are often used as signed distance function. One level set function is used to distinguish two different regions. N level set function can distinguish 2^N different regions. Two level set function based optimization for breast cancer detection is described in [33]. 3D FDTD of [34] is used to solve forward problem in the proposed approach of [33]. Level set based optimization steps are given below. Now, this algorithm is implemented to find a solution to

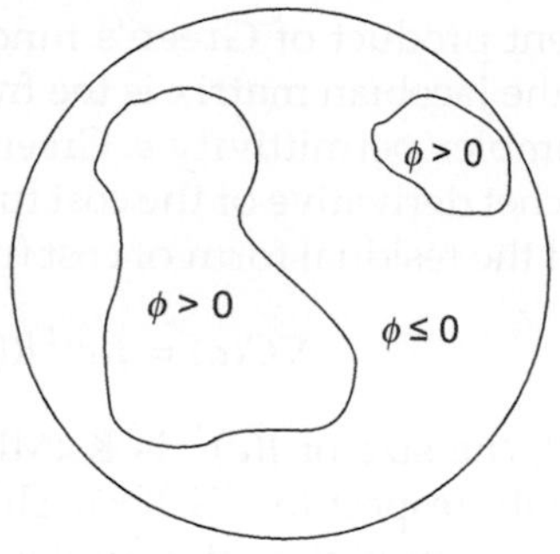

FIGURE 2.6
Level set function to distinguish two different regions.

the inverse problem. A combination of evolution and optimization is used in [30,33].

2.3.1 Single 3D Level Set Function Based Optimization

Single 3D level set function based optimization is described in [30]. Single level set function is shown in Figure 2.6. The scenario of Figure 2.6 is given as an equation.

$$\epsilon(r) = \epsilon^{fib}(r)H(\phi(r)) + \epsilon^{fat}(r)(1 - H(\phi(r))) \tag{2.9}$$

In equation (2.9), $\phi(r)$ is level set function, H(·) is the unit step function, ϵ^{fib} is the complex permittivity of the fibro-glandular tissues, ϵ^{fat} is the complex permittivity of the fatty tissues. Region $\phi > 0$ is represented by $H(\phi)$ and Region $\phi \leq 0$ is represented by $1 - H(\phi)$. Equations (2.10) and (2.11) represent linear relationships among Debye parameters [30].

$$\epsilon_\infty = 0.3265\epsilon_s + 1.6326 \tag{2.10}$$

$$\sigma_s = 0.0151\epsilon_s - 0.0365 \tag{2.11}$$

Above equations are used to reduce number of variables per voxel. Now, cost function of equation (2.8) is minimized in level set based optimization. The adjoint solution of level set optimization is computationally heavy. This computational cost is avoided by calculating jacobian matrix. The jacobian matrix of cost function equation (2.8) is calculated using equation (2.12).

$$G_r(r|r') \circ E_r^t(r') = J(\epsilon) \tag{2.12}$$

In equation (2.12), $G_r(r|r')$ is the MF×K Green's function matrix, where K is the number of voxels. $E_r^t(r')$ is the MF×K total field matrix. M is the number of measurements, F is the number of frequencies. The Jacobian matrix is element by element product of Green's function matrix and total field matrix. Each row of the Jacobian matrix is the frechet derivative of the residuals with respect to complex permittivity ϵ. Green function calculations are given in [17,30]. The frechet derivative of the cost function is calculated using the Jacobian matrix and the residual form of cost function by using equation (2.13).

$$\nabla C(\epsilon) = J(\epsilon)^T R(\epsilon) \tag{2.13}$$

In equation (2.13), the size of $J(\epsilon)^T$ is K×MF. The size of partial derivative of cost function with respect to ϵ is K×1. This method of calculating frechet derivative reduces computational complexity as compared to the adjoint method. This method results in only single FDTD simulation at every iteration. Therefore, this method reduces computational burden by half at every iteration. The partial derivative of equation (2.9) with respect to ϕ is computed by using equation (2.14).

$$\frac{\partial \epsilon}{\partial \phi} = (\epsilon^{fib}(r) - \epsilon^{fat}(r))\delta(\phi(r)) \tag{2.14}$$

The partial derivative of equation (2.9) with respect to static permittivity of fibro-glandular tissues ϵ_s^{fib} is computed by using equation (2.15).

$$\frac{\partial \epsilon}{\partial \epsilon_s^{fib}} = H(\phi(r))\frac{\partial \epsilon^{fib}}{\partial \epsilon_s^{fib}} \tag{2.15}$$

The partial derivative of equation (2.9) with respect to static permittivity of fatty tissues ϵ_s^{fat} is computed by using equation (2.16).

$$\frac{\partial \epsilon}{\partial \epsilon_s^{fat}} = (1 - H(\phi(r)))\frac{\partial \epsilon^{fat}}{\partial \epsilon_s^{fat}} \tag{2.16}$$

The partial derivative of cost function with respect to level set function ϕ is calculated by using equation (2.17).

$$\frac{\partial C}{\partial \phi} = \nabla C(\epsilon)\frac{\partial \epsilon}{\partial \phi} \tag{2.17}$$

The partial derivative of cost function with respect to ϵ_s^{fib} is computed by using equation (2.18).

$$\frac{\partial C}{\partial \epsilon_s^{fib}} = \nabla C(\epsilon)\frac{\partial \epsilon}{\partial \epsilon_s^{fib}} \tag{2.18}$$

The partial derivative of cost function with respect to ϵ_s^{fat} is computed by using equation (2.19).

$$\frac{\partial C}{\partial \epsilon_s^{fat}} = \nabla C(\epsilon)\frac{\partial \epsilon}{\partial \epsilon_s^{fat}} \tag{2.19}$$

The partial derivatives obtained above are used to implement gradient based descent optimization approach as shown below.

$$\phi^{n+1} = \phi^{n} - \alpha_{\phi}\frac{\partial C}{\partial \phi} \tag{2.20}$$

$$\left(\epsilon_s^{fib}\right)^{n+1} = \left(\epsilon_s^{fib}\right)^{n} - \alpha_{\epsilon_s}^{fib}\frac{\partial C}{\partial \epsilon_s^{fib}} \tag{2.21}$$

$$\left(\epsilon_s^{fat}\right)^{n+1} = \left(\epsilon_s^{fat}\right)^{n} - \alpha_{\epsilon_s}^{fat}\frac{\partial C}{\partial \epsilon_s^{fat}} \tag{2.22}$$

Where n is the iteration number. The step sizes α_{ϕ}, $\alpha_{\epsilon_s}^{fib}$, and $\alpha_{\epsilon_s}^{fat}$ are individually chosen. A priori information related to breast tissues is useful in deciding above parameters.

2.3.2 Two 3D Level Set Function Based Optimization

Shape and dielectric property reconstruction both are important in 3D reconstructions. 3D level set based optimization is more suitable for 3D reconstruction because it can reconstruct shape and dielectric property both. Two level set functions are used in Figure 2.7 to identify four different regions. In Figure 2.7, $(\phi \geq 0, \psi \geq 0)$, $(\phi \geq 0, \psi < 0)$, $(\phi < 0, \psi \geq 0)$ and $(\phi < 0, \psi < 0)$ represent healthy fatty tissues, healthy fibro-glandular tissues, malignant fatty tissues and malignant fibro-glandular tissues, respectively. The permittivity profile of Figure 2.7 is expressed in terms of two level set functions as equation (2.23).

$$\epsilon(r) = \epsilon^{tum}(1 - H(\phi)) + H(\phi)[\epsilon^{fib}H(\psi) + \epsilon^{fat}(1 - H(\psi))] \tag{2.23}$$

In equation (2.23), ϵ^{tum}, ϵ^{fib} and ϵ^{fat} are complex permittivity of tumour, fibro-glandular and fatty tissues, respectively. ϵ^{tum}, ϵ^{fib} and ϵ^{fat} are expressed in terms of single pole Debye model. *H*() is unit step or heavy-side function. In

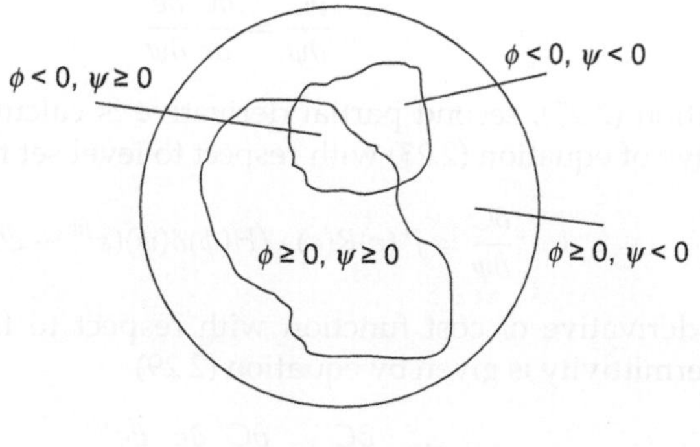

FIGURE 2.7
Application of two level set functions to distinguish four different regions (in 2D).

equation (2.23), ϕ and ψ are two level set functions. 3D level set based optimization always starts with an initial guess about solution. Signed distance function of initial guess is required. Steps to calculate signed distance function are given below.

- Find the edges of initial guess
- Find the positive distance inside the edge boundary
- Find the negative distance outside the edge boundary
- Normalize the distance

Signed distance function is between -1 to 1 after performing above steps. Now, this signed distance function is updated using iterative optimization approach. Equations (2.10) and (2.11) represent linear relationships among Debye parameters. Partial derivative of equation (2.8) (cost function) with respect to permittivity is given below.

$$\frac{\partial C}{\partial \epsilon} = J^T(\epsilon)R(\epsilon) \tag{2.24}$$

In equation (2.24), $J^T(\epsilon)$ is transpose of Jacobian matrix, $R(\epsilon)$ is residual. Jacobian matrix is calculated by element wise multiplication of Green's function matrix with total electric field matrix [30]. Partial derivative of cost function with respect to level set function ϕ is calculated by using equation (2.25).

$$\frac{\partial C}{\partial \phi} = \frac{\partial C}{\partial \epsilon}\frac{\partial \epsilon}{\partial \phi} \tag{2.25}$$

In equation (2.25), second partial derivative is calculated by taking partial derivative of equation (2.23) with respect to level set function ϕ.

$$\frac{\partial C}{\partial \phi} = J^T(\epsilon)R(\epsilon) \cdot \delta(\phi)(\epsilon^{fib}H(\psi) + \epsilon^{fat}(1 - H(\psi)) - \epsilon^{tum}) \tag{2.26}$$

Similarly, Partial derivative of cost function with respect to level set function ψ is calculated by using equation (2.27).

$$\frac{\partial C}{\partial \psi} = \frac{\partial C}{\partial \epsilon}\frac{\partial \epsilon}{\partial \psi} \tag{2.27}$$

In equation (2.27), second partial derivative is calculated by taking partial derivative of equation (2.23) with respect to level set function ψ.

$$\frac{\partial C}{\partial \psi} = J^T(\epsilon)R(\epsilon) \cdot (H(\phi)\delta(\psi)(\epsilon^{fib} - \epsilon^{fat})) \tag{2.28}$$

Partial derivative of cost function with respect to fibro-glandular tissue's static permittivity is given by equation (2.29).

$$\frac{\partial C}{\partial \epsilon_s^{fib}} = \frac{\partial C}{\partial \epsilon}\frac{\partial \epsilon}{\partial \epsilon^{fib}}\frac{\partial \epsilon^{fib}}{\partial \epsilon_s^{fib}} \tag{2.29}$$

Second partial derivative of equation (2.29) is calculated by taking partial derivative of equation (2.23) with respect to ϵ^{fib}. Third partial derivative of equation (2.29) is calculated using two steps. In first step, equations (2.10) and (2.11) are substituted in equation (2.1). In second step, partial derivative of resultant equation is taken with respect to ϵ_s^{fib}. Equation (2.30) is obtained by substituting partial derivatives in equation (2.29).

$$\frac{\partial C}{\partial \epsilon_s^{fib}} = J^T(\epsilon)R(\epsilon) \cdot H(\phi)H(\psi)\frac{\partial \epsilon^{fib}}{\partial \epsilon_s^{fib}} \tag{2.30}$$

Partial derivative of cost function with respect to fatty tissue's static permittivity is given by equation (2.31).

$$\frac{\partial C}{\partial \epsilon_s^{fat}} = \frac{\partial C}{\partial \epsilon}\frac{\partial \epsilon}{\partial \epsilon^{fat}}\frac{\partial \epsilon^{fat}}{\partial \epsilon_s^{fat}} \tag{2.31}$$

Equation (2.32) is obtained after calculating second and third partial derivatives of equation (2.31).

$$\frac{\partial C}{\partial \epsilon_s^{fat}} = J^T(\epsilon)R(\epsilon) \cdot H(\phi)(1 - H(\psi))\frac{\partial \epsilon^{fat}}{\partial \epsilon_s^{fat}} \tag{2.32}$$

Now, Four update equations are derived using equations (2.26), (2.28), (2.30) and (2.32).

$$\phi^{n+1} = \phi^n - \alpha_\phi \frac{\partial C}{\partial \phi} \tag{2.33}$$

$$\psi^{n+1} = \psi^n - \alpha_\psi \frac{\partial C}{\partial \psi} \tag{2.34}$$

$$\left(\epsilon_s^{fib}\right)^{n+1} = \left(\epsilon_s^{fib}\right)^n - \alpha_{\epsilon_s^{fib}} \frac{\partial C}{\partial \epsilon_s^{fib}} \tag{2.35}$$

$$\left(\epsilon_s^{fat}\right)^{n+1} = \left(\epsilon_s^{fat}\right)^n - \alpha_{\epsilon_s^{fat}} \frac{\partial C}{\partial \epsilon_s^{fat}} \tag{2.36}$$

Algorithm cannot converge to solution for larger values of step size. It becomes slower due to smaller step size. Equations (2.33), (2.34), (2.35) and (2.36) are updated using four stage reconstruction strategy and frequency hopping [30, 32]. Four stage reconstruction used in the thesis is modified to reduce computations. The first stage is an initial guess of class 3 numerical breast phantom internal structure. The second stage is reconstruction of both tissues by using equations (2.34), (2.35) and (2.36). In the third stage tumour location and shape are reconstructed by using equations (2.33) and (2.34). In the last stage, the tumour permittivity value is decided by using equation (2.33).

2.3.3 Implementation Overview

Level set based optimization steps are given below.

1. Convert system in matrix form.
2. Calculate scattered electric field using known ϵ.
3. Identify different regions to be reconstructed.
4. Decide number of level set functions to be used.
5. Start with the initial guess.
6. Calculate signed distance function.
7. Calculate initial cost function.
8. Calculate total electric field using 3D FDTD.
9. Calculate Jacobian matrix.
10. Calculate required partial derivatives of cost function.
11. Now, update all equations such that the cost function is minimized.
12. If stopping criteria is satisfied then stop; otherwise, repeat steps 8 to 12 by using reconstructed results of current iteration.

The above steps are implemented to reconstruct static permittivity values by minimizing cost function.

2.4 3D Level Set Based Regularized Optimization

In case of ill posed and noise affected inverse scattering problem, regularization is very useful [35–37]. Tikhonov and total variation regularization techniques are evaluated in this section. Details of both techniques are given in reference [37].

2.4.1 Tikhonov Regularization

Tikhonov regularization is a very well known technique. Cost function is updated to include regularization term. Now, the cost function of equation 2.37 is obtained by adding Tikhonov regularization term in equation (2.8).

$$C(\epsilon) = \frac{1}{2}\left(\sum_{i=1}^{FM} |R_i|^2 + \lambda \|X_1\|^2\right) \tag{2.37}$$

In equation (2.37), λ is regularization parameter, and $\|X_1\|$ is norm of column vector X_1. Column vector X_1 contains static permittivity values for all voxels. Two things are achieved by regularization: First, small residue is obtained for accurate solution. Second, small solution is achieved so the solution is not affected much by perturbation. Partial derivate of cost function with respect to unknown parameter is given by equation (2.38).

$$\frac{\partial C}{\partial \epsilon} = J^T(\epsilon)R(\epsilon) + \lambda X_1 \tag{2.38}$$

In equation (2.38), $J^T(\epsilon)$ is the transpose of Jacobian matrix. It is element by element multiplication of Green's function matrix and total electric field matrix, $R(\epsilon)$ is residual.

2.4.2 Total Variation Regularization

Tikhonov regularization performs well in a situation where the solution has smooth changes. It will not perform well in a case where the solution has abrupt changes. Total variation regularization term is defined as shown in equation (2.39).

$$TV(X) = \sum_{j=1}^{n-1} |X_{j+1} - X_j| = \|L_1X\|_1 \tag{2.39}$$

In equation (2.39), $\|L_1X\|_1$ is L^1 norm of $\|L_1X\|$. L_1 is a derivative matrix as shown by equation (2.40).

$$L_1 = \begin{bmatrix} -1 & 1 & 0 & \cdot & \cdot & 0 \\ 0 & -1 & 1 & 0 & \cdot & 0 \\ 0 & 0 & -1 & 1 & 0 & \cdot \\ \cdot & \cdot & 0 & \cdot & \cdot & \cdot \\ \cdot & \cdot & \cdot & \cdot & \cdot & \cdot \\ \cdot & \cdot & \cdot & 0 & -1 & 1 \\ 0 & 0 & 0 & 0 & 0 & -1 \end{bmatrix} \tag{2.40}$$

Now, equation (2.41) is obtained by replacing Tikhonov regularization term with total variation regularization term.

$$C(\epsilon) = \frac{1}{2}\sum_{i=1}^{FM} |R_i|^2 + \lambda\|L_1X\|_1 \tag{2.41}$$

L_1 norm is non differentiable. In order to obtain partial derivative diagonal matrix W is used. Equation (2.42) is obtained by using the procedure of [37].

$$\frac{\partial C}{\partial \epsilon} = J^T(\epsilon)R(\epsilon) + \lambda L_1^T W L_1 x \tag{2.42}$$

$W_{j,j} = 1/|x_{j+1} - x_j|$, where $(x_{j+1} - x_j)$ is jth element of vector L_1x. Tolerance can be set on values of W to accommodate non differentiability of L_1 norm.

$$w_{j,j} = \begin{cases} \dfrac{1}{|X_{j+1} - X_j|}, & |X_{j+1} - X_j| \geq \epsilon \\ \frac{1}{\epsilon}, & |X_{j+1} - X_j| < \epsilon \end{cases} \tag{2.43}$$

TABLE 2.1
Values of Debye Parameters for Different Breast Tissues

Tissues	ϵ_∞	$\Delta\epsilon$	$\sigma_s(s/m)$
Adipose (fatty)	4.09	3.54	0.0842
Fibro-glandular	18.6	35.6	0.817
Skin	15.3	24.8	0.741
Tumour (assumed)	23.2	41	0.93
Immersion medium	2.6	0	0

Diagonal matrix W is calculated by using equation (2.43) in the iterative process. Cost function and it's partial derivative with respect to permittivity are changed to include regularization. Other implementation details are same as previous section.

2.4.3 Simulation Parameters and Noise Consideration

Values of Debye parameters are given for different breast tissues in Table 2.1 [4,5,16,17]. These values are valid for 0.5 GHz to 3 GHz. For simplicity, only two major type of tissues are considered in the class 3 numerical breast phantom. Inverse problem is solved after adding white Gaussian noise to scattered electric field.

$$Ax = b + n \tag{2.44}$$

In equation 2.44, n is additive white gaussian noise column vector. RMSE in complex permittivity is calculated by using equation 2.45.

$$RMSE = \sqrt{\frac{\sum_{i=1}^{K}(\epsilon_i - \hat{\epsilon}_i)^2}{K}} \tag{2.45}$$

In equation 2.45, ϵ_i is an original permittivity value. $\hat{\epsilon}_i$ is reconstructed permittivity value. K is total number of cells used in the model.

2.5 Results and Discussion

Inverse scattering problem is solved for two regularization schemes to compare performance of both. SNR is 20 dB for all reconstructions. Original profile of static permittivity (ϵ_s) with 2 cm.×2 cm.×2 cm. tumour is shown in Figure 2.8.

Reconstructed profile of static permittivity without regularization is shown in Figure 2.9. By comparing Figure 2.9 with Figure 2.8, it is clear tha

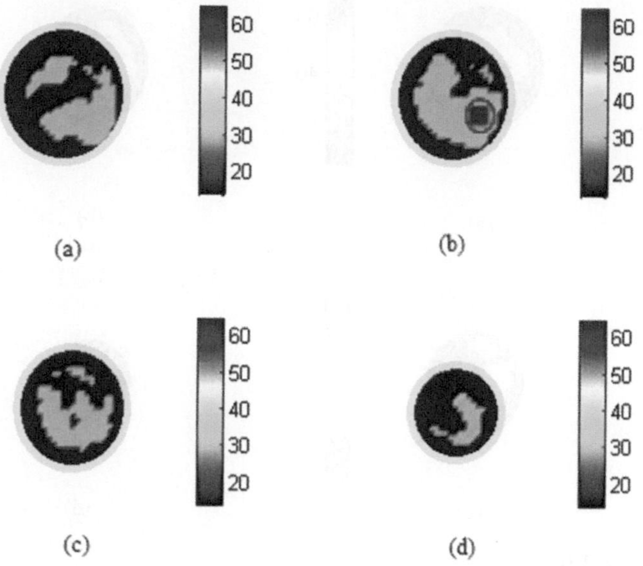

FIGURE 2.8
Coronal cross section of original static permittivity (ϵ_S) profile at (a) 1.5 cm. (b) 3 cm. (c) 4.5 cm. (d) 6 cm. (Brown dot in (b) represents 2 cm.×2 cm.×2 cm. tumour).

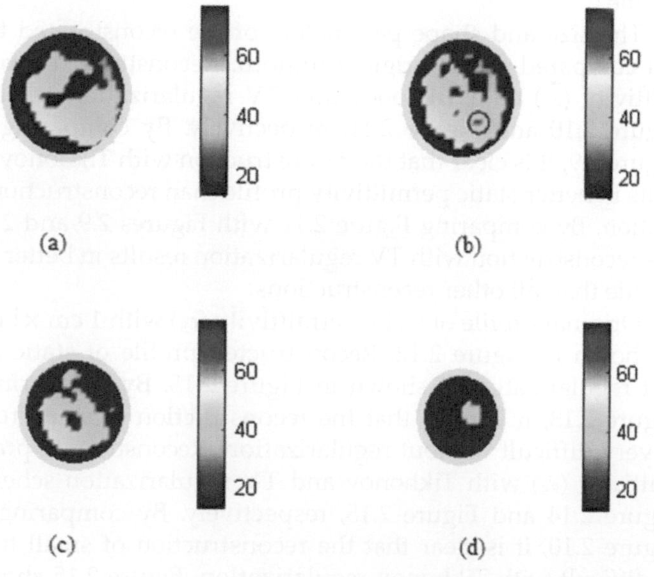

FIGURE 2.9
Coronal cross section of reconstructed static permittivity (ϵ_S) profile without regularization at (a) 1.5 cm. (b) 3 cm. (c) 4.5 cm. (d) 6.5 cm. (Brown dot in (b) represents tumour).

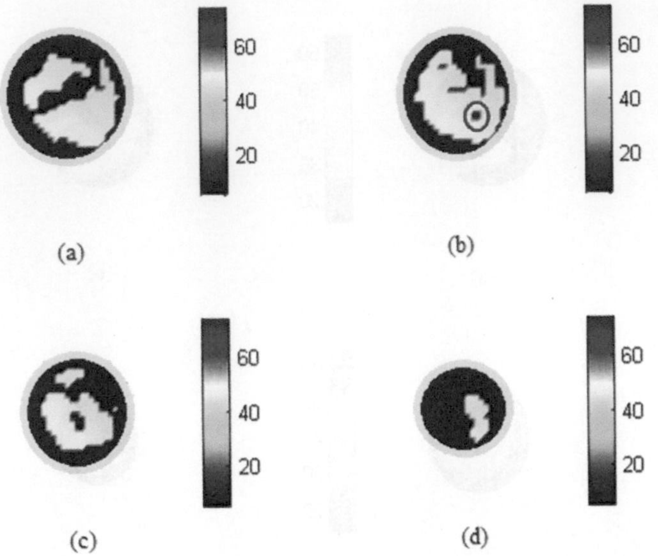

FIGURE 2.10
Coronal cross section of reconstructed static permittivity (ϵ_s) profile with Tikhonov regularization at (a) 1.5 cm. (b) 3 cm. (c) 4.5 cm. (d) 6.5 cm. (Brown dot in (b) represents tumour).

the reconstruction without regularization results in a poor static permittivity profile.

The size and shape parameters of the reconstructed tumour are different compared to the original tumour. Reconstructed profiles of static permittivity (ϵ_s) with Tikhonov and TV regularization schemes are shown in Figure 2.10 and Figure 2.11, respectively. By comparing Figure 2.10 with Figure 2.9, it is clear that the reconstruction with Tikhonov regularization results in better static permittivity profile than reconstruction without regularization. By comparing Figure 2.11 with Figures 2.9 and 2.10, it is clear that the reconstruction with TV regularization results in better static permittivity profile than all other reconstructions.

Original profile of static permittivity (ϵ_s) with 1 cm.×1 cm.×1 cm. tumour is shown in Figure 2.12. Reconstructed profile of static permittivity without regularization is shown in Figure 2.13. By comparing Figure 2.9 with Figure 2.13, it is clear that the reconstruction of small tumour parameters is very difficult without regularization. Reconstructed profiles of static permittivity (ϵ_s) with Tikhonov and TV regularization schemes are shown in Figure 2.14 and Figure 2.15, respectively. By comparing Figure 2.14 with Figure 2.10, it is clear that the reconstruction of small tumour parameters is difficult with Tikhonov regularization. Figure 2.15 shows that the reconstruction of small tumour parameters is very good with TV regularization The original profile of static permittivity (ϵ_s) with 0.5 cm.×0.5 cm.×0.5 cm. tumour is shown in Figure 2.16. The reconstructed profile of static permittivity

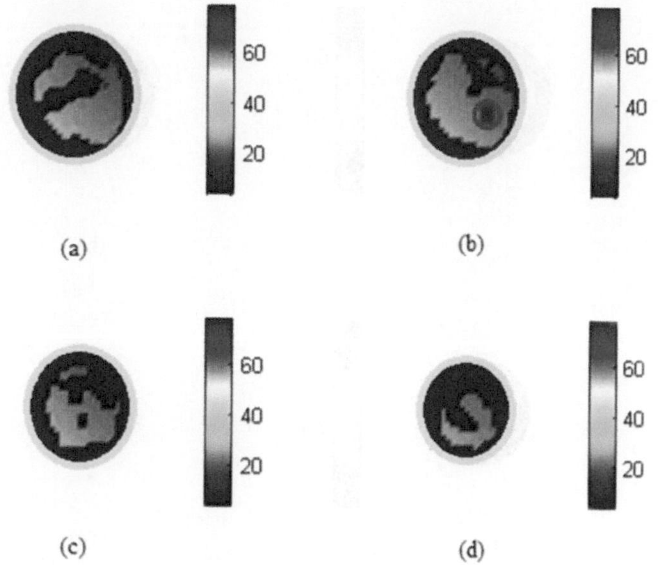

(a) (b)

(c) (d)

FIGURE 2.11
Coronal cross section of reconstructed static permittivity (ϵ_s) profile with TV regularization at (a) 1.5 cm. (b) 3 cm. (c) 4.5 cm. (d) 6.5 cm. (Brown dot in (b) represents tumour).

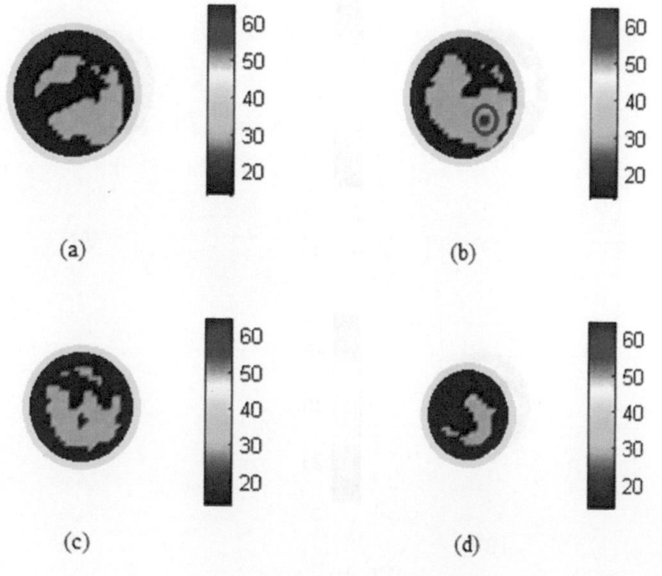

(a) (b)

(c) (d)

FIGURE 2.12
Coronal cross section of original static permittivity (ϵ_s) profile at (a) 1.5 cm. (b) 3 cm. (c) 4.5 cm. (d) 6.5 cm. (Brown dot in (b) represents 1 cm.×1 cm.×1 cm. tumour).

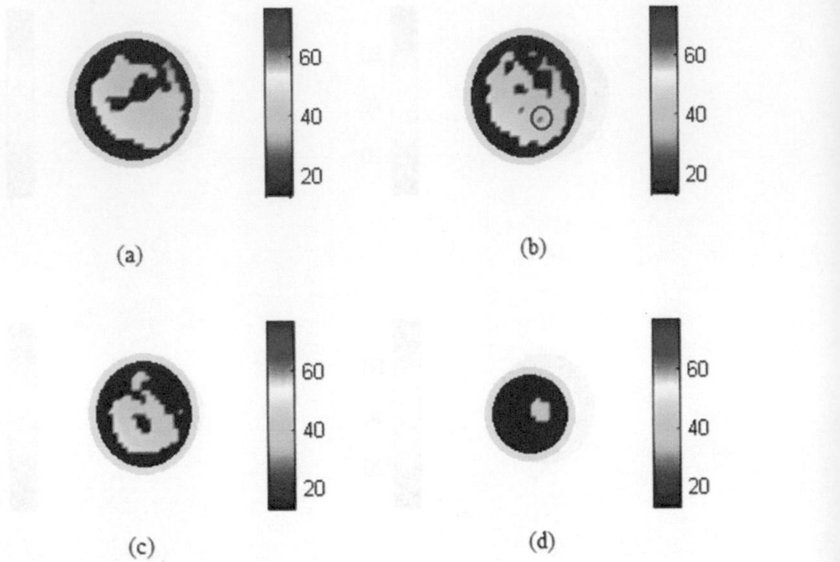

FIGURE 2.13
Coronal cross section of reconstructed static permittivity (ϵ_S) profile without regularization at (a) 1.5 cm. (b) 3 cm. (c) 4.5 cm. (d) 6.5 cm. (Brown dot in (b) represents tumour).

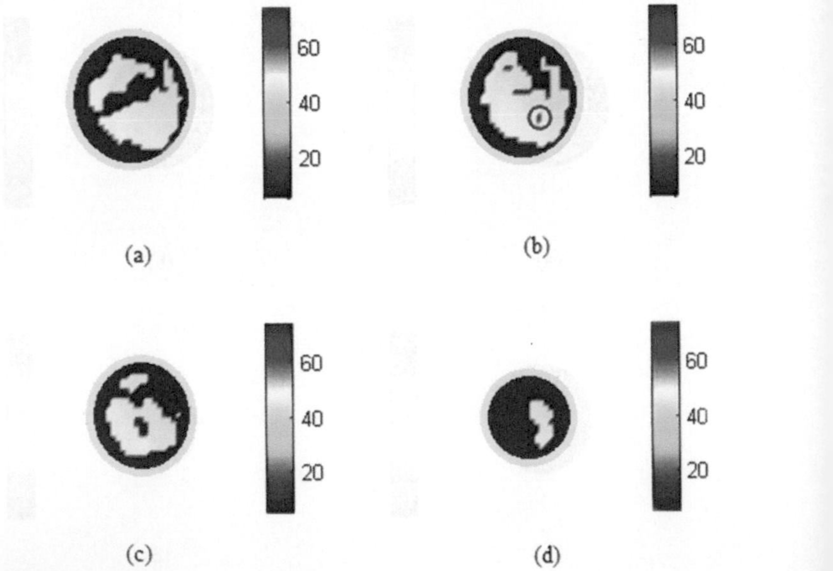

FIGURE 2.14
Coronal cross section of reconstructed static permittivity (ϵ_S) profile with Tikhonov regularization at (a) 1.5 cm. (b) 3 cm. (c) 4.5 cm. (d) 6.5 cm. (Brown dot in (b) represents tumour).

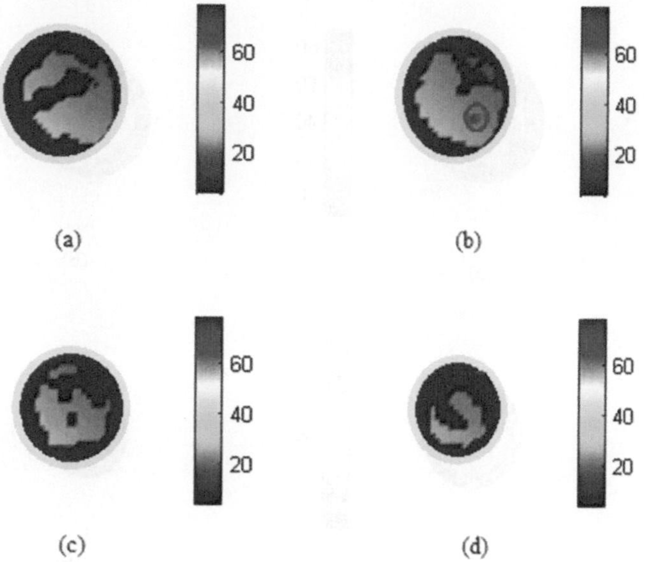

FIGURE 2.15
Coronal cross section of reconstructed static permittivity (ϵ_s) profile with TV regularization at (a) 1.5 cm. (b) 3 cm. (c) 4.5 cm. (d) 6.5 cm. (Brown dot in (b) represents tumour).

without regularization is shown in Figure 2.17. By comparing Figure 2.17 with Figure 2.16, it is clear that the reconstruction of very small tumour parameters is impossible without regularization. Reconstructed profiles of static permittivity (ϵ_s) with Tikhonov and TV regularization schemes are shown in Figure 2.18 and Figure 2.19, respectively. By comparing Figure 2.18 with Figure 2.16, it is clear that the reconstruction of very small tumour parameters is almost impossible with Tikhonov regularization. By comparing Figure 2.19 with Figure 2.16, it is clear that the reconstruction of very small tumour parameters is difficult with TV regularization. The location of a very small tumour is not properly detected with TV regularization. RMSE versus SNR graph is shown in Figure 2.20 for three cases. Cost function versus number of iterations graph is shown in Figure 2.21.

RMSE values clearly show that the performance of total variation regularization is better than the Tiknonov regularization. A comparison of different algorithms is given below. Details of Gauss-Newton, conjugate gradient and genetic algorithms are given in [38], [17,40], and [39], respectively.

Table 2.2 (below) clearly shows that the performance of 3D level set method is better than all other methods. 3D level set method has a shape optimization feature which results in less error as compared to other methods. Multiple frequency inverse scattering problem formulation is quite effective due to the inclusion of more information. Level set based methods solve value and shape optimization problems very efficiently by following

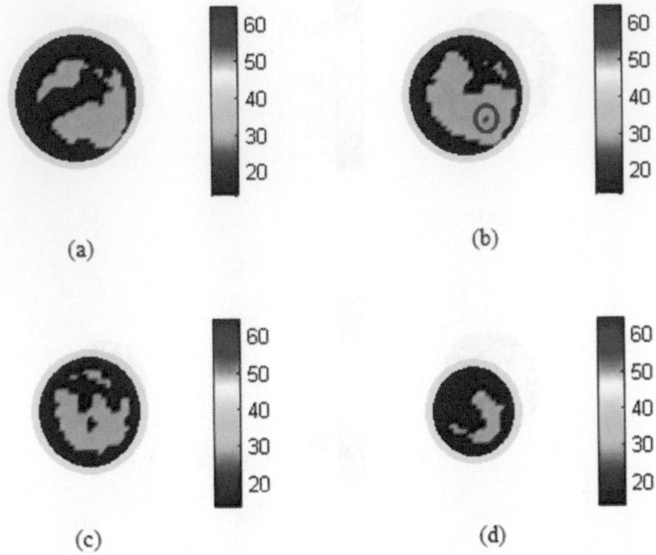

FIGURE 2.16
Coronal cross section of original static permittivity (ϵ_s) profile at (a) 1.5 cm. (b) 3 cm. (c) 4.5 cm. (d) 6.5 cm. (Brown dot in (b) represents 0.5 cm.×0.5 cm.×0.5 cm. tumour).

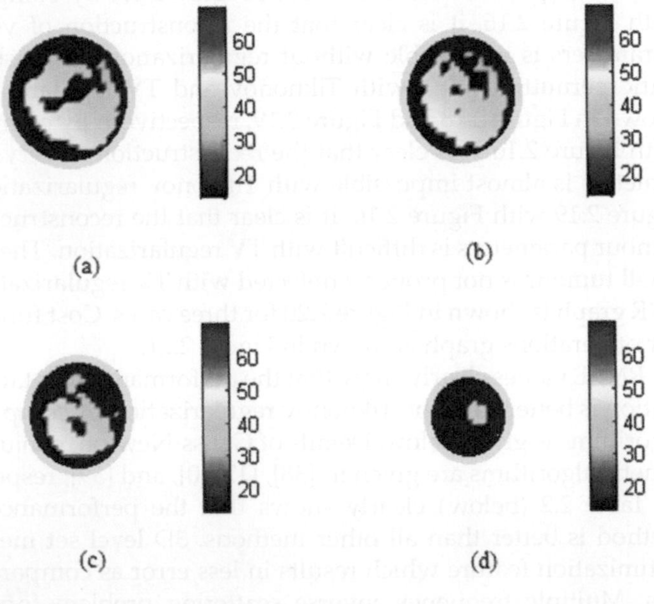

FIGURE 2.17
Coronal cross section of reconstructed static permittivity (ϵ_s) profile without regularization a
(a) 1.5 cm. (b) 3 cm. (c) 4.5 cm. (d) 6.5 cm.

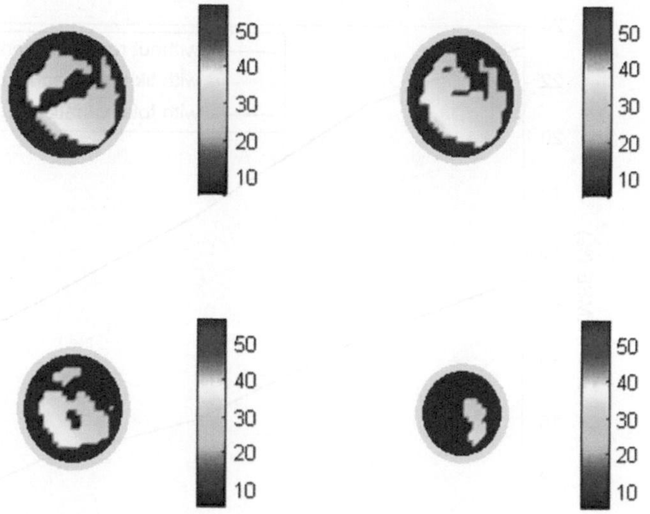

FIGURE 2.18
Coronal cross section of reconstructed static permittivity (ϵ_s) profile with Tikhonov regularization at (a) 1.5 cm. (b) 3 cm. (c) 4.5 cm. (d) 6.5 cm.

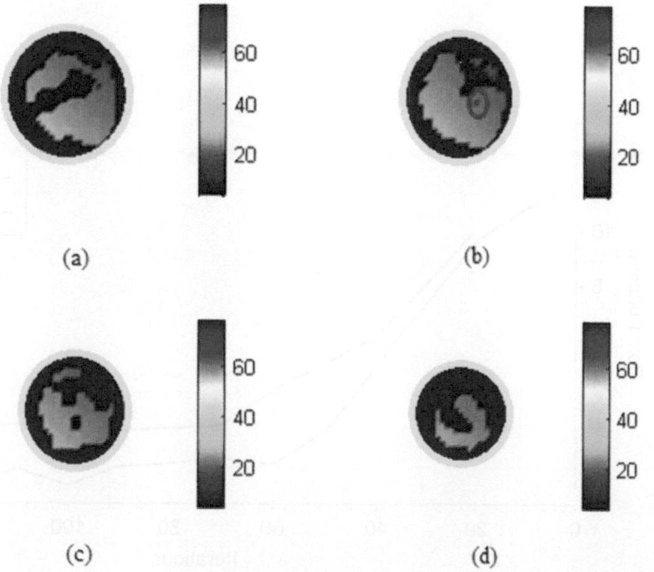

FIGURE 2.19
Coronal cross section of reconstructed static permittivity (ϵ_s) profile with TV regularization at (a) 1.5 cm. (b) 3 cm. (c) 4.5 cm. (d) 6.5 cm. (Brown dot in (b) represents tumour).

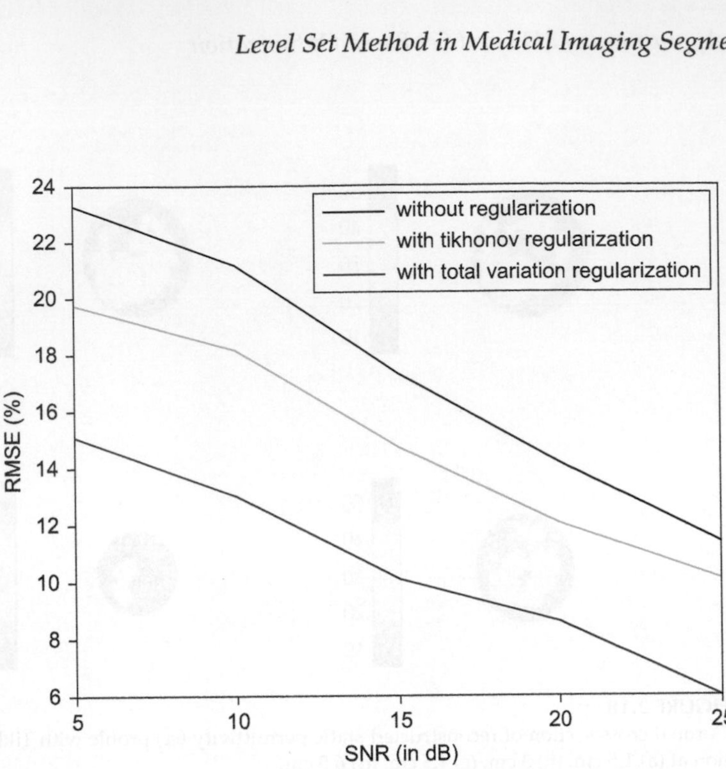

FIGURE 2.20
RMSE in static permittivity (ϵ_s) vs. SNR.

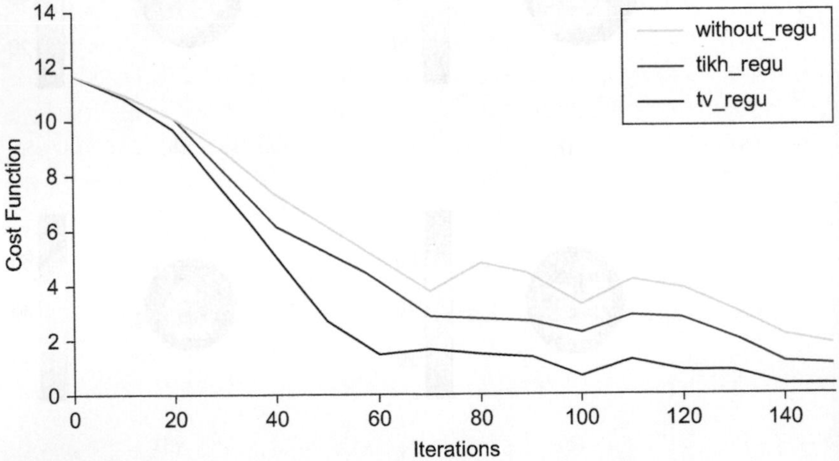

FIGURE 2.21
Cost vs. No. of Iterations.

TABLE 2.2
Comparison of RMSE for Different Algorithms

Methods	RMSE(%)
Gauss-Newton	24.14
Conjugate gradient method	21.62
Genetic algorithm	17.71
Level Set method	12.43

normal direction. Shape, size, and location detection of a breast tumour is possible by using 3D level set based methods. It is very difficult to reconstruct a static permittivity profile without regularization. It is difficult to reconstruct the exact shape, size and location of a tumour as its size decreases at 20 dB SNR. Tikhonov regularization improves reconstruction results but its performance degrades for a very small sized tumour. The performance of TV regularization is better than Tikhonov regularization for medium, small and very small breast tumours. TV regularization reconstructs the shape and size of a very small tumour but it fails to reconstruct the exact location of a very small tumour. Total variation regularization performs better than Tikhonov regularization because there are abrupt changes in the solution. L_1 norm performs better than L_2 norm in the 2D modified level set method [31]. The above conclusion is also true for our 3D level set based optimization. Oscillations are reduced by using regularization schemes during cost function minimization which makes convergence faster. 3D level set based optimization with TV regularization is quite effective for 5 dB to 25 dB SNR. Level set based optimization performs better than traditional optimization schemes due to its natural merging and breaking features. 30 dB SNR is required for better microwave image reconstruction in [30]. In this work, 20 dB SNR is required for better microwave image reconstruction and tumour detection. Shape and values both are reconstructed simultaneously in 3D level set based regularized optimization. As shown in this chapter, the potential 3D level set optimization based medical image segmentation is very promising. Future work should include the improving the computational efficiency of level set based optimization for medical image segmentation.

References

1. Ferlay, Jacques, Isabelle Soerjomataram, Rajesh Dikshit, Sultan Eser, Colin Mathers, Marise Rebelo, Donald Maxwell Parkin, David Forman, and Freddie Bray. "Cancer incidence and mortality worldwide: sources, methods and major patterns in GLOBOCAN 2012," *International Journal of Cancer*, Vol. 136, no. 5, pp. 359–386, March 2015.

2. Elise C. Fear, Paul M. Meaney, and Maria A. Stuchly. "Microwaves for breast cancer detection," *IEEE Potentials*, Vol. 22, no. 1, pp. 12–18, 2003.
3. Campbell, A. M., and D. V. Land. "Dielectric properties of female human breast tissue measured in vitro at 3.2 GHz," *Physics in Medicine and Biology*, Vol. 37, no. 1, pp. 193–210, 1992.
4. Lazebnik, Mariya, Leah McCartney, Dijana Popovic, Cynthia B. Watkins, Mary J. Lindstrom, Josephine Harter, Sarah Sewall et al. "A large-scale study of the ultra-wideband microwave dielectric properties of normal breast tissue obtained from reduction surgeries," *Physics in Medicine and Biology*, Vol. 52, no. 10, pp. 2637–2656, 2007.
5. Lazebnik, Mariya, Dijana Popovic, Leah McCartney, Cynthia B. Watkins, Mary J. Lindstrom, Josephine Harter, Sarah Sewall et al. "A large-scale study of the ultra-wideband microwave dielectric properties of normal, benign and malignant breast tissues obtained from cancer surgeries," *Physics in Medicine and Biology*, Vol. 52, no. 20, pp. 6093–6115, 2007.
6. Robert A. Jesinger, MD, MSE "Breast Anatomy for the Interventionalist," *Techniques in Vascular and Interventional Radiology*, Elsevier, Vol. 17, no. 1, pp. 3–9, March 2014.
7. Douglas Hanahan and Robert A. Weinberg, "Hallmarks of Cancer: The Next Generation," Elsevier, *Cell Press*, Vol. 144, no. 5, pp. 646–674, March 2011.
8. Zhou, Chuan, Heang-Ping Chan, Nicholas Petrick, Mark A. Helvie, Mitchell M. Goodsitt, Berkman Sahiner, and Lubomir M. Hadjiiski. "Computerized image analysis: estimation of breast density on mammograms," *Medical Physics*, Vol. 28, no. 6, pp. 1056–1069, 2001.
9. Vacek, Pamela M., and Berta M. Geller. "A prospective study of breast cancer risk using routine mammographic breast density measurements," *Cancer Epidemiology and Prevention Biomarkers*, Vol. 13, no. 5, pp. 715–722, 2004.
10. Boyd, Norman F., Gina A. Lockwood, Jeff W. Byng, David L. Tritchler, and Martin J. Yaffe. "Mammographic densities and breast cancer risk," *Cancer Epidemiology and Prevention Biomarkers*, Vol. 7, no. 12, pp. 1133–1144, 1998.
11. Vachon, Celine M., Carla H. Van Gils, Thomas A. Sellers, Karthik Ghosh, Sandhya Pruthi, Kathleen R. Brandt, and V. Shane Pankratz. "Mammographic density, breast cancer risk and risk prediction," *Breast Cancer Research*, Vol. 9, no. 6, pp. 217–225, 2007.
12. Freer, Phoebe E. "Mammographic breast density: impact on breast cancer risk and implications for screening," *Radiographics*, Vol. 35, no. 2, pp. 302–315, 2015.
13. Nelson, Heidi D., Ellen S. O'meara, Karla Kerlikowske, Steven Balch, and Diana Miglioretti. "Factors Associated With Rates of False-Positive and False-Negative Results From Digital Mammography Screening: An Analysis of Registry DataFalse-Positive and False-Negative Digital Mammography Screening Results," *Annals of Internal Medicine*, Vol. 164, no. 4, pp. 226–235, 2016.
14. Zastrow, E., S. K. Davis, M. Lazebnik, F. Kelcz, B. D. Van Veen, and S. C. Hagness, "Development of anatomically realistic numerical breast phantoms with accurate dielectric properties for modelling microwave interactions with the human breast," *IEEE Transactions on Biomedical Engineering*, Vol. 55, no. 12, pp. 2792-2800, 2008.
15. Lazebnik, M., M. Okoniewski, J. H. Booske, and S. C. Hagness, "Highly accurate Debye models for normal and malignant breast tissue dielectric properties at

microwave frequencies," *IEEE Microwave and Wireless Components Letters*, Vol. 17, no. 12, pp. 822–824, 2007.
16. David W. Winters, Jacob D. Shea, Panagiotis Kosmas, Barry D. VanVeen, Susan C. Hagness, "Three-dimensional microwave breast imaging: dispersive dielectric properties estimation using patient-specific basis functions," *IEEE Transactions on Medical Imaging*, Vol. 28, no. 7, pp. 969–981, July 2009.
17. J. D., Shea, P. Kosmas, S. C. Hagness, and B. D. Van Veen, "Three-dimensional microwave imaging of realistic numerical breast phantoms via a multiple-frequency inverse scattering technique," *Medical Physics*, Vol. 37, no. 8, pp. 4210–4226, 2010.
18. S. Osher, J.A. Sethian, "Fronts propagating with curvature-dependent speed: algorithms based on Hamilton-Jacobi formulations," *Journal of Computational Physics*, Vol. 79, pp. 12–49, 1988.
19. S. Osher and R. Fedkiw, "Level set methods and dynamic implicit surfaces," *Applied Mathematical Sciences*, 2003 Springer-Verlag New York Inc.
20. Fadil Santosa, "A level-set approach for inverse problems involving obstacles," *EASIM: Control, Optimization and calculus of variations*, Vol. 1, pp. 17–33, January 1996.
21. Oliver Dorn, Eric L Miller and Carey M Rappaport, "A shape reconstruction method for electromagnetic tomography using adjoint fields and level sets," *Inverse Problems*, Vol. 16, No. 5, October 2000.
22. Martin Burger, "A level set method for inverse problems," *Inverse Problems*, Volume 17, Number 5, August 2001.
23. R. Ferraye, J.-Y. Dauvignac, C. Pichot, "An inverse scattering method based on contour deformations by means of a level set method using frequency hopping technique," *IEEE Transactions on Antennas and Propagation*, Vol. 51, No. 5, pp. 1100–1113, July 2003.
24. Martin burger and stanley j. osher, "A survey on level set methods for inverse problems and optimal design," *European Journal of Applied Mathematics*, Vol. 16, No. 2, pp. 263–301, April 2005.
25. Oliver Dorn and Dominique Lesselier, "Level set methods for inverse scattering," *Inverse Problems*, Volume 22, Number 4, June 2006.
26. Natalia Irishina, Oliver Dorn, Miguel, "A level set evolution strategy in microwave imaging for early breast cancer detection," *Computers & Mathematics with Applications*, Elsevier, Volume 56, Issue 3, pp. 607–618, August 2008.
27. Natalia Irishina, Miguel Moscoso, Oliver Dorn, "Microwave Imaging for Early Breast Cancer Detection Using a Shape-based Strategy," *IEEE Transactions on Biomedical Engineering*, Vol. 56, No.4, pp. 1143–1153, January 2009.
28. Alireza Aghasi, Misha Kilmer, and Eric L. Miller, "Parametric Level Set Methods for Inverse Problems," *SIAM Journal on Imaging Sciences*, Vol. 4, No. 2, 618–650, 2011.
29. Oguz Semerci, Eric L. Miller, "A Parametric Level-Set Approach to Simultaneous Object Identification and Background Reconstruction for Dual-Energy Computed Tomography," *IEEE transactions on Image Processing*, Vol. 21, No. 5, pp. 2719–2734, February 2012.
30. Timothy J. Colgan, Susan C. Hagness, Barry D. Van Veen, "A 3-D Level Set Method for Microwave Breast Imaging," *IEEE Transactions on Biomedical Engineering*, Vol. 62, No. 10, pp. 2526–2534, Oct. 2015.
31. Mohammad Reza Eskandari, Mojtaba Dehmollaian, Reza Safian, "Simultaneous Microwave Imaging and Parameter Estimation Using Modified Level-Set

Method," *IEEE Transactions on Antennas and Propagation* Vol. 64, No. 8, pp. 3554–3564, June 2016.
32. Natalia Irishina, "Microwave medical imaging using level set techniques," PhD Thesis, University of Carlos, Spain, 2009.
33. H. N. Patel and D. K. Ghodgaonkar, "3D level set based optimization of inverse scattering problem for microwave breast imaging", IEEE MTT-S International Microwave Bio Conference, 15-17 May 2017, Gothenburg, Sweden, pp. 1–4.
34. H. N. Patel and D. K. Ghodgaonkar, "Study of effect of numerical breast phantom heterogeneity on dielectric profile reconstruction using microwave imaging," *Progress In Electromagnetics Research* M, Vol. 58, pp. 135–145, 2017.
35. Hua, Ping, Eung Je Woo, John G. Webster, and Willis J. Tompkins. "Iterative reconstruction methods using regularization and optimal current patterns in electrical impedance tomography," *IEEE Transactions on Medical Imaging*, Vol. 10, no. 4, pp. 621–628, 1991.
36. Zhang, Hua, Jing Huang, Jianhua Ma, Zhaoying Bian, Qianjin Feng, Hongbing Lu, Zhengrong Liang, and Wufan Chen. "Iterative reconstruction for X-ray computed tomography using prior-image induced nonlocal regularization," *IEEE Transactions on Biomedical Engineering*, Vol. 61, no. 9, pp. 2367–2378, 2014.
37. Zhao, Shan, and Imad L. Al-Qadi. "Development of regularization methods on simulated ground-penetrating radar signals to predict thin asphalt overlay thickness," *Signal Processing, Elsevier*, Vol. 132, pp. 261–271, March 2017.
38. Jurgen De Zaeytijd, Ann Franchois, Christelle Eyraud, and Jean-Michel Geffrin, "Full-Wave Three-Dimensional Microwave Imaging With a Regularized Gauss-Newton Method-Theory and Experiment," *IEEE Transactions on Antennas and Wave Propagation*, Vol. 55, no. 11, pp. 3279–3292, November 2007.
39. Park, C. S. and B. S. Jeong, "Reconstruction of a high contrast and large object by using the hybrid algorithm combining a Levenberg-Marquardt algorithm and a genetic algorithm," *IEEE Transactions on Magnetics*, Vol. 35, no. 3, pp. 1582–1585, May 1999.
40. Rubk, T., P. M. Meaney, P. Meincke, and K. D. Paulsen, "Nonlinear microwave imaging for breast-cancer screening using Gauss-Newton's method and the CGLS inversion algorithm," *IEEE Transactions on Antennas and Propagation*, Vol. 55, no. 8, pp. 2320–2331, August 2007.

3

A Modified Global and Elastic ICP Shape Registration for Medical Imaging Applications

Hossam Abd El Munim and Aly A. Farag

CONTENTS

3.1 Introduction

Medical shapes registration and alignment [1–4] is an important complex problem in medical imaging. Model based segmentation is one of the most important applications that makes use of shape alignment. This process aims to find a transformation that moves a model towards a target image or shape [5] maximizing a similarity measure. Such similarity specifies how a source shape is close to a target image or model.

The iterative closest point algorithm [6] is based on finding the mappings based on the minimum distance criterion. Different shape registration methods based on this technique are provided in the literature (e.g. [7]). It is used in registering either *2D* or *3D* objects.

Many literature algorithms like those in [8–10] suffer serious problems including scale variations and dependency on initialization. Elastic deformations cannot be covered efficiently as well.

Images are registered in [11] using the iterative closest point technique. The hierarchical B-spline approach is involved to match these surfaces. The registration depends on the points that represent the source and target images as well as the control points, which create a huge matrix equation system. Solving such a system of equations is sometimes impossible.

In [19], object contours are extracted from the image to be matched with a database to mark some joints of the human body. Features are extracted using edge detectors for computing the similarity measures.

Implicit functions are used to match shapes in [5, 12]. The signed distance transform is computed over the domains of the source and target shapes. The sum of squared differences is formulated by matching scaled distances which are rotation and translation invariant. The registration parameters are estimated using the gradient descent approach in a variational framework. The technique was used to segment 2D and 3D images with prior shape models. Unfortunately, these approaches cannot cover in-homogenous scaling parameters.

Maximization of mutual information was involved for shape matching and registration in [22]. Signed distance functions were used as images to represent shapes. Mutual information measures the amount of information matching between the source and target shape images. Global motion parameters were estimated by maximizing the mutual information. The local deformations were represented by the incremental free form deformations (IFFD) approach. The control points minimize a sum of squared differences energy function. This method complicated the problem because a large number of control points might be required to cover detailed local deformations. The gradient descent optimization has a problem with these large number of variables associated with different levels of the IFFD.

The vector level set functions were firstly used for shape-based segmentation in [17]. The implicit function components represent the vector projections from any point in space to the closest point on the shape boundary. Positive sign labels points inside the shape while outside points are given negative implicit values. A dissimilarity measure is used to handle the problem of in-homogeneous scaling in a variational shape registration framework.

In this chapter, we present a global and elastic shape registration technique using the iterative closest point algorithm. The global motion is described by an affine transformation, while local deformations are handled by the incremental free form deformations. In both cases, a closed form solution is illustrated to estimate the mapping motion directly. The elastic motion uses control points which are computed by a closed form solution for energy minimization as a point-based registration problem. Sum of least squares and smoothing constraints are demonstrated to formulate an energy function which is quadratic in terms of control point deformations. We will show that the multi-level resolution control lattice approach gives exact and accurate mappings compared to the single high resolution level case. The minimization of the energy function results in a linear system of size dependence only on the number of control points, which makes the solution possible and reasonable. Different synthetic and real shapes registration will be demonstrated to illustrate the efficiency of the approach through the following application.

Many medical image application require building a detailed 3D model of the organ under investigation. These details can be achieved using different imaging radiology like CT scans and MRI's. CT scans are expensive, and the radiation dose is considered to be high; therefore it is not accepted as a routine practice. To achieve this goal, we need to build a system that gives detailed volumetric information about the human jaw. This system will start from that surface model which is divided into individual crowns (the teeth upper parts). Each crown will be matched with a **database** of different individual teeth types. So, a database of anatomical structures is of great interest for such a problem.

The generation of robust, accurate and accessible 3D anatomical models is now a landmark for future research and understanding in the medical world. Diverse 3D anatomical libraries provide a passive means by which the motivations of education, simulation and experimentation may all greatly benefit. Thus, an efficient technique for creating a diverse, 3D anatomical library is a viable medical resource with a great emphasis on autonomy. A reliable and autonomous procedure for obtaining 3D anatomical models provides an efficient means for enrolling large amounts of subjects into a 3D library that can be made available to students and professionals in the medical field.

The focus of this application is to outline the framework for autonomously building a 3D library of human teeth. Currently, research in this field includes a tooth library generated by Nagasawa and Yoshida *et.al.* [16], using X-ray images of 55 human teeth that were obtained by 3D micro-CT.

Real extracted human teeth of different types are fixed over wax rods. Then, we use Cone-beam CT to scan the wax and teeth. Total 280 teeth have been processed in this fashion. A point-based 3D shape registration method has been further applied to align all subjects enrolled into the library, providing a more uniform orientation for ease of use. Thus, an autonomous algorithm is proposed for reconstructing human teeth, enrolling each into a comprehensive library and further carrying out global, 3D registration. This framework will be outlined in detail and some preliminary results will be given.

The rest of this book chapter is organized as follows: Global shape registration is presented in Section 3.2; elastic deformations are estimated in Section 3.3; experimental results and validation are demonstrated in Section 3.4; and a Conclusion is made in Section 3.5.

3.2 Point-Based Global Shape Registration and Alignment

This section aims to formulate the registration between two different surface models based on explicit point mappings [19–21]. A source and target surface models are represented by $\mathbf{M_s}$ and $\mathbf{M_t}$, respectively. A transformation $\mathbf{A}$ that moves points from $\mathbf{M_s}$ to $\mathbf{M_t}$ needs to be estimated. The transformation has a set of parameters which will be estimated to minimize a certain energy function. We consider affine transformation with the following homogeneous format:

$$\mathbf{A} = \begin{pmatrix} a_1 & a_2 & a_3 & a_4 \\ a_5 & a_6 & a_7 & a_8 \\ a_9 & a_{10} & a_{11} & a_{12} \\ 0 & 0 & 0 & 1 \end{pmatrix} \tag{3.1}$$

Here we consider that $x_i \in \mathbf{M_s}, i = 1, 2, \ldots, N_s$ and $y_i \in \mathbf{M_t}$ is the closest point to $\mathbf{A}x_i$ on the target shape where N_s is the number of points on the source surface. Both $x_i = (x_{i1}\ x_{i2}\ x_{i3}\ 1)^T$ and $y_i = (y_{i1}\ y_{i2}\ y_{i3}\ 1)^T$ are put in the homogeneous vector notation of size 4×1. Consider the Euclidean distance between the moved point and its closet position to be the dissimilarity measure as follows:

$$d_i = ||\mathbf{A}x_i - y_i||. \tag{3.2}$$

The summation of squared differences is computed as the following objective energy function:

$$E = E(a_1, a_2, \ldots, a_{12}) = \sum_{i=1}^{N_s} \frac{1}{2} (\mathbf{A}x_i - y_i)^T (\mathbf{A}x_i - y_i) \tag{3.3}$$

We divided by 2 just to remove numbers from the derivative equation as follows. The transformation parameters $\{a_k\}$ are required to minimize the above functional. Taking the derivative of the energy with respect to a_k will result in:

$$\frac{\partial E}{\partial a_k} = \sum_{i=1}^{N_s} (\mathbf{A}x_i - y_i)^T (\mathbf{A}_{a_k} x_i) \tag{3.4}$$

where $\mathbf{A}_{a_k}$ is the derivative of the transformation matrix $\mathbf{A}$ with respect to the parameter a_k. So, any element $\mathbf{A}_{a_k}(m,n)$ in row m and column n of the derivative matrix can be written in the following format:

$$\mathbf{A}_{a_k}(m,n) = \begin{cases} 1 & if\, k == 4(m-1)+n \\ 0 & \text{otherwise} \end{cases} \tag{3.5}$$

Taking derivatives with respect to all the 12 parameters will result in a linear system of equations as shown below:

$$\Psi_G \Theta_G = \Lambda_G \tag{3.6}$$

where $\Theta_G = (a_1 a_2 \dots a_{11} a_{12})^T$. The column vector Λ has 12 elements defined as follows:

$$\Lambda_G = \Sigma_{i=1}^{N_s} (x_{i1}y_{i1}\; x_{i2}y_{i1}\; x_{i3}y_{i1}\; y_{i1}\; x_{i1}y_{i2}\; x_{i2}y_{i2}\; x_{i3}y_{i2}\; y_{i2}\; x_{i1}y_{i3}\; x_{i2}y_{i3}\; x_{i3}y_{i3}\; y_{i3})^T \tag{3.7}$$

The square matrix Ψ_G has 12×12 elements in Eq. 3.8.

$$\Psi_G = \Sigma_{i=1}^{N_s}$$

$$\times \begin{pmatrix} x_{i1}^2 & x_{i1}x_{i2} & x_{i1}x_{i3} & x_{i1} & 0 & 0 & 0 & 0 & 0 & 0 & 0 & 0 \\ x_{i1}x_{i2} & x_{i2}^2 & x_{i2}x_{i3} & x_{i2} & 0 & 0 & 0 & 0 & 0 & 0 & 0 & 0 \\ x_{i1}x_{i3} & x_{i2}x_{i3} & x_{i3}^2 & x_{i3} & 0 & 0 & 0 & 0 & 0 & 0 & 0 & 0 \\ x_{i1} & x_{i2} & x_{i3} & 1 & 0 & 0 & 0 & 0 & 0 & 0 & 0 & 0 \\ 0 & 0 & 0 & 0 & x_{i1}^2 & x_{i1}x_{i2} & x_{i1}x_{i3} & x_{i1} & 0 & 0 & 0 & 0 \\ 0 & 0 & 0 & 0 & x_{i1}x_{i2} & x_{i2}^2 & x_{i2}x_{i3} & x_{i2} & 0 & 0 & 0 & 0 \\ 0 & 0 & 0 & 0 & x_{i1}x_{i3} & x_{i2}x_{i3} & x_{i3}^2 & x_{i3} & 0 & 0 & 0 & 0 \\ 0 & 0 & 0 & 0 & x_{i1} & x_{i2} & x_{i3} & 1 & 0 & 0 & 0 & 0 \\ 0 & 0 & 0 & 0 & 0 & 0 & 0 & 0 & x_{i1}^2 & x_{i1}x_{i2} & x_{i1}x_{i3} & x_{i1} \\ 0 & 0 & 0 & 0 & 0 & 0 & 0 & 0 & x_{i1}x_{i2} & x_{i2}^2 & x_{i2}x_{i3} & x_{i2} \\ 0 & 0 & 0 & 0 & 0 & 0 & 0 & 0 & x_{i1}x_{i3} & x_{i2}x_{i3} & x_{i3}^2 & x_{i3} \\ 0 & 0 & 0 & 0 & 0 & 0 & 0 & 0 & x_{i1} & x_{i2} & x_{i3} & 1 \end{pmatrix} \tag{3.8}$$

Solving the above linear system will compute the parameters of the affine transformation that minimizes the distance between the two shape models. This process is repeated on the transformed surface until the change in the transformed points is not significant.

3.3 Point-Based Elastic Shape Registration

Our objective is to find a function that gives the point mappings between the two given domains (source and target). Let us define the 2D shape registration as follows:

A map $\mathbf{C}^s(p) : [0,1] \in R \rightarrow R^2$ defines a planar source curve with a parameter p. The target is defined by $\mathbf{C}^t(p) : [0,1] \in R \rightarrow R^2$. The Cartesian coordinates of the point vector can be defined by $\mathbf{C}(p) = [x\ y]^T$ where $0 \leq x \leq X$ and $0 \leq y \leq Y$.

3.3.1 Finding Mappings

Assume that $\mathbf{C}^t(p)$ is the mapping point of $\mathbf{C}^s(p)$ (the criteria for finding mappings will come in the following sections). The output will be a C^0 function $f : R^2 \rightarrow R^2$ with $f(\mathbf{C}^s(p)) = \mathbf{C}^t(p)$, $\forall p \in [0,1]$. Different interpolation functions have been proposed to handle this problem [11]. We choose the free form deformation *FFD* model, based on B-splines [13,14], which is a powerful tool for modeling deformable objects and has been previously applied to the tracking and motion analysis problems. The basic idea is to deform the shape by manipulating a mesh of control points. The resulting deformation controls the shape of the object and produces a smooth and continuous transformation.

Consider a lattice of control points $\mathbf{P} = \mathbf{P}_{m,n}$; $m = 1, \ldots, M$. $n = 1, \ldots, N$, each point on the source shape will have the following form of deformation:

$$\mathbf{L}(p) = \sum_{k=0}^{3} \sum_{l=0}^{3} B_k(u) B_l(v) \delta \mathbf{P}_{i+k,j+l} \tag{3.9}$$

where $\delta\mathbf{P} = \delta\mathbf{P}_{m,n}$ is the control point deformation, $i = \lfloor (x.(M-1)/X) \rfloor + 1$, $j = \lfloor (y.(N-1)/Y) \rfloor + 1$, $u = x.M/X - \lfloor (x.M/X) \rfloor$, $v = y.N/Y - \lfloor (y.N/Y) \rfloor$, and the spline basis functions (B) are defined in [14]. So the cubic B-spline is used as an approximation function for our interpolation problem. We propose the following energy to measure the difference between the deformed contour and its target points based on the Euclidean distance:

$$E(\delta\mathbf{P}) = \int_0^1 \|\mathbf{C}^s(p) + \mathbf{L}(p) - \mathbf{C}^t(p)\|^2 dp \tag{3.10}$$

Also, we need to avoid any undesired distortion in the shape and preserve the regularity of the registration grid flow. Another weighted term (by $\lambda \in R^+$) is added for smoothness constrain as follows [15]:

$$E(\delta\mathbf{P}) = \int_0^1 \|\mathbf{C}^s(p) + \mathbf{L}(p) - \mathbf{C}^t(p)\|^2 dp + \lambda \int_0^1 (\|\mathbf{L}_p\|^2 + \|\mathbf{L}_{pp}\|^2) dp \tag{3.11}$$

where $\mathbf{L}_p$ and $\mathbf{L}_{pp}$ are the first and second derivatives respectively of the deformation vector with respect to the parameterizations p. The above objective function is required to be minimal to calculate the control points locations and hence the deformation field at each point in the domain. Gradient descent and calculus of variation are used to optimize the given function as follows:

$$\frac{\partial E}{\partial \delta \mathbf{P}} = 2\int_0^1 (\mathbf{L}(p) - \mathbf{C}(p))^T \frac{\partial \mathbf{L}}{\partial \delta \mathbf{P}} dp + 2\lambda \int_0^1 \left(\mathbf{L}_p^T \frac{\partial \mathbf{L}_p}{\partial \delta \mathbf{P}} + \mathbf{L}_{pp}^T \frac{\partial \mathbf{L}_{pp}}{\partial \delta \mathbf{P}} \right) dp \tag{3.12}$$

where $\mathbf{C}(p) = \mathbf{C}^t(p) - \mathbf{C}^s(p)$. A detailed illustration for the local deformation derivatives are found in [22].

By setting the above equation to zero, we get a linear system of the control points coordinates:

$$\int_0^1 (\mathbf{C}(p))^T \frac{\partial \mathbf{L}}{\partial \delta \mathbf{P}} dp = \int_0^1 \mathbf{L}^T \frac{\partial \mathbf{L}}{\partial \delta \mathbf{P}} dp + \lambda \int_0^1 \left(\mathbf{L}_p^T \frac{\partial \mathbf{L}_p}{\partial \delta \mathbf{P}} + \mathbf{L}_{pp}^T \frac{\partial \mathbf{L}_{pp}}{\partial \delta \mathbf{P}} \right) dp \tag{3.13}$$

The left hand side is free from the coordinates of the control points while the other side is linearly a function of these unknowns. The following linear equation holds:-

$$\Psi \Theta = \Lambda \tag{3.14}$$

where $\Theta = [\delta \mathbf{P}_{1,1}^x, \dots, \delta \mathbf{P}_{M,N}^x, \delta \mathbf{P}_{1,1}^y, \dots, \delta \mathbf{P}_{M,N}^y]^T$ and x, y are the coordinates of the embedding space. The other matrices elements are calculated as follows:

$$\Psi_{r,c} = \int_0^1 (\mathbf{L}^{r,c})^T \frac{\partial \mathbf{L}}{\partial \theta_r} dp + \lambda \int_0^1 \left((\mathbf{L}_p^{r,c})^T \frac{\partial \mathbf{L}_p}{\partial \theta_r} + (\mathbf{L}_{pp}^{r,c})^T \frac{\partial \mathbf{L}_{pp}}{\partial \theta_r} \right) dp \tag{3.15}$$

$$\Lambda_r = \int_0^1 (\mathbf{C}(p))^T \frac{\partial \mathbf{L}}{\partial \theta_r} dp \tag{3.16}$$

where $\theta_r \in \Theta$ and $\mathbf{L}^{r,c}$ stands for the coefficient of the control point vector calculated from the cubic spline interpolation. Row and column are represented by *r and c* respectively.

The resulting matrix equation size depends on the number of control points and the space dimensions. Size of the data points of the curve does not have any impact on the matrices sizes which guarantees its computational efficiency (this is a huge advantage over the work proposed in [11] where number of linear equations is equal to number of data points). Also note that the smoothing constrains do not add extra load to the solution of the matrix equation.

3.3.2 A Coarse to Fine Strategy (Incremental Free Form Deformation)

The derived energy function is required to be minimized by moving the grid positions to get the correct mapping over shape boundaries. A very small error can be achieved when using a high resolution control lattice because the number of degrees of freedom increases. However this is not enough. Such sudden movement will result in unnecessary crossovers of the domain

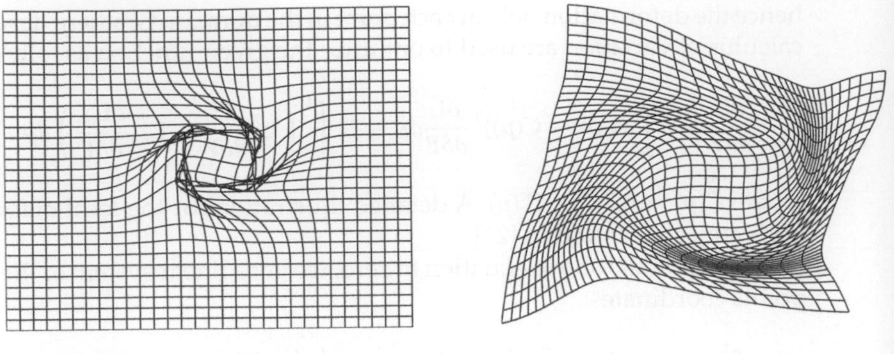

FIGURE 3.1
The grid local deformations using a resolution of 12 × 12 is given in the left image while multi level deformation result is demonstrated in the right panel.

grid lines and the registration process will be meaningless. This will result in changing and corrupting the object topology. A better way is to move the grid step by step towards the target.

For illustration purposes, assume a square to represent some source shape. Another shape is obtained by rotating the square by an angle of $\pi/2$ (this will stand for the target). Mappings between the source and target shapes are established by the rotation effect. A control lattice is constructed and computed using the above formula for the point-based registration. When using a relatively high resolution of 12 × 12 lattice, foldovers occur as shown in Figure 3.1 (top left image). To avoid this, a coarse to fine strategy is used (equivalent to the incremental free form deformations used in [22]). We start with a resolution of 4 × 4 and solve for the deformation. Iteratively we increase the resolution as 5 × 5, 6 × 6, and so on and so forth. In each step, the control points positions are computed and the contour moves to the new position until a satisfactory error distance is obtained. The result is smooth and the mapping is achieved accurately. The final grid deformation is shown in the right image. This process handles extremely well the error and gives impressive infinitesimal energy function and smooth grid deformations at the same time.

3.3.3 Iterative Closest Point (ICP) Algorithm for Elastic Registration

The iterative closest point (ICP) algorithm is a widely applied method for the registration of two data sets of points. For two Euclidean point sets, assume that the source point set is $\mathbf{C}^s$ and the target point is $\mathbf{C}^t$. The source point set is assumed to change or deform according to a certain known form of transformation and the target will remain fixed. The ICP algorithm can be described (as in Algorithm 1) [6]:

Algorithm 1 Conventional Elastic Shape Registration using ICP.

input: *Source and Target Contours* $(\mathbf{C}^s, \mathbf{C}^t)$

1: Initialize transformation parameters.
2: For every point in $\mathbf{C}^s$ determine its closest point in $\mathbf{C}^t$.
3: Compute the transformation parameters that minimize the sum of square differences between the mappings.
4: Based on the new parameters, update the source points $\mathbf{C}^s$ to the new positions.
5: If the change in the source points is less than a certain threshold terminate; otherwise go to step #2

output: *Final Deformed Source Contour, and Point Mappings.*

Transformation parameters will represent the way that the source data set moves to be registered to the target.

The conventional ICP drawbacks are well known. For elastic registration, it is difficult to find a deformation function to keep the topology of the registered objects. Another issue is that the closest point is not unique. According to [11], a coarse to fine strategy using the B-splines overcomes these problems for covering the local deformations. Below we will use a similar algorithm with our closed form solution for the point-based registration problem.

3.3.4 A Coarse to Fine Strategy with the ICP

Now we will illustrate the whole algorithm for shape registration. Assume that $N_x^i \times N_y^i$ is the resolution of the control point lattice initially denoted by i. The resolution at any time will be $N_x \times N_y$. The basic steps will be as in Algorithm 2:

Algorithm 2 The ICP Elastic Shape Registration using the IFFD.

input: *Source and Target Contours* $(\mathbf{C}^s, \mathbf{C}^t)$

1: Set $N_x = N_x^i$ and $N_y = N_y^i$
2: Construct a control lattice of size $N_x \times N_y$ and initialize its point deformation vectors to zeros.
3: For each point in $\mathbf{C}^s$, determine its corresponding closest point in $\mathbf{C}^t$.
4: Solve Eq. 3.16 to get the new deformation of each control point and hence calculate its new position.
5: Based on the new lattice, update the source points $\mathbf{C}^s$ by calculating the new deformation field using Eq. 3.9.
6: Set $N_x = N_x + 1$ and $N_y = N_y + 1$.
7: Check the stopping criteria. Either the objective function goes below a certain threshold or a number of maximum resolution levels is reached, otherwise go to step #2.

output: *Final Deformed Source Contour, Point Correspondences.*

3.4 Experimental Results and Discussions

3.4.1 Teeth Dataset Description

We have collected about 280 teeth from the School of Dentistry, University of Louisville, Louisville, KY, USA. Images were acquired by i-CAT Cone-beam scanner manufactured by Imaging Science International (Hatfield, PA). The CT protocol includes 3-8 mA (Pulse mode) and 120 kVp scanner settings. Primary reconstruction takes 1 minute for standard 20 second scan. The spatial resolution for each dataset is $0.2 \times 0.2 \times 0.2 mm^3$. Figure 3.2 shows different CT slices of a set of different real extracted teeth fixed over wax that takes the shape of the jaw. Wax appears in dark while bone tissues show up in bright areas.

The teeth dataset is first segmented by a variational model for surface evolution based on region statistics [17]. Since not all the slices contain teeth areas in each dataset, in order to reduce the computation complexity, the first slice and last slice containing teeth areas are automatically found. Then the central slice in between is extracted to have all the teeth areas. The centroid of each single tooth is automatically computed as the initial seeds of the 3D level set segmentation. The closed surfaces (a sphere for each tooth) centered at initial seeds, are propagated toward the desired 3D tooth region boundaries through the iterative evolution of the implicit surface. The bone tissue is considered the object while wax regions are considered as a background. Black regions are excluded from the process. The Expectation Maximization Algorithm is used initially to set the initial surfaces of the level set function (see [18] for details).

Figure 3.3 (a) shows the geometrical locations of all the twelve teeth, which are numbered from 1 to 12 clockwise. Figures 3.3 (b), (c) and (d) show the 3D segmentation and model visualization of the 12-teeth dataset from top, front and bottom views, respectively.

Figure 3.4 shows different 3D teeth models, including the twelve ones (in Figure 3.3) from (1) to (12), and more results from (13) to (40).

3.4.2 Global Alignment Results

As we mentioned above, our goal is to construct a 3D model of the jaw. So, using 3D tooth models will be more appropriate if they are vertically aligned. Because of this, registration of different models should be incorporated. Our registration approach depends on measuring distance between surfaces based on their cloud of points. Initially, each 3D model is aligned to a virtual model that contains only two points. The two points lie at the center of the top and bottom squares of the cube that contains the 3D volume. That alignment does not include any scaling. Figure 3.4 shows results

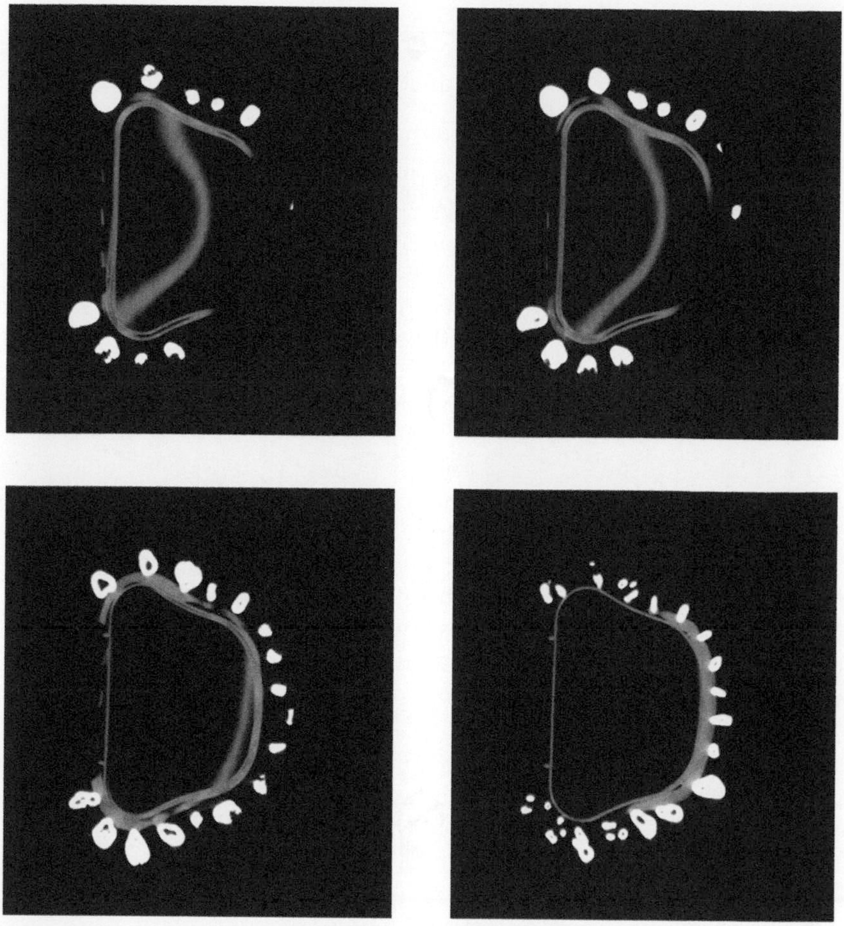

FIGURE 3.2
Different CT slices of a set of different real extracted teeth fixed over wax that takes the shape of the jaw. Wax appears in dark, whereas bone tissues show up in bright areas.

of segmented models lined up vertically to make them reasonable for the modeling process. After this step, 3D models will almost have no rotation and translation differences but still have scale differences. We carry out our proposed registration approach between the different models and the first tooth model. This is the typical approach used in building shape models [18]. Registration results are shown in Figure 3.5. It shows that the proposed registration approach can cover scales, rotation, and translations successfully between different models. Apparently, the proposed registration techniques does not need any implicit representation of the surfaces. Actually, computing distance transforms to implicitly represent shapes is a slow process [22].

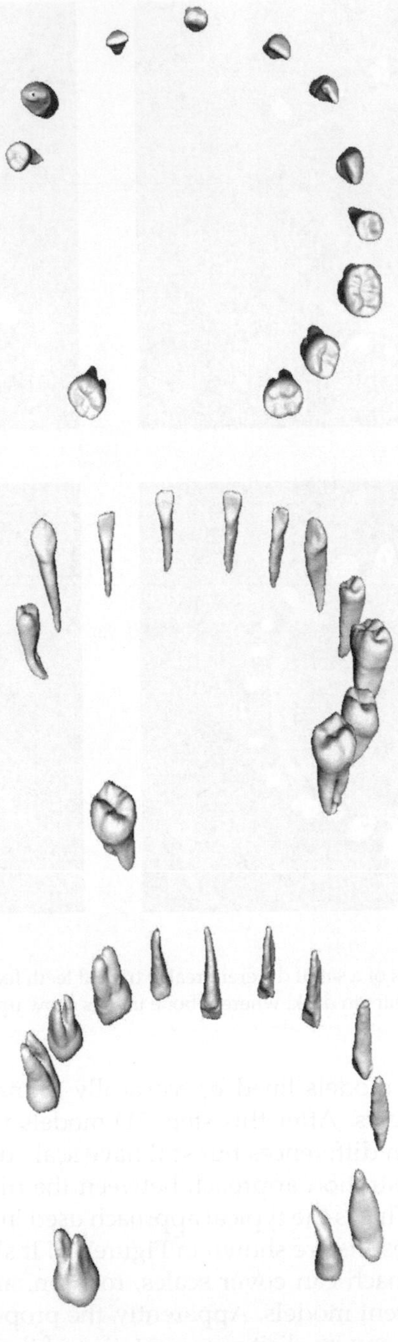

FIGURE 3.3
3D segmentation and model visualization of a-12 teeth set, from top, front, and bottom views.

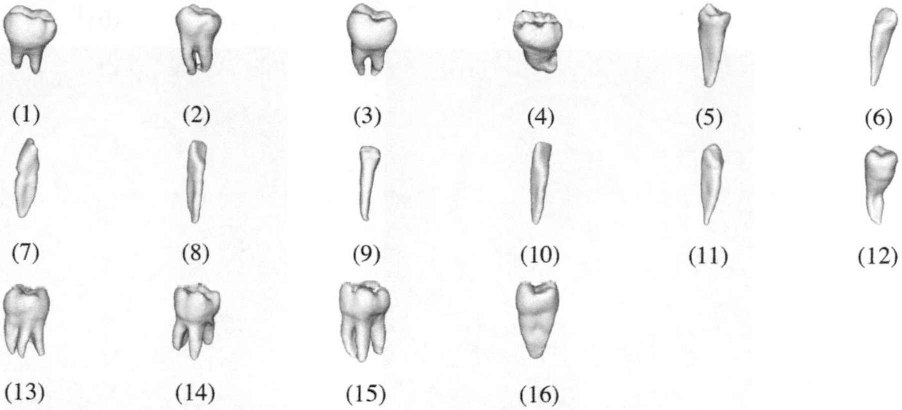

FIGURE 3.4
3D modeling of each single tooth as shown in Figure 3.3 after segmentation from (1) to (16).

In addition, we do not need any mutual information maximization in this process, and hence, we claim that ours is faster.

3.4.3 Elastic Registration Results

We start our experimental results by demonstrating an example for the point-based registration algorithm. We deformed an MRI image by constructing a 12×12 lattice of control points over its grid. The control points are moved randomly in a certain direction resulting in deforming the image grid points together as shown in Figure 3.6 (1.b). Point mappings are constructed by

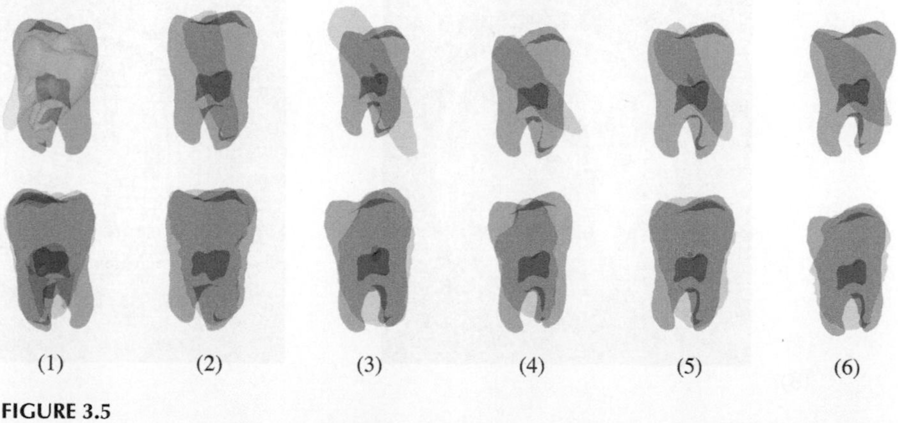

FIGURE 3.5
Six source models are visualized in light blue while the corresponding targets are shown in light red. First and third rows show initial positions. Final registration results are demonstrated in the second and fourth rows, respectively.

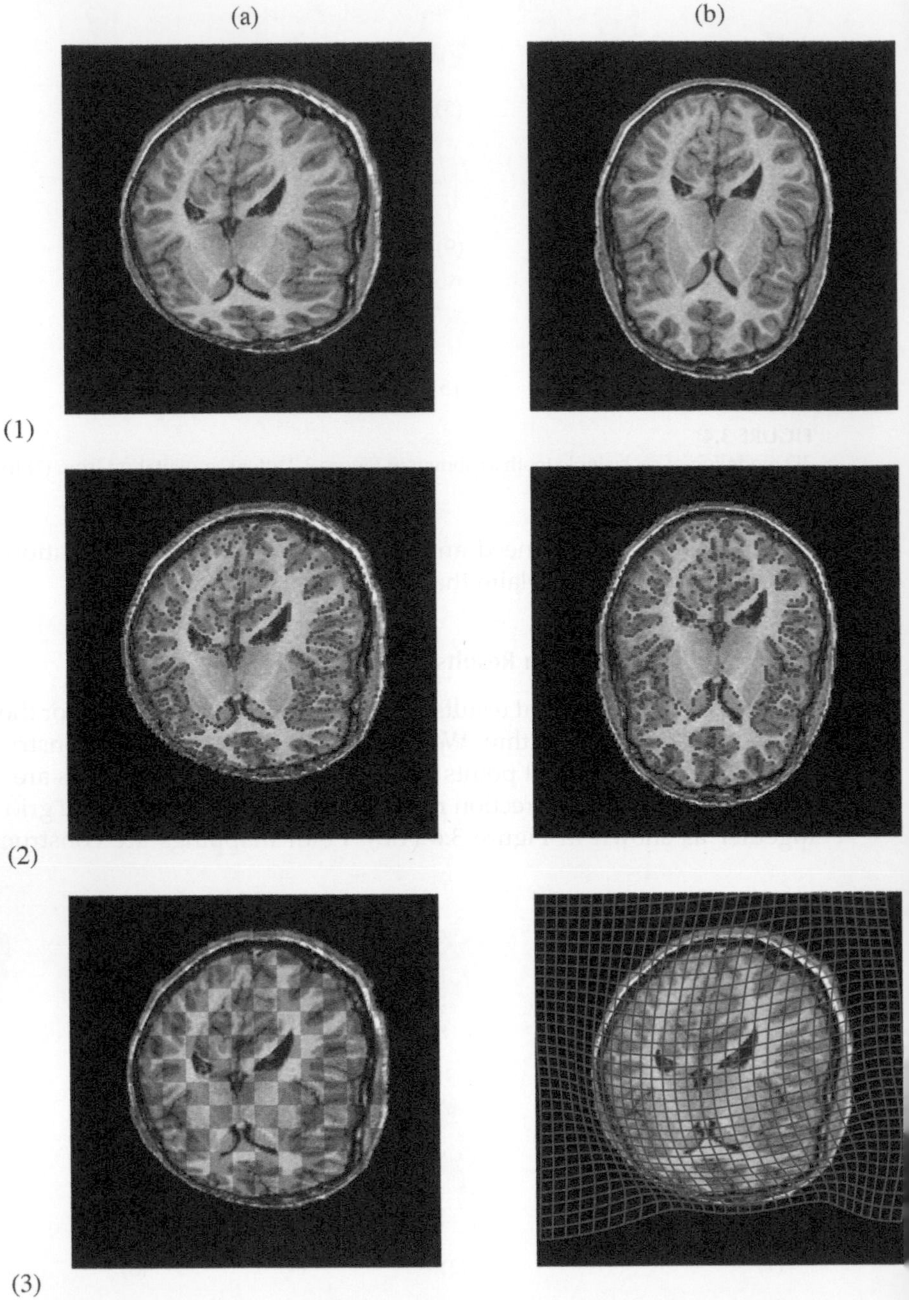

FIGURE 3.6
A largely deformed image of an MRI slice (1.b) is shown in (1.a). Source and target edge points are visualized in the second row images. Final deformed grid and checkerboard images are shown at the bottom row images.

taking the edge contours of the original and deformed images (point illustration is given in (2.a) and (2.b)). So each point is associated with its target priori because the control points new position are already known. Now, the situation is reversed. Given the edge contours of the source and target images, we need to calculate the deformation grid using our point-based algorithm. Our approach successfully covers the deformation at each point with the coarse to fine strategy. A final average pixel error of 0.2 is achieved. As we notice from the graph on the bottom, the average error dramatically gets reduced when increasing the resolution of the control lattice. The deformed image is gathered with its target in a checkerboard illustration as shown in (3.b). Having a closer look at the ventricles shows that the deformation is very accurate since, the two parts coming from different images have no transition. Edges are connected along the squares in all parts of the checkerboard image.

To show the difference between our approach and the conventional ICP algorithm [6], [7], we demonstrate the registration of two humanoid models in Figure 3.7. The ICP fails to establish correct point mappings. Our approach does the job efficiently because the whole grid moves slowly and step by step towards the target.

In all experiments, shapes are priori registered globally using the abovementioned approach. Different scales, rotations, and translations are estimated for each case. Different elastic shape registration experiments are demonstrated in Figure 3.8. The algorithms demonstrated in Sec. 3.3.4 is used for registration. In all experiments, an initial lattice resolution of 7×7 is established and then the level is increased until a satisfactory deformation is achieved. Examples (1) to (4) are dedicated to teeth deformations. The first registration example does not have complicated local difference

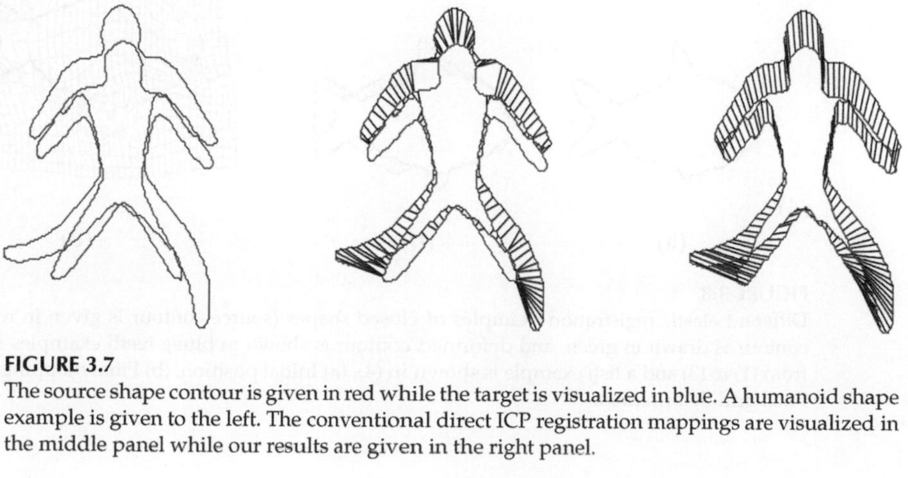

FIGURE 3.7
The source shape contour is given in red while the target is visualized in blue. A humanoid shape example is given to the left. The conventional direct ICP registration mappings are visualized in the middle panel while our results are given in the right panel.

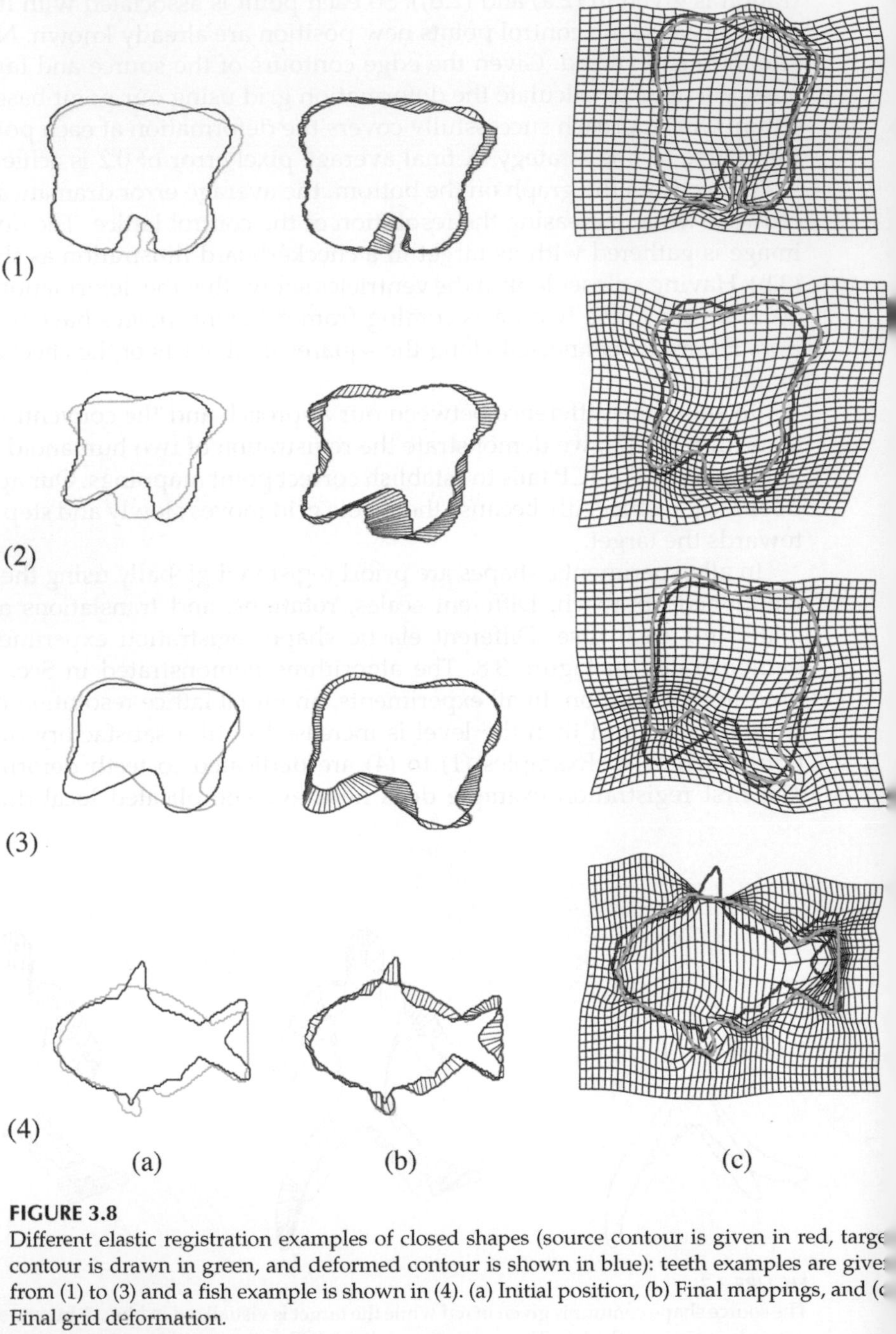

FIGURE 3.8
Different elastic registration examples of closed shapes (source contour is given in red, targe contour is drawn in green, and deformed contour is shown in blue): teeth examples are giver from (1) to (3) and a fish example is shown in (4). (a) Initial position, (b) Final mappings, and (c Final grid deformation.

details between the given shapes. This does not require a high level of resolution. More complicated differences in the tags and roots areas can be noticed in examples (2), (3), and (4). Large number of resolution levels are used to successfully achieve these local deformations. Another more complicated deformation example is shown for the fish in (5). Investigating the point mappings in each case, we find that: our algorithm gives exact physical dense mappings and the grid deformations do not have crossovers which shows the necessity of the coarse to fine strategy and the smoothness constrains.

Our approach does not only work for closed shapes but it can also handle open structures registration problem efficiently as shown in Figure 3.9. Another issue is the registration of shapes that include multiple parts. The registration of two brain structures, for example, is shown in Figure 3.10. Open and multiple parts shapes are parameterized in different ways. End points of the open shape are different $\mathbf{C}(0) \neq \mathbf{C}(1)$ while in closed shapes $\mathbf{C}(0) = \mathbf{C}(1)$. For the multiple parts case, each individual curve is parameterized independently then gathered together to handle the entire shape.

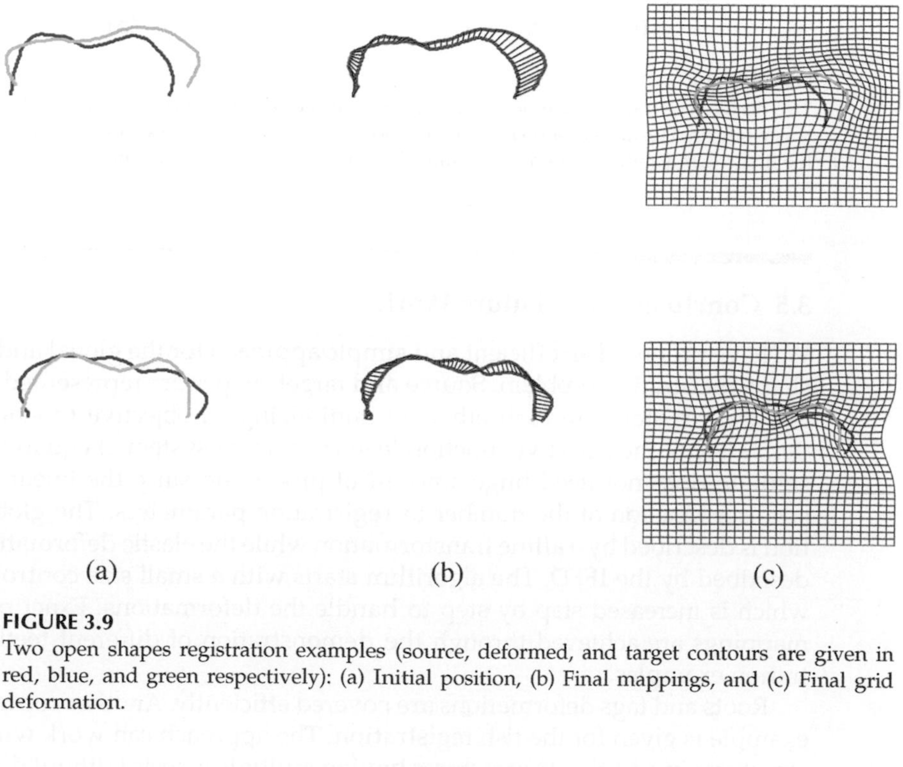

(a) (b) (c)

FIGURE 3.9
Two open shapes registration examples (source, deformed, and target contours are given in red, blue, and green respectively): (a) Initial position, (b) Final mappings, and (c) Final grid deformation.

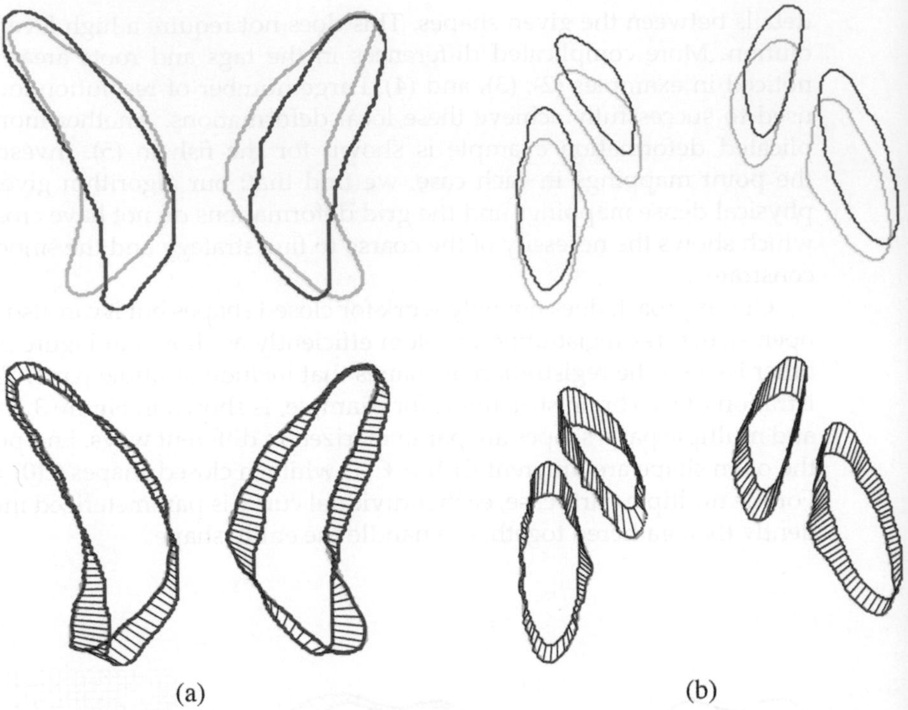

FIGURE 3.10
Two elastic registration examples are given. Source and target shapes are visualized in the first row while final results are shown in the second row. A brain ventricle shape is demonstrated in the first column and a hippocampus example is shown in the second column.

3.5 Conclusion and Future Work

We have proposed an efficient and simple approach for the global and elastic shape registration problem. Source and target shapes are represented explicitly and registered to each other by minimizing an objective function. The derivative of the objective function leads to a linear system of equations. The solution does not need huge amount of processing since the linear system size is a function of the number of registration parameters. The global motion is described by a affine transformation while the elastic deformations are described by the IFFD. The algorithm starts with a small size control lattice which is increased step by step to handle the deformations. Exact physical mappings are achieved through the demonstration of different teeth registration examples.

Roots and tags deformations are covered efficiently. Another complicated example is given for the fish registration. The approach can work with open structures in addition to structures having multiple objects without difficulty.

Only 2D examples are demonstrated but future work will be geared towards considering 3D applications. Image registration is of great interest and will be considered for future research.

Also, we have presented a system for building a database of real human teeth 3D models. Teeth are scanned using Cone-beam CT with a resolution of $0.2 \times 0.2 \times 0.2 mm^3$. Level set segmentation is used to extract 3D teeth models from the wax in a variational framework. Different teeth models have been registered to minimize global differences represented in scales, rotations, and translations using a point-based least squares technique.

In the future, shape models and active appearance models can be built based on our database for either single tooth type or a whole jaw that contains all types. Principal component analysis can be performed to handle the modeling process. Up till now, our database includes 280 teeth models. Moreover, we aim to enlarge the database to include scans from different genders, races, ages,...etc. Also, we will make 3D teeth surface meshes available for researchers and dentistry students to use.

References

1. A.A. Farag, H.E. Abd El Munim, J.H. Graham, A.A. Farag: A *Novel Approach for Lung Nodules Segmentation in Chest CT using Level Sets*, IEEE Trans. on Image Processing, 22(12):5202–5213, 2013.
2. A.H. Yousef and H.E. Abd El Munim, "An accelerated shape based segmentation approach adopting the pattern search optimizer, Ain Shams Engineering Journal," 2016, http://dx.doi.org/10.1016/j.asej.2016.11.002.
3. A.H. Yousef and H.E. Abd El Munim, "A GPU-Based Elastic Shape Registration Approach in Implicit Spaces," *Journal of Real-Time Image Processing*, pp. 1–13, August, 2017.
4. R. Veltkamp and M. Hagedoorn, "State of the Art in Shape Matching,"*Technical Report*, UU-CS-19999-27, Utrecht University, Sept. 1999.
5. Nikos Paragios, Mikael Rousson and Visvanathan Ramesh, "Matching Distance Functions: A Shape-to-Area Variational Approach for Global-to-Local Registration,"*European Conference in Computer Vision*, Copenhagen, Denmark, Jun. 2002.
6. P. Besl and N. Mckay, "A Method for Registration of 3-D Shapes,"*IEEE Tr. on PAMI*, 14(2):239–256, 1992.
7. Z. Zhang, "Iterative Point Matching for Registration of Free-form Curves and Surfaces," *Ph.D. International Journal of Computer Vision*, vol. 13, no. 2, pp. 119–152, 1994.
8. I. Cohen and I. Herlin, "Curve Matching Using Geodesic Paths,"*In IEEE CVPR*, pp 741–746, Santa Barbara, USA, 1998.
9. A. Fitzgibbon, "Robust Registration of 2D and 3D Points Sets,"*In Proceeding of The British Machine Vision Conference (BMVC)*, vol. 2, pp 411–420, University of Manchester, UK, 2001.

10. D. Kozinska, O. Tretika, J. Nissanov, and C. Ozturk, "Multidimensional Alignment Using the Euclidean Distance Transform, "*Graphical Models and Image Processing*, pp 6:373–385, 1997.
11. Z. Xie and G. E. Farin, "Image Registration Using Hierarchical B-Splines,"*IEEE Transaction on Visualization and Computer Graphics*, Vol. 10, NO. 1, 2004.
12. M. Rousson, N. Paragios and R. Deriche. "Implicit Active Shape Models for 3D Segmentation in MRI Imaging," *Medical Image Computing and Computer Assisted Intervention (MICCAI)*, Part 1, pp 209–216, Saint-Malo, France, September 26-29, 2004.
13. T. Sederberg and S. Parry, "Free-Form Deformation of Solid Geometric Models,"*in ACM SIGGRAPH*, 1986, pp. 151–160.
14. D. Rueckert, L. Sonoda, C. Hayes, D. Hill, M. Leach, and D. Hawkes, "Nonrigid Registration Using Free-Form Deformations: Application to Breast MR Images,"*IEEE Transactions on Medical Imaging*, vol. 8, pp. 712–721, 1999.
15. Tim McInerney and Demetri Terzopoulos, "Deformable Models in Medical Image Analysis: A Survey," *In Medical Image Analysis*, 1(2):91–108, 1996.
16. Sakae Nagasawa, Takamitsu Yoshida, Kaoru Tamura, Masatoshi Yamazoe, Yoshinori Arai Keigo Hayano, Hirohito Yamada, Etsuo Kasahara, and Michio Ito, "Construction of database for three-dimensional human tooth models and its ability for education and research - carious tooth models," *Dental Materials Journal*, vol. 29, 2010.
17. H. E. Abd El Munim and A. A. Farag, "A Shape-Based Segmentation Approach: An Improved Technique Using Level Sets ," *(ICCV'05)*, pp. 930–935.
18. H. E. Abd El Munim and A. A. Farag, "Curve/Surface Representation and Evolution using Vector Level Sets with Application to the Shape-based Segmentation Problem ," *PAMI*, Vol. 29, No. 6, pp. 945–958, June 2007.
19. G. Mori and J. Malik,, "Recovering 3D Human Body Configurations Using Shape Contexts, "*PAMI*, VOL. 28, NO. 7, pp. 1052–1062, July 2006.
20. N. Hasler, H. Ackermann, B. Rosenhahn, T. Thormahlen, and H. Seidel, "Multilinear pose and body shape estimation of dressed subjects from image sets,"*CVPR* Page(s): 1823–1830.
21. R. Sagawa, K. Akasaka, Y. Yagi, H. Hamer, and L. Van Gool, "Elastic convolved ICP for the registration of deformable objects,"*ICCV*, Page(s): 1558–1565, Kyoto Japan, Sep. 27 to Oct. 4, 2009.
22. Xiaolei Huang, N. Paragios, and D.N. Metaxas, "Shape registration in implicit spaces using information theory and free form deformations ," *TPAMI*, Vol. 28 Issue 8, Aug. 2006 Page(s): 1303–1318.

4

Robust Nuclei Segmentation Using Statistical Level Set Method with Topology Preserving Constraint

Shaghayegh Taheri, Thomas Fevens, and Tien D. Bui

CONTENTS

4.1 Introduction

Pathology is a medical specialty which concerns laboratory examination of cells and tissue samples with the purpose of diagnosis and characterization of diseases. More specifically, cytopathological and histopathological examinations of a biopsy or surgical specimen are two main branches of anatomical pathology that are commonly applied to diagnose various diseases, including cancer. Cytopathology (or cytology) refers to the microscopic investigation of samples at the cellular level and is mainly advantageous when quick preparation, staining, and interpretation procedures are needed. Despite the fact that cytopathological imagery are highly beneficial as they provide great cellular detail at low cost, cytopathological examinations alone are not sufficient for accurate diagnosis purposes. For instance, they cannot indicate whether the cancer cells are spreading into and damaging surrounding tissues. Therefore, to obtain higher diagnostic accuracy, the preliminary cytopathological tests must be confirmed by the so-called histopathological (or histological) assessments for which the overall tissue architecture is evaluated. Pathologists usually make diagnostic interferences by visual inspection of cells based on their morphological features and architecture, such as shape, position, size, number, etc. Although still being considered as the gold standard, manual examination of biological images is tedious work which requires many hours of human labor. This highlights the requirement for an automatic system that accurately measures these features in a few seconds.

Recently, computerized methods, including automatic detection, segmentation, and classification of objects in cyto-histopathological specimens, have drawn increased attention in the field of digital pathology as the result of developments in digital whole slide scanners and computer hardware. Due to the essential role of the nucleus in cellular functionality, automatic segmentation of cell nuclei is a fundamental prerequisite for all histopathological and cytopathological automated systems. Moreover, it substantially facilitates the segmentation of the cytoplasm and the surrounding tissues. Despite the considerable amount of research that has been dedicated to this topic, nuclei segmentation in cyto-histopathological imagery is still one of the most challenging tasks for several reasons. First, because of the staining process the presence of noise is almost ineluctable. Second, final segmentation results may be affected by nonuniform illumination of the image, resulting from the thickness of the sample or microscope setup. Finally and most importantly, in 2D projection images, nuclei commonly appear to overlap each other and the separation of severely overlapping regions is not trivial.

4.2 Background and Related Work

Although a large variety of nuclei segmentation approaches have been recently developed by researchers, their overall strategies typically include the same routines; i.e., Preprocessing, Nuclei detection/localization, Nuclei segmentation and Nuclei Refinement. Nuclei Refinement is a post-processing step, which usually refers to the task of detaching the aggregated nuclei or merging the over-segmented nuclei.

For instance, nuclei seeds are first identified using the extended H-maxima transform [1]. Seeds then serve as the starting points in watershed segmentation. Finally, clumps of nuclei are separated using a distance transform, considering the fact that nuclei are fairly round. Nuclei are first segmented from the background using local thresholding [2]. The watershed algorithm is then performed to separate the overlapping nuclei, followed by a re-emerging step to avoid over-segmentation. Adaptive thresholding [3] and active contours [4] are utilized respectively to segment the foreground clustered nuclei. Subsequently, distance transform, H-minima transform and watershed algorithm are applied for marker extraction and nuclei separation.

4.2.1 Preprocessing

Prior to the main segmentation stage (e.g. nuclei detection and segmentation), a few preprocessing steps are normally required to compensate for unfavorable acquisition conditions and inconsistencies in the preparation of slides such as nonuniform illumination, nonuniform color, and noise [5]. The illumination correction can be achieved using either white shading correction or estimating the illumination pattern according to the series of images. Furthermore, many nuclei segmentation approaches perform color normalization in a different color space rather than the conventional RGB color model, including HSV, Lab, LUV, or MDC [6]. Finally, thresholding, morphological operation, and Gaussian smoothing are the common noise reduction methods frequently used in literature.

4.2.2 Nuclei Detection

Nuclei detection can be regarded as identification of cell nuclei by means of locating the set of points referred to as "seeds" or "markers," normally one per nucleus and close to its center. This step is of great importance because the final segmentation results highly rely on how precisely the initial seeds are determined. Nuclei of most cells are generally rounded or slightly elliptical in shape, as observed in histopathological and cytopathological imagery. Therefore, many nuclei detection techniques in literature have been developed according to the prior knowledge of the nucleus shape. In most cases, nuclei detection involves extracting the local maxima of a response map, where the mapping function highlights regions with certain prior aspects.

Among earlier approaches, Distance Transform [7] has been commonly employed in conjunction with H-maxima/H-minima transforms [1, 3, 4, 8]. The distance transform (DT) is a simple operator which is normally applied to the binarized images. The resulting image is obtained by replacing the intensity of each pixel with its distance from the nearest background pixel. One great drawback of the use of distance transform is being highly sensitive to the noise, thereby leading to over-seeding and over-segmentation.

The classical Hough transform and its variations [9, 10] have been extensively used for nuclei detection [11, 12]. There are several limitations associated with the Hough transform. First, the transform is computationally expensive, being of order $O(KBN)$, where K is the number of pixels in the image, B is the number of circular bins, and N is the width of the neighborhood. Moreover, since the transform is applied to the gradient image, the efficiency of the transform relies on how correctly nuclei edges are extracted. It also means that the transform is sensitive to noise. As an alternative, Radon Transform [13,14] seems to be more robust to noise, yet it suffers from the lack of efficiency.

In [15], Esteves et al. thoroughly investigated the application of Local Convergence Filters (LCF), initially proposed by [16–18], in nuclei detection. LCF refers to the wide range of filters that are commonly designed to find convex objects as they reveal locations in the image where the gradient vectors converge within a local region (support region).

4.2.3 Nuclei Segmentation

As mentioned earlier, nuclei segmentation is an essential requirement in computer-aided cyto-histological diagnosis. Generally speaking, image segmentation is the process of subdividing an image into multiple regions or categories, usually with the aim of simplifying further analysis. In this process each pixel of the image is assigned to one of the available categories such that (1) pixels that are assigned to the same category have similar characteristics whereas (2) adjacent pixels assigned to different categories are disparate from each other regarding those characteristics. Since the primary concentration of this paper is on pathology specimen images, only the common segmentation approaches to this area of research are briefly discussed.

Thresholding is the simplest and perhaps the most common segmentation technique that classifies pixels into two categories based on a certain threshold intensity value [2,19]. Another group of segmentation schemes frequently used in this context are those ones that mainly rely on morphological operations to perform segmentation [1, 20].

A very common region-based segmentation approach in medical image analysis, and particularly in nuclei segmentation, is the so called watershed algorithm. This is the method of choice, mainly because of its intrinsi capability of separating overlapping objects [1–4, 12, 21, 22]. For this reason, in the next section we will review a common mathematical definition of watershed, based on the concept of topographical distance [23].

4.2.3.1 Watershed Segmentation Method

Intuitively, a grayscale image can be viewed as a topographic surface in which the elevation of each location in the landscape indicates the intensity value of the corresponding pixel. Assuming that the landscape is gradually being immersed in water, then the catchment basins around the local minima or valleys start to get filled with water. Also, catchment basins are separated from the adjacent catchment by locating a watershed line (or watershed) at the points where water coming from two catchment basins is about to merge. Finally, as the water reaches to the highest point, the process is stopped and the resulting watersheds form the final segmentation boundaries. To be more explicit, let I represent a digital grayscale image, then the lower slope $LS(\mathbf{p})$ of I at pixel $\mathbf{p}$ is defined as:

$$LS(\mathbf{p}) = \max_{\mathbf{q} \in N(\mathbf{p})} \left(\frac{I(\mathbf{p}) - I(\mathbf{q})}{d(\mathbf{p}, \mathbf{q})} \right) \tag{4.1}$$

where $N(\mathbf{p})$ denotes the neighbors of pixel $\mathbf{p}$ including $\mathbf{p}$, and $d(\mathbf{p}, \mathbf{q})$ is the Euclidean distance between pixels $\mathbf{p}$ and $\mathbf{q}$. Also, when $\mathbf{p} = \mathbf{q}$ the lower slope is defined to be zero. Accordingly, the set of lower neighbors of pixel $\mathbf{p}$ denoted by $\Gamma(\mathbf{p})$ is:

$$\Gamma(\mathbf{p}) = \left\{ \mathbf{q} \in N(\mathbf{p}) \;\middle|\; \frac{I(\mathbf{p}) - I(\mathbf{q})}{d(\mathbf{p}, \mathbf{q})} = LS(\mathbf{p}) \right\} \tag{4.2}$$

Pixel $\mathbf{q}$ is said to belong to the upstream of pixel $\mathbf{p}$, if there exists a path $\pi = (\mathbf{p}_0, .., \mathbf{p}_l)$ of steepest slope from $\mathbf{p}_0$ to $\mathbf{p}_l$, that means: $\forall i = 0, .., l-1, \mathbf{p}_{i-1} \in \Gamma(\mathbf{p}_i)$. For each local minima m_i in the image, the corresponding catchment basin $CB(m_i)$ is the set of all points in the upstream of m_i. Finally, watershed pixels are the pixels for which there is at least two paths of steepest slope toward different local minima.

Despite its simplicity, high speed and inclusive segmentation, the traditional watershed transform has the major drawback of over-segmentation, since the method is highly sensitive to noise and irrelevant local minima. Thus several alternatives such as marker controlled watersheds and hierarchical watersheds have been developed to improve the method. A comprehensive study of different watershed definitions and algorithms was given by Roerdink and Meijster [24].

While there have been various attempts on the field of nuclei segmentation in literature, optimization techniques are being considered as more principled, systematic, and flexible methods. Generally speaking, these methods may be categorized mainly into spatially discrete and spatially continuous settings. In the discrete setting, the input image is converted into a directed graph such that pixels of the image are treated as the graph nodes and the segmentation is obtained by means of finding the minimal (cost) cut in the graph. Continuous optimization methods, on the other hand, aim at minimizing an energy functional which mostly involves solving partial differential equations. In what follows, we will briefly discuss some major contributions to this field.

4.2.4 Curve Evolution and Level-Set Techniques

In the variational frameworks, the segmentation of an image $u_C : \Omega \in \mathbb{R}^2 \rightarrow \mathbb{R}$ is achieved through the minimization of an appropriate energy functional $E(C)$ subject to some constraints, in such a way that the local or global minima occurs at the boundary of the desired objects. This is obtained by deforming a closed curve $C : [0\ 1] \rightarrow \Omega$ in the direction of negative energy gradient, described by the following gradient descent:

$$\frac{\partial C}{\partial t} = -\frac{\partial E(C)}{\partial C} \tag{4.3}$$

Here, the evolution of the curve is expressed in an explicit manner. Using the alternative implicit representation, in which contours are regarded as the zero level curve of some embedding function ϕ:

$$C = \{(x,y) \in \Omega \mid \phi(x,y) = 0\}, \tag{4.4}$$

one can reformulate equation (4.3) as:

$$\frac{\partial \phi}{\partial t} = -\frac{\partial E(\phi)}{\partial \phi} \tag{4.5}$$

The level-set methods originally developed by Osher and Sethian [25] are conceptually simple, yet powerful mathematical tools for numerically analyzing and computing the motion of curves and surfaces. The level-set approach suggests that rather than directly evaluating the motion of a curve in the plane, we can find an embedding surface such that at each time, the evolving curve exactly fits the intersection between the moving surface and the $x - y$ plane. For this reason, the curve is commonly referred to as the zero level-set or zero level-curve of the surface.

To be more precise, through the introduction of a Lipschitz continuous function $\phi(x,y,t) : \Omega \rightarrow \mathbb{R}$, the level-set representation of a curve is given as follows:

$$C = \{(x,y) \in \Omega \mid \phi(x,y) = 0\}, \quad \begin{cases} \phi(x,y,t) = 0 & \text{on the curve} \\ \phi(x,y,t) > 0 & \text{inside the curve} \\ \phi(x,y,t) < 0 & \text{outside the curve} \end{cases} \tag{4.6}$$

One typical example of such function is the signed distance function of curve

Level-set based techniques have become increasingly popular in the field of Geometric Partial Differential Equations and variational image segmentation, as they bring several advantages: In case of 2D plane curves, calculations are done in a fixed rectangular grid, making the level-set formulation perfectly suited for dealing with gray level images. Moreover, unlike the explicit parametrization methods, they can handle the automatic changes in topology i.e. merging and splitting of the segmented regions. Further, the issue of self-intersection of curves in parametric deformable models no longer exists.

4.2.4.1 Edge-Based and Region-Based Active Contours

Earlier works in the variational framework were mainly based upon the classical snakes, also called active contours models [26]:

$$E(C) = -\int |\nabla I(C)|^2 ds + \nu_1 \int |C_s|^2 ds + \nu_2 \int |C_{ss}|^2 ds \tag{4.7}$$

Where parameter s is the arc-length along the curve and C_s and C_{ss} stand for the first and second derivative of the curve with respect to s. One main difficulty of using the explicit representation of snakes in (4.7) is that they are not capable of handling the topological changes; therefore not capable of detecting multiple objects in the image simultaneously. Besides, because of the explicit parametrization of the evolution, a re-parameterization procedure is required every few iterations. With some slight modifications, the Geodesic Active Contours model [27] proposed a level-set formulation for the Snake model, which resolves the issues arising from the explicit parametrization:

$$\begin{aligned} \frac{\partial \phi}{\partial t} &= |\nabla \phi| \; div \left(g(I) \frac{\nabla \phi}{|\nabla \phi|} \right) \\ &= g(I)|\nabla \phi| \; div \left(\frac{\nabla \phi}{|\nabla \phi|} \right) + \nabla g(I).\nabla \phi \end{aligned} \tag{4.8}$$

The classical snakes and the geodesic active contours are considered as "edge-based" active contours as they both rely on an edge detector function (of $|\nabla I|$) to stop the evolving curve. As a result, they can only detect objects with distinct boundaries. Also, since they are locally optimized the segmentation result highly depends on the initialization and there is always a high chance of getting trapped in the false local minimum. Furthermore, in cases with complex topology e.g. multiple holes and bridges, the edge-based active contours will not suffice to properly segment the image. In contrast to the "edge-based" methods that mainly depend on local features such as gradient, "region-based" active contours use the global or regional information of the image for the stopping procedure which makes them more robust to noise compared with the edge-based techniques. In this context, the Mumford-Shah (MS) energy model [28] and its well-established piecewise constant approximation, also known as "Cartoon Limit," have been broadly used as the region-based variational approaches to the task of image segmentation.

In Mumford-Shah model, segmentation of a given image $u_C : \Omega \in \mathbb{R}^2 \rightarrow \mathbb{R}$ into a number of sub-regions is considered as the problem of computing the optimal piecewise smooth approximation $u : \Omega \rightarrow \mathbb{R}$ of the image, such that u varies smoothly or slowly within each region, and it varies discontinuously or rapidly across the boundaries of the regions. Accordingly, the piecewise smooth approximation is obtained by minimizing the following energy functional:

$$E^{MS}(u, C) = \int_{\Omega \backslash C} |u - u_C|^2 dxdy + \mu \int_{\Omega \backslash C} |\nabla u|^2 dxdy + \nu |C| \tag{4.9}$$

Where constants $\mu \geq 0$ and $\nu \geq 0$ are weighting parameters, C is the boundary of an open subset ω of Ω, i.e. $\omega \in \Omega$ *and* $C = \partial\omega$, and the total length of the boundaries of regions |C|, penalizes the smoothness of the segmentation curve. If we assume that the segmentation curve C partitions image into two regions u_1 and u_2 referring to inside the curve and outside the curve, i.e. foreground and background regions, equation (4.9) can be re-written as follows:

$$\begin{aligned} E^{MS}(u_1, u_2, C) = & \int_{inside\ C} |u_1 - u_C|^2 dxdy + \mu_1 \int_{inside\ C} |\nabla u_1|^2 dxdy \\ & + \int_{outside\ C} |u_2 - u_C|^2 dxdy + \mu_2 \int_{outside\ C} |\nabla u_2|^2 dxdy + \nu |C| \end{aligned} \tag{4.10}$$

The numerical solution of MS equation was facilitated by the level-set method which can be found in [29] in more details. Accordingly, the level-set representation of the above equation can be written as:

$$\begin{aligned} E^{MS}(u_1, u_2, \phi) = & \int |u_1 - u_C|^2 H(\phi) dxdy + \mu_1 \int |\nabla u_1|^2 H(\phi) dxdy \\ & + \int |u_2 - u_C|^2 (1 - H(\phi)) dxdy \\ & + \mu_2 \int |\nabla u_2|^2 (1 - H(\phi)) dxdy + \nu \int |\nabla H(\phi)| dxdy. \end{aligned} \tag{4.11}$$

where $H(z)$ is the Heaviside function of variable z:

$$H(z) = \begin{cases} 1 & \text{if } z \geq 0 \\ 0 & \text{if } z < 0 \end{cases} \tag{4.12}$$

The Mumford-Shah paradigm in its original form has a nontrivial solution that requires much computation time because it involves solving three Euler Lagrange equations simultaneously [29]. As an alternative, Chan and Ves in [30] proposed a piecewise constant model along with its level-set formulation and demonstrated that the model is equivalent to the two-phase piecewise constant approximation of MS. Assuming that image u_C is composed c two regions u_1 and u_2 having constant intensities c_1 and c_2 respectively, the "Chan-Vese" (CV) model is written as:

$$E^{CV}(c_1, c_2, C) = \lambda_1 \int_{inside\ C} |c_1 - u_C|^2\, dxdy + \lambda_2 \int_{outside\ C} |c_2 - u_C|^2\, dxdy \\ + \nu\,.\, Length(C). \tag{4.13}$$

Using the level-set framework, the above energy can be written as:

$$\begin{aligned} E^{CV}(c_1, c_2, \phi) = \lambda_1 &\int_\Omega |c_1 - u_C|^2\, H(\phi(x,y))\, dxdy \\ &+ \lambda_2 \int_\Omega |c_2 - u_C|^2\, (1 - H(\phi(x,y)))\, dxdy \\ &+ \nu \int_\Omega \delta(\phi(x,y))\, |\nabla\phi(x,y)|\, dxdy. \end{aligned} \tag{4.14}$$

Here $H(\cdot)$ and $\delta(\cdot)$ respectively denote the Heaviside function defined in equation (4.12) and one-dimensional Dirac delta function, i.e. $\delta(z) = dH(z)/dz$. The Gradient descent equations of the above functional are then formed by employing the Euler-Lagrange derivation:

$$\frac{\partial\phi}{\partial t} = \delta(\phi)\left[-(c_1 - u_C)^2 + (c_2 - u_C)^2 + \nu\, div\left(\frac{\nabla\phi}{|\nabla\phi|}\right)\right]. \tag{4.15}$$

$$c_1(\phi) = \frac{\int_\Omega u_C(x,y) H(\phi(x,y))\, dxdy}{\int_\Omega H(\phi(x,y))\, dxdy}. \tag{4.16}$$

$$c_2(\phi) = \frac{\int_\Omega u_C(x,y)(1 - H(\phi(x,y)))\, dxdy}{\int_\Omega (1 - H(\phi(x,y)))\, dxdy}. \tag{4.17}$$

A possible regularization of functions $H(\cdot)$ and $\delta(\cdot)$ is suggested by [30]:

$$H(z) = \frac{1}{2} + \frac{1}{\pi}\, arctan\left(\frac{z}{\epsilon}\right), \quad \delta(z) = \frac{dH(z)}{dz}, \tag{4.18}$$

where ϵ is a small number.

4.2.4.2 Optimum Choice of Smoothness Parameter

The smoothness parameter has a critical role in segmentation results. Choosing very small values of ν will lead to over segmentation, since small edges created by the noise are also segmented. On the other hand, choosing very large values of ν will not produce some of the important edges. In [31], the optimum choice of parameter ν is suggested to be:

$$\nu = \beta\sigma^2 \tag{4.19}$$

$$\sigma^2 = \frac{\int_{\Omega} (u - \bar{u})^2 dxdy}{\int_{\Omega} dxdy} \tag{4.20}$$

where, σ^2 denotes the variance of image u, $\bar{u}$ is the mean value of u and β is a constant factor which depends on the amount of noise in the original image.

4.3 Methodology

The proposed framework is a region-based segmentation method, which consists of three major modules. First, to extract the desired stains, the image is passed through a color deconvolution unit [32]. Afterward, the generalized fast radial symmetry transform, also known as GFRS [33], followed by non-maxima suppression is used to specify the initial seed points and their corresponding GFRS ellipses. Later, the resulting ellipses, which may be interpreted as the initial nuclei borders (one per nucleus) serve as the initial curves in a level-set variational framework. Finally, nuclei borders are evolved through the use of a statistical level-set approach along with topology preserving criteria that successfully carries out the task of segmentation and separation of nuclei at the same time. Indeed, the topology preserving constraint [34] prevents the evolving regions from re-emerging into each other. The flow chart in Figure 4.1 demonstrates the presented framework. In the following sections, we give more detail of the steps of the framework outlined above.

4.3.1 Color Deconvolution

In order to improve the visualization of cell and tissue sections and highlight the desired structures, biological specimens are usually stained with a certain number of dyes. The most widely used staining protocol is the combination of Hematoxylin and Eosin (H&E). Hematoxylin stains nuclei blue, whereas Eosin is employed to stain red blood cells, cytoplasm and extracellular structures magenta or red. Whole slide digital scanners currently available use the Red-Green-Blue-based (RGB-based) imaging sensors, thus a stain separation method is needed to calculate the contribution of each stain. Ruifrok and Johnston [32] proposed an unmixing algorithm for up to three stains that

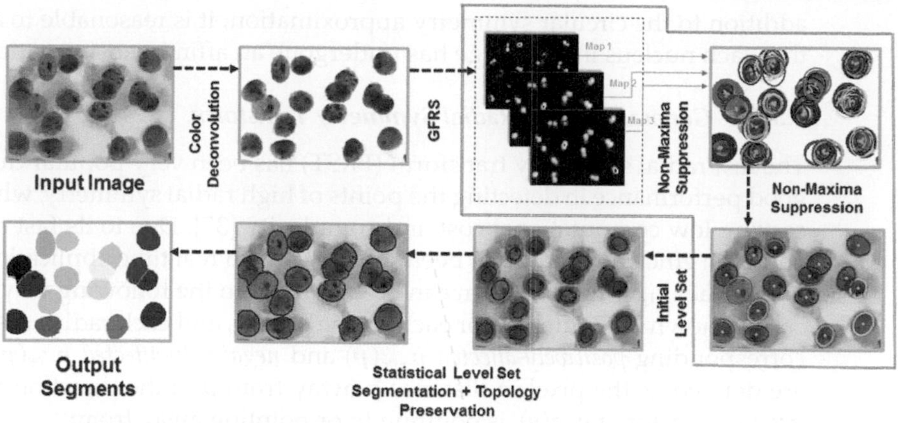

FIGURE 4.1
Proposed nuclei segmentation pipeline.

reveals uncorrelated information about stain concentration even when the stains have overlapping spectral absorption.

Given the reference optical densities, each stain can be characterized by a 3 × 1 vector, $OD = [s_r\ s_g\ s_b]^T$. After dividing each OD vector by its total length, the normalized OD matrix, **S**, can be formed:

$$\begin{array}{cc} & \begin{array}{ccc} \textit{stain } 1 & \textit{stain } 2 & \textit{stain } 3 \end{array} \\ \mathbf{S} = & \left(\begin{array}{ccc} s_{r,1} & s_{r,2} & s_{r,3} \\ s_{g,1} & s_{g,2} & s_{g,3} \\ s_{b,1} & s_{b,2} & s_{b,3} \end{array} \right) \begin{array}{c} R \\ G \\ B \end{array} \end{array}$$

Assuming that **X** is a 3 × 1 vector containing the amount of each stain at a particular pixel (x, y), then the following linear equation yields a 3 × 1 vector representing the amount of staining s_1, s_2, s_3 at pixel (x, y):

$$\mathbf{X}(x, y) = \mathbf{S}^{-1}\mathbf{Y}(x, y) = \mathbf{D}\mathbf{Y}(x, y) \tag{4.21}$$

where **Y** is a 3 × 1 vector denoting the OD values at pixel (x, y).

4.3.2 Nuclei Detection

Cell nuclei vary in size and shape during different phases of metabolism. Moreover they may deviate significantly from spherical symmetry in response to many different factors. For instance, it has been observed that diseases like cancer may cause significant elongation in nuclei shape. Therefore, in order to precisely locate the cell nuclei, it is necessary to incorporate techniques that can handle the elongation in shape of the nuclei. For this reason, in addition to the circular symmetry approximation, it is reasonable to assume that each nucleus in the image has undergone an affine transformation.

4.3.2.1 Generalized Fast Radial Symmetry Transform

The fast radial symmetry transform (FRST) has been very popular due to its good performance in detecting the points of high radial symmetry, while preserving low computational cost and complexity [35]. Due to its fast runtime and high efficiency, FRST has been widely used in real time applications, e.g. object tracking. The transform can be explained in the following way:

As shown in Figure 4.2, for each image pixel $\boldsymbol{p}$, and each radius $n \in N$, the corresponding *positively-affected* $\boldsymbol{p}_{+ve}(\boldsymbol{p})$ and *negatively-affected* $\boldsymbol{p}_{-ve}(\boldsymbol{p})$ pixels are defined as the pixels a distance n away from $\boldsymbol{p}$ in the direction that the gradient vector at $\boldsymbol{p}$, $g(\boldsymbol{p})$, is pointing to or pointing away from:

$$\boldsymbol{p}_{\pm ve}(\boldsymbol{p}) = \boldsymbol{p} \pm round\left(\frac{g(\boldsymbol{p})}{||g(\boldsymbol{p})||}n\right) \tag{4.22}$$

Using affected points $\boldsymbol{p}_{+ve}(\boldsymbol{p})$ and $\boldsymbol{p}_{-ve}(\boldsymbol{p})$, the *orientation projection image* O_n and *magnitude projection image* M_n are formed:

$$O_n(\boldsymbol{p}_{\pm ve}(\boldsymbol{p})) = O_n(\boldsymbol{p}_{\pm ve}(\boldsymbol{p})) \pm 1 \tag{4.23}$$

$$M_n(\boldsymbol{p}_{\pm ve}(\boldsymbol{p})) = M_n(\boldsymbol{p}_{\pm ve}(\boldsymbol{p})) \pm ||g(\boldsymbol{p})|| \tag{4.24}$$

where O_n and M_n are initially zero. At each positively affected point, images O_n and M_n are incremented by 1 and $||g(\boldsymbol{p})||$ respectively and at each negatively affected point, O_n and M_n are decremented by the same quantities. Finally, radial symmetry transform at radius n is defined as the convolution

$$S_n = F_n * A_n \tag{4.25}$$

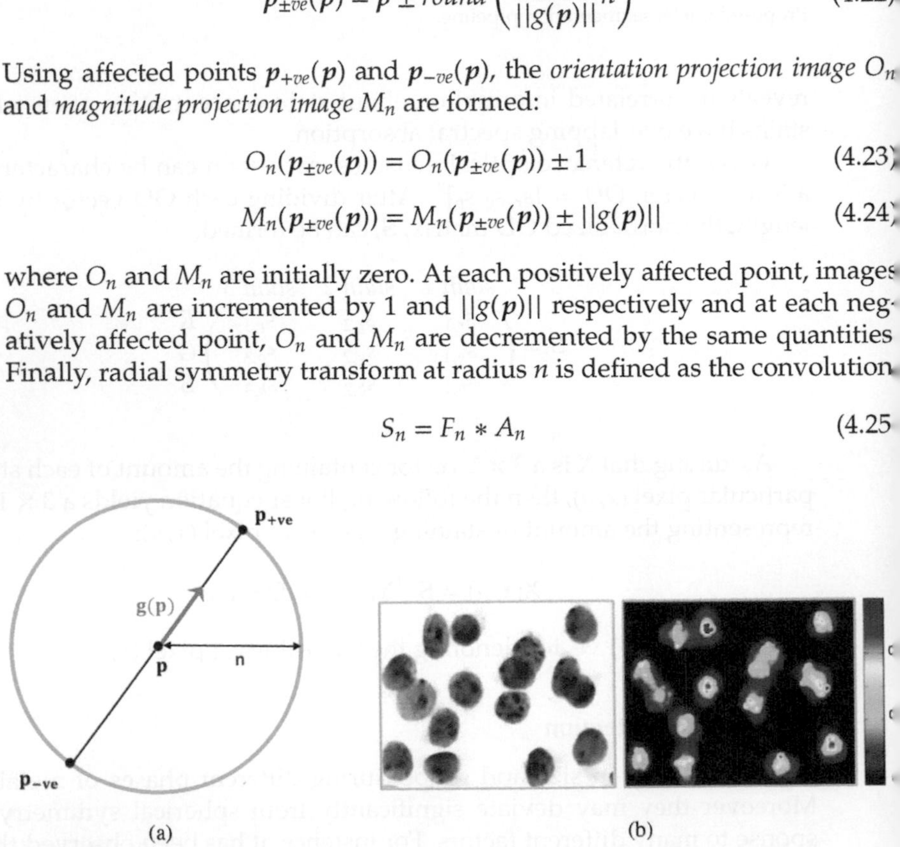

FIGURE 4.2
Fast Radial Symmetry Transform: (a) Point $\boldsymbol{p}$ and the corresponding affected pixels $\boldsymbol{p}_{+ve}$ and $\boldsymbol{p}_{-}$ shown with black dots. (b) A grayscale image and its FRST transform.

where A_n is a Gaussian kernel, F_n and $\tilde{O}_n$ are:

$$F_n(p) = \frac{M_n(p)}{k_n}\left(\frac{|\tilde{O}_n(p)|}{k_n}\right)^{\alpha} \qquad \tilde{O}_n = \begin{cases} O_n(p) & if\ O_n(p) < k_n \\ k_n & otherwise \end{cases} \tag{4.26}$$

and k_n and α are the scaling factor at radius n and radial strictness parameter respectively. The total transform over a set of radii $N = \{n_1, n_2, \ldots\}$ is defined as the average of all radially symmetric transforms S_n, $n \in N$.

Although the fast radial symmetry (FRS) [35] has been regarded as an efficient method which provides impressive results with a relatively low computational cost, it is not invariant with respect to the affine transformations. The fast radial symmetry was extended by Ni *et al.* [33] to the generalized fast radial symmetry (GFRS) for affine invariance systematically by considering the rotation (R) and scaling (S) matrices:

$$R = \begin{pmatrix} \cos(\theta) & -\sin(\theta) \\ \sin(\theta) & \cos(\theta) \end{pmatrix}, \quad S = \begin{pmatrix} a & 0 \\ 0 & b \end{pmatrix}, \tag{4.27}$$

where θ, a, b denote the orientation, major and minor axes, respectively. Accordingly, the total affine transformation matrix G and the voting vector $\hat{V}$ are determined, respectively, by $G = R\,S$ and

$$\hat{V} = G\,M\,G^{-1}\,M^{-1}\,g(p)\,, \quad M = \begin{pmatrix} 0 & 1 \\ -1 & 0 \end{pmatrix}. \tag{4.28}$$

In the same manner with FRST, for each radius n, the associated affected pixels are formed, as stated by Ni *et al.* [33], merely by replacing the gradient vector with the voting vector at point p:

$$p_{\pm ve}(p) = p \pm \text{round}\left(\frac{\hat{V}(p)}{||\hat{V}(p)||}n\right). \tag{4.29}$$

4.3.3 Nuclei Segmentation: Statistical Approach to Level-Set Segmentation

The segmentation problem can be addressed within the framework of Bayesian inference by maximizing a posterior probability. Assuming that $\mathcal{P}(\Omega)$ represents the optimal partition of the image $u : \Omega \to \mathbb{R}$ into disjoint regions: $\Omega_1, \ldots, \Omega_N$, Bayes' rule suggests that [36]:

$$p(\mathcal{P}(\Omega)|u) \propto p(u|\mathcal{P}(\Omega))\,p(\mathcal{P}(\Omega)), \tag{4.30}$$

where the conditional probability $p(u|\mathcal{P}(\Omega))$ represents the image information based on the partitioning $\mathcal{P}(\Omega)$, whereas the second term is the a priori probability of the optimal partitioning $\mathcal{P}(\Omega)$ which corresponds to the geometric aspects of the partition and shape priors.

Assuming that regions are independent and different locations (x, y) within the same region Ω_i are independent and identically distributed with the probability density function p_i, the posterior probability $p(u|\mathcal{P})$ can be extended to:

$$p(u|\mathcal{P}(\Omega)) = p(u|\{\Omega_1, \ldots, \Omega_N\}) = \prod_{i=1}^{N} \prod_{(x,y)\in\Omega_i} (p_i(u(x,y)))^{dxdy}, \tag{4.31}$$

where the bin volume $dxdy$ is introduced to guarantee the correct continuum limit.

4.3.3.1 Investigation of the Model in Two-Phase Setting

Rather than directly maximizing the posterior probability, it is more feasible to minimize its negative logarithm. Assuming that regions are independent and different locations (x, y) within the same region Ω_i are independent and identically distributed, maximizing the posterior probability in equation (4.30) comes down to minimizing the following energy functional:

$$E(u, C) = \int_{\Omega} -\log\, p_1(u(x,y))\, dxdy + \int_{\Omega\backslash C} -\log\, p_2(u(x,y))\, dxdy + \nu\, |C|, \tag{4.32}$$

where the total length of the boundaries of regions $|C|$, penalizes the smoothness of the segmentation curve. Pursuing the level-set scheme, the level-set representation of the above functional is

$$\begin{aligned} E(\phi) = \int_{\Omega} \big(& -H(\phi(x,y)) \log\, p_1(u(x,y)) \\ & - (1 - H(\phi(x,y))) \log\, p_2(u(x,y)) + \nu |\nabla H(\phi(x,y))| \big)\, dxdy, \end{aligned} \tag{4.33}$$

and the corresponding gradient descent,

$$\frac{\partial \phi}{\partial t} = \delta(\phi) \left(\log\, \frac{p_1(u(x,y))}{p_2(u(x,y))} + \nu\, \text{div} \frac{\nabla \phi}{|\nabla \phi|} \right), \tag{4.34}$$

is formed, where functions $H(\cdot)$ and $\delta(\cdot)$ are the Heaviside and Dirac delta functions, respectively. To further narrow down the statistical approach, the probabilistic model p_i needs to be specified. A reasonable choice of such parametric models is the Gaussian distribution function with parameters μ_i and σ_i^2:

$$p(s \mid \mu_i, \sigma_i^2) = \frac{1}{\sqrt{2\pi}\sigma_i} \exp\left(-\frac{(s - \mu_i)^2}{2\sigma_i^2} \right). \tag{4.35}$$

In addition to the parametric models such as Gaussian approximation, non-parametric density estimates are also applicable to the statistical segmentation scheme. As pointed out by [37], the Parzen density estimate can be simply obtained by smoothing the discrete histogram of the region with a Gaussian kernel.

4.3.3.2 Adding Topology Constraint

Although the automatic handling of topology changes is generally being considered as a great advantage of level-set based schemes, such flexibility becomes undesirable in applications where the number of components to be segmented and their topological arrangement are known in advance, as in the case of nuclei segmentation with predefined seed points. To address this problem, a topology preserving level-set method (TLSM) was proposed by Han *et al.* [34] that can be generally applied to all level-set based approaches, within a narrow band. TLSM provides an effective strategy to prevent automatic topology changing while maintaining the other advantages of level-set over the previously stated parametric approaches. The advantages of TLSM include the ability of generating nonintersecting curves, facilitating the computation by using fixed grid points, and handling sharp corners.

The key idea of TLSM is to monitor the sign of level-set function at every iteration and examine a potential sign change to see whether it occurs at a so called "simple point" or at a "non-simple point." In accordance with the digital topology context, a simple point is a point whose deletion does not change the topology of the binarized level-set function. This verification of the candidate point can be obtained through the connected component labeling within the 3×3 neighborhood of the point, using the concepts of Geodesic Neighborhood and Topological Numbers [34,38] in 2D settings. Even though the topology constraint computations are only being done within a narrow band of the zero level-set, calculation of topological numbers at every iteration, decelerate the segmentation process. Consequently, we have used a 511×1 look up table containing every combination of pixels in a 3×3 neighborhood.

4.3.3.3 Roundness Energy

In applications where the nuclei are a priori known to have a fairly circular structure without elongation, in these cases we suggest adding a new roundness energy to the existing energy functional. One way to measure the shape roundness is to calculate the inner product of the gradient vector and the vector connecting each point (x,y) to a specified center point (x_c, y_c). In our case this center point could be easily obtained using Fast Radial Symmetry Transform (FRST). In order to get the desired segmentation as round as possible, we need to maximize $\cos \angle(\vec{r}, \nabla \vec{H}(\phi))$:

$$E_R = \iint \cos \angle(\vec{r}, \nabla H(\phi)) = \iint \frac{\vec{r} \,.\, \nabla \vec{H}(\phi)}{||\vec{r}|| \,.\, ||\nabla \vec{H}(\phi)||} dxdy$$
$$= \iint \frac{(x - x_C).\phi_x + (y - y_C).\phi_y}{\sqrt{(x - x_C)^2 + (y - y_C)^2}} \delta(\phi) dxdy. \tag{4.36}$$

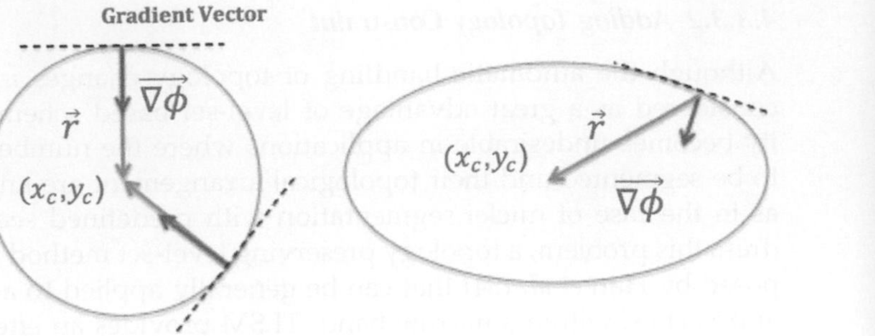

FIGURE 4.3
Illustration of roundness measurement.

Using the Euler Lagrange Equation the gradient descent is obtained:

$$\frac{\partial \phi_R}{\partial t} = -\nabla E = \frac{1}{\sqrt{(x - x_C)^2 + (y - y_C)^2}} \delta(\phi). \quad (4.37)$$

Next, the total energy of the curve can be formed using:

$$E = E^{Region} + \beta E^{Roundness} + \nu|C|. \quad (4.38)$$

Finally, the gradient descent equation with shape roundness prior is determined by:

$$\frac{\partial \phi}{\partial t} = \delta(\phi)\left(log\,\frac{p_1(u(x,y))}{p_2(u(x,y))} + \beta \frac{1}{\sqrt{(x - x_C)^2 + (y - y_C)^2}} + \nu\, div \frac{\nabla \phi}{|\nabla \phi|} \right) \quad (4.39)$$

An illustration of the roundness measure is given in Figure 4.3.

4.3.3.4 The Proposed Method

The overview of the proposed nuclei segmentation pipeline is presented in Algorithm 1. An important property of the proposed method is that all the computations are required only in a narrow band within the curve. The proposed framework does not add too much computational complexity to the regular level-set based narrow band implementation. In fact, at the first stage of the pipeline, computation of GFRS ellipses is of the order $O(Kl)$, where K is the total number of pixels and l is the number of affine transformations (in this paper $l = 36$). All the other computations are linear with the total number of pixels. To compute the gradient descent of equation (4.34) we have implemented two commonly used finite difference schemes: Forward Time Centered Space (FTCS) and Alternating Directional Implicit (ADI). More details on the numerical approximations of these schemes can be found in [31].

Algorithm 1 Proposed Method

1. Convert RGB image to grayscale using color deconvolution method in section 4.3.1.
2. Calculate GFRS transforms of the image $MAP = \{MAP_1, MAP_2, \ldots, MAP_l\}$, where l is the total number of affine transformations. If the overall nuclei symmetry in the dataset is circular use the FRST transform to obtain $MAP = \{MAP_1\}$.
3. Apply non-maxima suppression on MAP to find the local maxima of each transform $S = \left\{ \{p_{11}, p_{12}, \ldots\}, \{p_{21}, p_{22}, \ldots\}, \ldots, \{p_{l1}, p_{l2}, \ldots\} \right\}$ and store their associated parameters A_i, B_i, θ_i. If you have used the FRST transform go to step (5).
4. Re-apply non-maxima suppression on S to obtain Initial seed ellipses $S_c = \{p_1, p_2, \ldots, p_k\}$, $A_c = \{a_1, a_2, \ldots, a_k\}$, $B_c = \{b_1, b_2, \ldots, b_k\}$, $\theta_c = \{\theta_1, \theta_2, \ldots, \theta_k\}$,
5. Initialize the level-set $\phi^0(.)$to the signed distance function of initial ellipses obtained from previous step. (Rescale parameters A_c and B_c.)
6. Update the level-set function within a narrow band $\mathbf{q}_i \in \{\mathbf{p}_i \, |\phi^m(\mathbf{p}_i)| < W_{nb}, \, i = 1, \ldots, N_{nb}\}$, at iteration $m + 1$:
   (a) Compute $\phi^{temp} = \phi^m(\mathbf{q}_i) + \Delta t \; \Delta\phi^m(\mathbf{q}_i)$ according to equation 4.34 or 4.39 (If you have used the FRST transform). Use Gaussian approximation or Parzen density estimation. If sign($\phi^{temp}(\mathbf{q}_i) =$ sign($\phi^m(\mathbf{q}_i)$: set $\phi^{m+1}(\mathbf{q}_i) = \phi^{temp}(\mathbf{q}_i)$, keep $B(\mathbf{q}_i)$ unchanged, and go to step (d) otherwise continue to the next step.
   (b) extract the 3×3 neighboring points of $\mathbf{q}_i$ and use topology look-up table to check if the point is simple or not. if $\mathbf{q}_i$ is simple set $\phi^{m+1}(\mathbf{y}_i) = \phi^{temp}(\mathbf{y}_i)$, $B(\mathbf{y}_i) = 1 - B(\mathbf{y}_i)$ and go to step (d) otherwise continue to the next step.
   (c) Set $\phi^{m+1}(\mathbf{q}_i) = \epsilon \, . \, sign(\phi^m(\mathbf{q}_i))$ and keep $B(\mathbf{q}_i)$ unchanged.
   (d) If $i \leq N_{nb}$, then set $i = i + 1$, otherwise go to step (8).
7. Re-initialize the level-set function to the signed distance function of the current curve.
8. Terminate the algorithm if the the zero level-set has stopped moving, otherwise set $m = m + 1$ and go back to step (6).

4.4 Results and Discussion

In this section, several examples of cyto-histopathological images are examined to validate the proposed method. Note that for the proposed method, all the boundary curves are evolved together using only one level-set function.

In Figures 4.4–4.6 three histopathological sections of benign and malignant specimens are segmented using three different methods: marker controlled watershed on image gradient, thresholding method along with nuclei separation, and the proposed energy-based method with Gaussian statistical model. For all three methods Hematoxylin and Eosin images are first deconvolved according to Ruifrok and Johnston [32]. Also the initial markers of watershed method are obtained using the GFRS algorithm [33].

In Figure 4.7 several magnified patches of segmented benign and malignant specimens are depicted in detail, using marker controlled watershed, thresholding along with nuclei separation, and the proposed energy-based method with Gaussian model. As can be seen from the figure, watershed and thresholding methods have failed to segment the entire nuclei area whereas the proposed curve evolution method has been greatly successful in reaching nuclei borders.

To validate our new method, we have also tested our proposed method on a set of 47 fluorescent microscopy images (U2OS cells) [39]. In all experiments, fixed parameters, e.g., major and minor axes (a and b) and smoothness parameter (ν), for all the images have been used. Also, since this data set contains small nuclei patches on the boundary with small GFRS responses, a simple mean thresholding and nonlinear diffusion are added to the segmentation pipeline. In Figure 4.8 we have compared the proposed method with the CellProfiler previously mentioned nuclei segmentation unit: Maximum correlation thresholding (MCT) segmentation combined with shape-based separation (CellProfiler Automatic strategy).

4.4.1 Robustness of the Overlapping Boundaries and Smoothness Parameter

For the sake of separating touching nuclei, conventional shape-based approaches usually take the advantage of points of high concavity. In our proposed method, however, nuclei boundaries automatically tend to occur at points of high curvature by minimizing the total curvature; and therefore by setting higher values of smoothness parameter ν. To get accurate and smooth boundaries within the overlapping regions, in the first few iterations we set the smoothness parameter to lower values in order for the curve to reach closer to nuclei boundaries; then we set the smoothness parameter to higher values. This will prevent the formation of jagged edges in overlapping regions. The effect of smoothness parameter on overlapping edges has been illustrated in Figures 4.9c and 4.9d. The smoothness parameter of Figure 4.9d is chosen twice that of Figure 4.9c.

4.4.2 Segmentation Evaluation Metrics

Considering segmentation as a form of a data clustering problem, we can use the similarity measurements commonly used for evaluating clustering results. We have used the Rand and Jaccard indices [39]. Let S and R be the

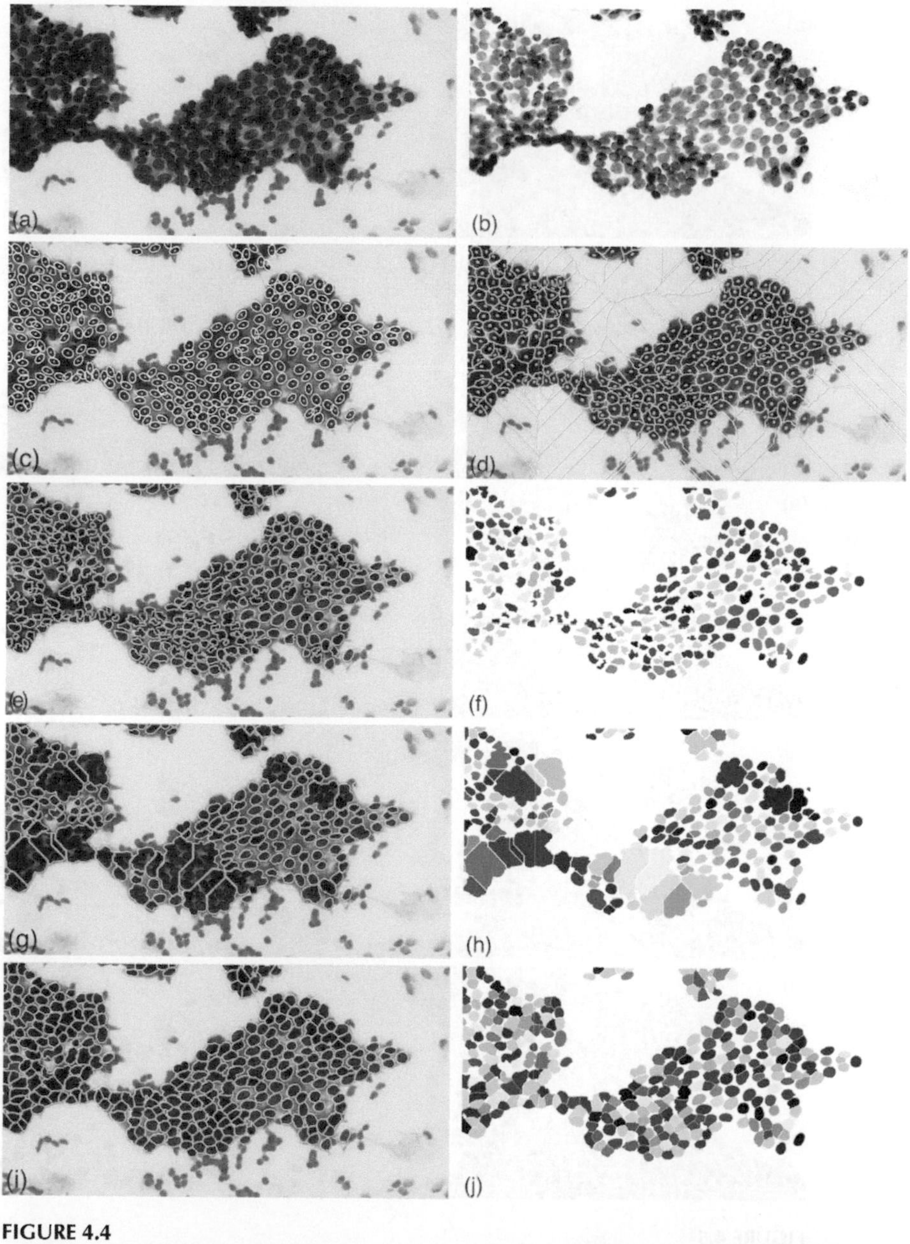

FIGURE 4.4
Comparison of different segmentation results on a benign H&E tissue section. (a) Original image (of size 1583 × 828, 40x magnification). (b) Original image after color deconvolution. (c) Initial ellipses obtained from GFRS. (d) Initial watershed markers based on initial ellipses in (c). (e,f) Watershed (gradient) segmentation of (d). (g,h) Maximum correlation thresholding (MCT) segmentation of (b) and shape-based separation (CellProfiler Automatic strategy, the desired range of cells diameter is set to [10 30]). (i,j) Proposed method. ($a = \{20\}, b = \{0.6, 0.8\} * a, \theta = k\pi/8, k = 0, 1, \ldots, 8$).

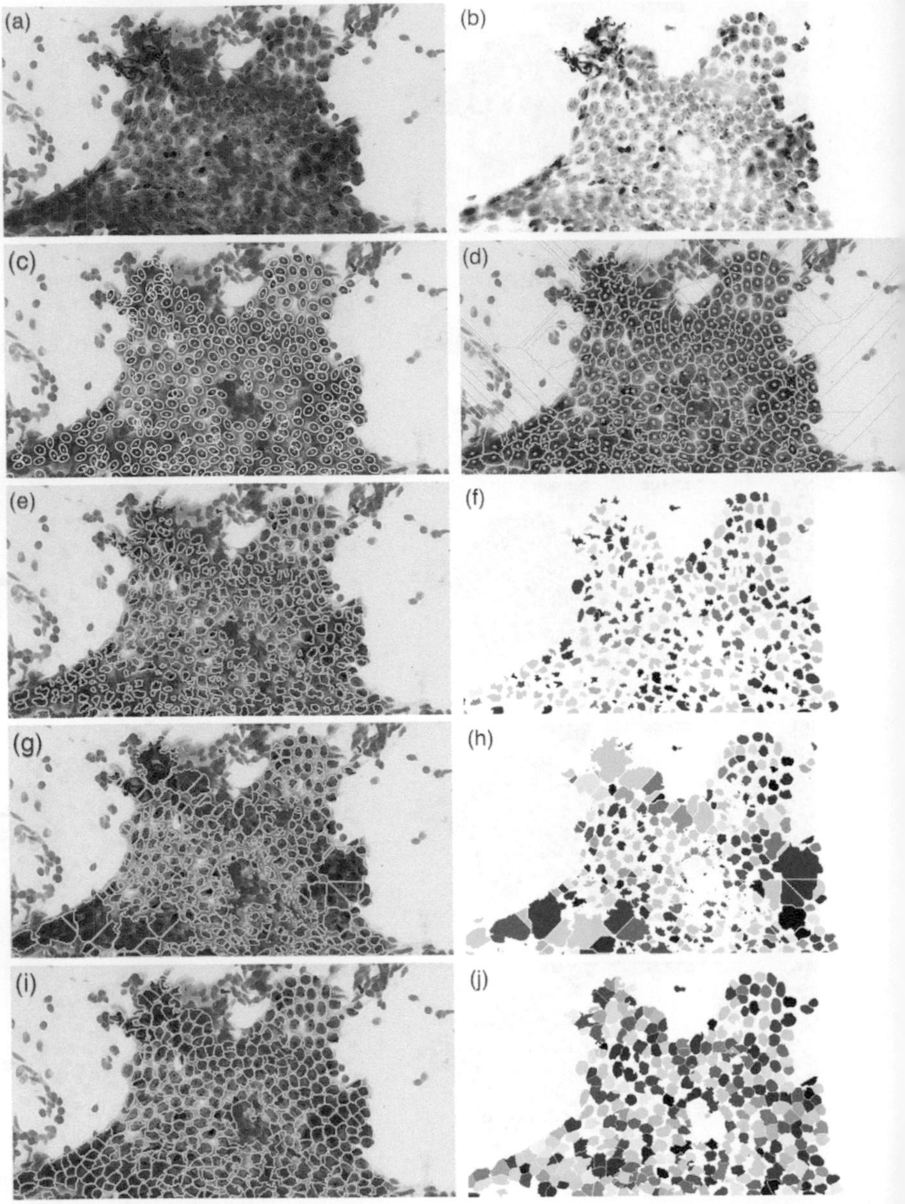

FIGURE 4.5
Comparison of different segmentation results on a benign H&E tissue section. (a) Original image (of size 1583 × 828, 40x magnification). (b) Original image after color deconvolution. (c) Initial ellipses obtained from GFRS. (d) Initial watershed markers based on initial ellipses in (c). (e,f) Watershed segmentation of (d). (g,h) Maximum correlation thresholding (MCT) segmentation of (b) and shape-based separation (CellProfiler Automatic strategy, the desired range of cell diameter is set to [10 30]). (i,j) Proposed method. ($a = \{20\}, b = \{0.6, 0.8\} * a, \theta = k\pi/8, k = 1, \ldots, 8$).

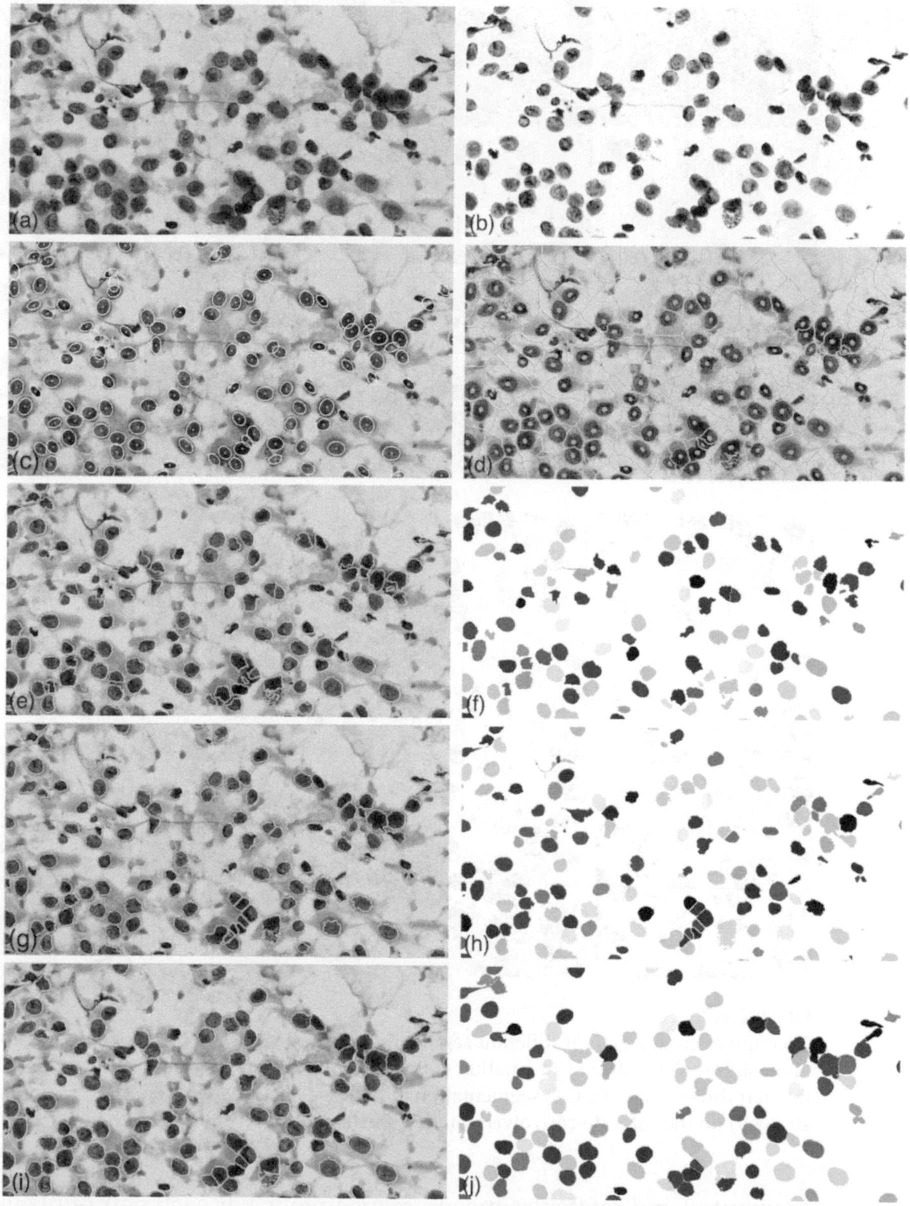

FIGURE 4.6
Comparison of different segmentation results on a malignant H&E tissue section. (a) Original image. (of size 1583 × 828, 40x magnification).(b) Original image after color deconvolution. (c) Initial ellipses obtained from GFRS. (d) Initial watershed markers based on initial ellipses in (c). (e,f) Watershed segmentation of (d). (g,h) Maximum correlation thresholding (MCT) segmentation of (b) and shape-based separation (CellProfiler Automatic strategy, the desired range of cells diameter is set to [10 30]). (i,j) Proposed method. ($a = \{20\}, b = \{0.6, 0.8\} * a, \theta = k\pi/8, k = 0, 1, \dots, 8$).

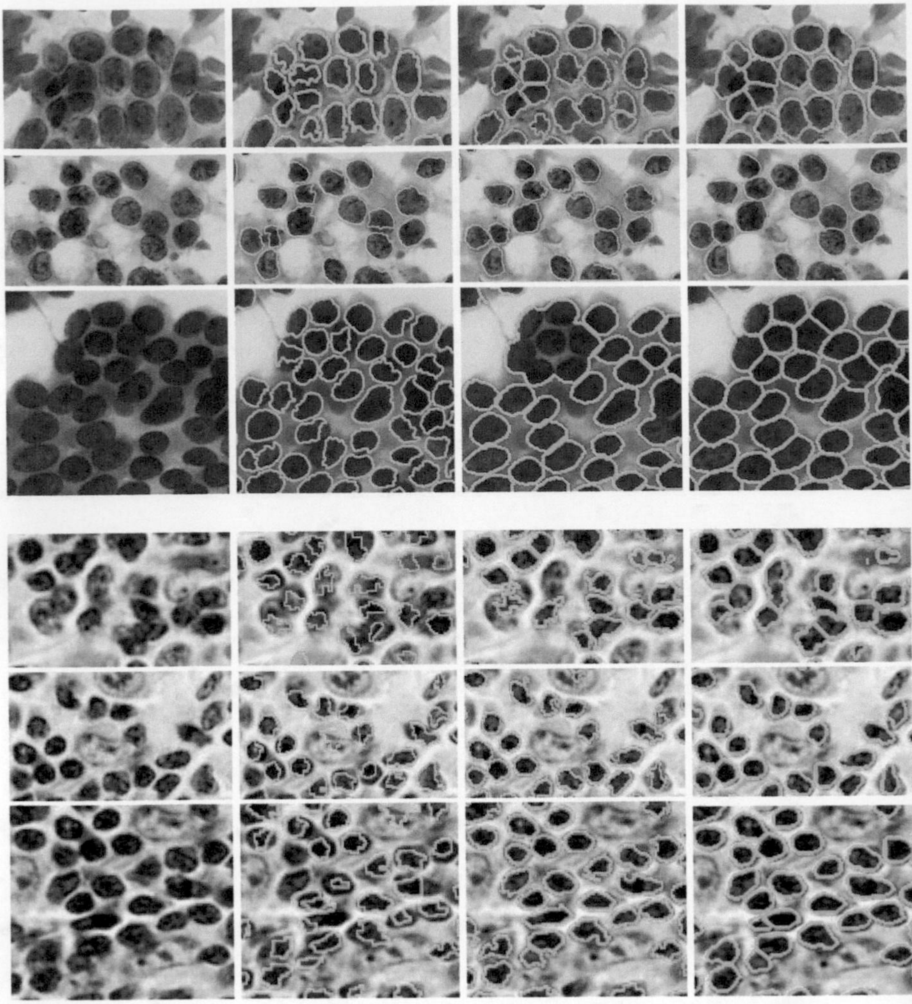

FIGURE 4.7
Qualitative comparison of different segmentation methods. First column: Original image. Second column: Watershed segmentation with GFRS initial markers. Third column: Maximum correlation thresholding (MCT) segmentation and shape-based separation (CellProfiler Automatic strategy) on the color de-convolved image. Fourth column: Proposed method.

segmented and reference images, respectively. For each pair of pixels p_i and p_j, , $i, j = 1, \ldots, n, i \neq j$, where n is the total number of pixels in R and S, there are four possible situations: True Positive (TP) : $R_i = R_j, S_i = S_j$; False Positive (FP) : $R_i \neq R_j, S_i = S_j$; False Negative (FN) : $R_i = R_j, S_i \neq S_j$; or True Negative (TN) : $R_i \neq R_j, S_i \neq S_j$.

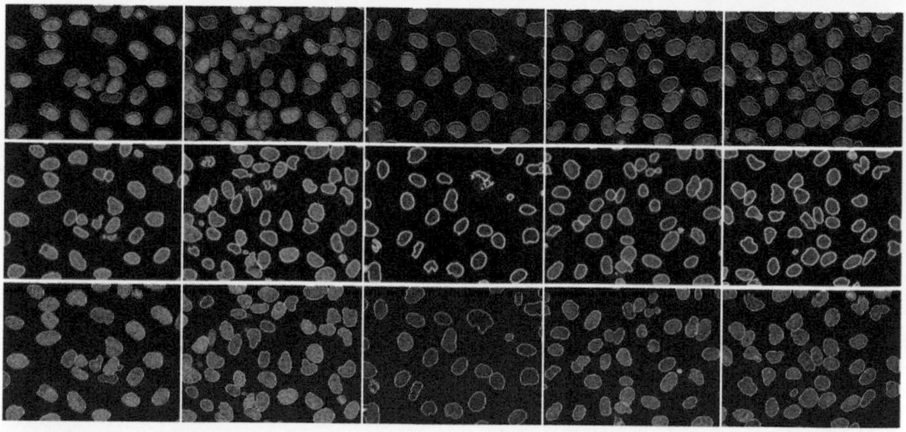

FIGURE 4.8
Fluorescence microscopy image segmentation. First row: The ground truth segmentation results presented in [39]. Second row: The CellProfiler [40] segmentation results using thresholding technique and shape prior for distinguishing clumped objects (the desired range of cells diameter is set to [80 120]). Third row: Segmentation results using the proposed method. ($a = \{50, 60\}$, $b = \{0.6, 0.8\} * a, \theta = k\pi/8, k = 0, 1, \ldots, 8$).

The Rand index (RI) which measures the percentage of the pairs of pixels where two clusters concur is defined as

$$RI(R, S) = (TP + TN)/(TP + FP + FN + TN). \tag{4.40}$$

Similarly, Jaccard index is defined as: $JI(R, S) = (TP + TN)/(FP + FN + TN)$. In addition to the Rand and Jaccard indices, we also count the number of split, merged, added and missing nuclei in accordance with the metrics [39]. As illustrated in Table 4.1, the proposed method yields in relatively high Rand and Jaccard indices (with the highest Jaccard index). Also, the average number of split, merged and missing nuclei are the minimum.

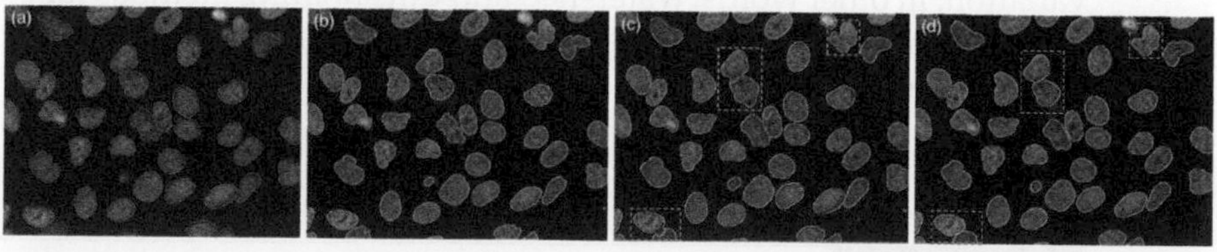

FIGURE 4.9
Effect of smoothness parameter. (a) Ground truth, (b) Cell profiler result, (c) Proposed method with $\nu = \nu_1$, and (d) Proposed method with $\nu = 2\nu_1$.

TABLE 4.1

Comparison of Different Segmentation Algorithms According to Published Results [39]. (Dataset : U2OS, Pixel Size: 1349 × 1030, Nr. Cells: 1831, Min Nr. Cells: 24, Max Nr. Cells: 63)

Algorithm	Rand Index	Jaccard Index	Split	Merged	Added	Missing
Expert Manual	95 %	2.4	1.6	1.0	0.8	2.2
RC Threshold	92 %	2.2	1.1	2.4	0.3	5.5
Ostu Threshold	92 %	2.2	1.1	2.4	0.3	5.6
Mean Threshold	96 %	2.2	1.3	3.4	0.9	3.6
Watershed (direct)	91 %	1.9	13.8	1.2	2.0	3.0
Watershed (gradient)	90 %	1.8	7.7	2.0	2.0	2.9
Active Masks	87 %	2.1	10.5	2.1	0.4	10.8
Merging Algorithm	96 %	2.2	1.8	2.1	1.0	3.3
Proposed Method	**95 %**	**2.5**	**0.5**	**0.79**	**0.57**	**0.19**

4.4.3 New or Breakthrough Work to Be Presented

In this work, we have addressed the two main problems of active contours for segmenting cyto-histopathological imagery. The main drawback of active contours is the problem of getting stuck in local minima. We have resolved this issue by locating the initial curves as close as possible to the desired objects by utilizing their radial or elliptical symmetric features. Furthermore, we have implicitly combined both boundary and region information through the use of a gradient-based transform (FRST or GFRS) and a region-based active contour. The second issue is that active contour method itself is not capable of separating severely overlapped cells and a separation method (e.g., concavity detection, distance transform,...) is needed at the ultimate stage By considering the topology criteria, initial curves no longer merge to each other and no more separation is required. Finally, a new roundness energy is introduced for applications where nuclei are a priori known to have a fairly circular structure without elongation. Experiments in the Results section (4.4 revealed that the statistical model (i.e. Gaussian or Parzen approximation) is much stronger than watershed and thresholding in the presence of intensity variation. In other words, watershed and thresholding methods failed to segment the entire nuclei area in regions with significant intensity variations and produced incomplete edges.

4.5 Conclusions

In this work, we presented a novel segmentation technique which effectively addresses the problem of segmenting touching or overlapping cell nuclei in cyto-histopathological images. The proposed framework is based upon a statistical level-set approach along with topology preserving criteria that successfully carries out the task of segmentation while preserving the separation of the nuclei. The proposed method is evaluated qualitatively on Hematoxylin and Eosin stained images, and quantitatively and qualitatively on fluorescent stained images. The results indicate that the method outperforms conventional nuclei segmentation approaches based on thresholding and watershed.

References

1. C. Wählby, I.-M. Sintorn, F. Erlandsson, G. Borgefors, and E. Bengtsson, "Combining intensity, edge and shape information for 2D and 3D segmentation of cell nuclei in tissue sections," *Journal of Microscopy*, vol. 215, no. 1, pp. 67–76, 2004.
2. S. Di Cataldo, E. Ficarra, A. Acquaviva, and E. Macii, "Automated segmentation of tissue images for computerized IHC analysis," *Computer Methods and Programs in Biomedicine*, vol. 100, no. 1, pp. 1–15, 2010.
3. C. Jung and C. Kim, "Segmenting clustered nuclei using H-minima transform-based marker extraction and contour parameterization," *IEEE Transactions on Biomedical Engineering*, vol. 57, no. 10, pp. 2600–2604, Oct 2010.
4. J. Cheng and J. Rajapakse, "Segmentation of clustered nuclei with shape markers and marking function," *IEEE Transactions on Biomedical Engineering*, vol. 56, no. 3, pp. 741–748, March 2009.
5. H. Irshad, A. Veillard, L. Roux, and D. Racoceanu, "Methods for nuclei detection, segmentation, and classification in digital histopathology: A review – current status and future potential," *IEEE Reviews in Biomedical Engineering*, vol. 7, pp. 97–114, 2014.
6. H. Kong, M. Gurcan, and K. Belkacem-Boussaid, "Partitioning histopathological images: an integrated framework for supervised color-texture segmentation and cell splitting," *IEEE Transactions on Medical Imaging*, vol. 30, no. 9, pp. 1661–1677, 2011.
7. A. Rosenfeld and J. L. Pfaltz, "Sequential operations in digital picture processing," *J. ACM*, vol. 13, no. 4, pp. 471–494, Oct. 1966. [Online]. Available: http://doi.acm.org/10.1145/321356.321357
8. C. Jung, C. Kim, S. W. Chae, and S. Oh, "Unsupervised segmentation of overlapped nuclei using bayesian classification," *IEEE Transactions on Biomedical Engineering*, vol. 57, no. 12, pp. 2825–2832, 2010.
9. D. Ballard, "Generalizing the Hough transform to detect arbitrary shapes," *Pattern Recognition*, vol. 13, no. 2, pp. 111–122, 1981. [Online]. Available: http://www.sciencedirect.com/science/article/pii/0031320381900091
10. R. O. Duda and P. E. Hart, "Use of the Hough transformation to detect lines and curves in pictures," *Commun. ACM*, vol. 15, no. 1, pp. 11–15, Jan. 1972. [Online]. Available: http://doi.acm.org/10.1145/361237.361242
11. E. Cosatto, M. Miller, H. Graf, and J. Meyer, "Grading nuclear pleomorphism on histological micrographs," in *19th International Conference on Pattern Recognition (ICPR)*, Dec 2008, pp. 1–4.

12. Y. M. George, B. M. Bagoury, H. H. Zayed, and M. I. Roushdy, "Automated cell nuclei segmentation for breast fine needle aspiration cytology," *Signal Processing*, vol. 93, no. 10, pp. 2804–2816, 2013.
13. O. Dzyubachyk, W. van Cappellen, J. Essers, W. Niessen, and E. Meijering, "Advanced level-set-based cell tracking in time-lapse fluorescence microscopy," *IEEE Transactions on Medical Imaging*, vol. 29, no. 3, pp. 852–867, March 2010.
14. F. Tek, A. Dempster, and I. Kale, "Blood cell segmentation using minimum area watershed and circle Radon transformations," in *Mathematical Morphology: 40 Years On*, ser. Computational Imaging and Vision, C. Ronse, L. Najman, and E. Decencière, Eds. Springer Netherlands, 2005, vol. 30, pp. 441–454. [Online]. Available: http://dx.doi.org/10.1007/1-4020-3443-1_40
15. T. Esteves, P. Quelhas, A. M. Mendonça, and A. Campilho, "Gradient convergence filters and a phase congruency approach for in vivo cell nuclei detection," *Machine Vision and Applications*, vol. 23, no. 4, pp. 623–638, 2012.
16. H. Kobatake and S. Hashimoto, "Convergence index filter for vector fields," *IEEE Transactions on Image Processing*, vol. 8, no. 8, pp. 1029–1038, 1999.
17. C. Pereira, H. Fernandes, A. Mendonça, and A. Campilho, "Detection of lung nodule candidates in chest radiographs," *Pattern Recognition and Image Analysis*, pp. 170–177, 2007.
18. J. Wei, Y. Hagihara, and H. Kobatake, "Detection of cancerous tumors on chest X-ray images-candidate detection filter and its evaluation," in *International Conference on Image Processing (ICIP)*, vol. 3. IEEE, 1999, pp. 397–401.
19. R. A. Russell, N. M. Adams, D. A. Stephens, E. Batty, K. Jensen, and P. S. Freemont, "Segmentation of fluorescence microscopy images for quantitative analysis of cell nuclear architecture," *Biophysical journal*, vol. 96, no. 8, pp. 3379–3389, 2009.
20. M. N. Gurcan, T. Pan, H. Shimada, and J. Saltz, "Image analysis for neuroblastoma classification: Segmentation of cell nuclei," in *28th Annual International Conference of the IEEE Engineering in Medicine and Biology Society (EMBS)*. IEEE, 2006, pp. 4844–4847.
21. F. Cloppet and A. Boucher, "Segmentation of complex nucleus configurations in biological images," *Pattern Recognition Letters*, vol. 31, no. 8, pp. 755–761, 2010.
22. O. Schmitt and M. Hasse, "Radial symmetries based decomposition of cell clusters in binary and gray level images," *Pattern Recognition*, vol. 41, no. 6, pp. 1905–1923, 2008.
23. F. Meyer, "Topographic distance and watershed lines," *Signal Processing*, vol. 38, no. 1, pp. 113–125, 1994.
24. J. B. Roerdink and A. Meijster, "The watershed transform: Definitions, algorithms and parallelization strategies," *Fundamenta Informaticae*, vol. 41, no. 1,2, pp. 187–228, Apr. 2000. [Online]. Available: http://dl.acm.org/citation.cfm?id=2372488.2372495
25. S. Osher and J. A. Sethian, "Fronts propagating with curvature-dependent speed: algorithms based on Hamilton-Jacobi formulations," *Journal of Computational Physics*, vol. 79, no. 1, pp. 12–49, 1988.
26. M. Kass, A. Witkin, and D. Terzopoulos, "Snakes: Active contour models," *International Journal of Computer Vision*, vol. 1, no. 4, pp. 321–331, 1988.
27. V. Caselles, R. Kimmel, and G. Sapiro, "Geodesic active contours," *International Journal of Computer Vision*, vol. 22, no. 1, pp. 61–79, 1997.

28. D. Mumford and J. Shah, "Optimal approximations by piecewise smooth functions and associated variational problems," *Communications on Pure and Applied Mathematics*, vol. 42, no. 5, pp. 577–685, 1989.
29. T. E. Chan and L. Vese, "A level set algorithm for minimizing the Mumford-Shah functional in image processing," in *IEEE Workshop on Variational and Level Set Methods in Computer Vision*. IEEE, 2001, pp. 161–168.
30. T. F. Chan and L. Vese, "Active contours without edges," *IEEE Transactions on Image Processing*, vol. 10, no. 2, pp. 266–277, 2001.
31. S. Gao and T. D. Bui, "A multistage image segmentation and denoising method–based on the Mumford and Shah variational approach," in *Image Analysis and Recognition*. Springer, 2004, pp. 82–89.
32. A. C. Ruifrok and D. A. Johnston, "Quantification of histochemical staining by color deconvolution," *Analytical and Quantitative Cytology and Histology*, vol. 23, no. 4, pp. 291–299, 2001.
33. J. Ni, M. Singh, and C. Bahlmann, "Fast radial symmetry detection under affine transformations," in *IEEE Conference on Computer Vision and Pattern Recognition (CVPR)*, June 2012, pp. 932–939.
34. X. Han, C. Xu, and J. L. Prince, "A topology preserving level set method for geometric deformable models," *IEEE Transactions on Pattern Analysis and Machine Intelligence*, vol. 25, no. 6, pp. 755–768, 2003.
35. G. Loy and A. Zelinsky, "Fast radial symmetry for detecting points of interest," *IEEE Transactions on Pattern Analysis and Machine Intelligence*, vol. 25, no. 8, pp. 959–973, August 2003.
36. D. Cremers, M. Rousson, and R. Deriche, "A review of statistical approaches to level set segmentation: integrating color, texture, motion and shape," *International Journal of Computer Vision*, vol. 72, no. 2, pp. 195–215, 2007.
37. T. Brox, M. Rousson, R. Deriche, and J. Weickert, "Colour, texture, and motion in level set based segmentation and tracking," *Image and Vision Computing*, vol. 28, no. 3, pp. 376–390, 2010. [Online]. Available: http://www.sciencedirect.com/science/article/pii/S0262885609001334
38. G. Bertrand, "Simple points, topological numbers and geodesic neighborhoods in cubic grids," *Pattern Recognition Letters*, vol. 15, no. 10, pp. 1003–1011, 1994. [Online]. Available: http://www.sciencedirect.com/science/article/pii/0167865594900329
39. L. Coelho, A. Shariff, and R. Murphy, "Nuclear segmentation in microscope cell images: A hand-segmented dataset and comparison of algorithms," in *IEEE International Symposium on Biomedical Imaging: From Nano to Macro (ISBI)*, June 2009, pp. 518–521.
40. A. E. Carpenter, T. R. Jones, M. R. Lamprecht, C. Clarke, I. H. Kang, O. Friman, D. A. Guertin, J. H. Chang, R. A. Lindquist, J. Moffat *et al.*, "Cellprofiler: image analysis software for identifying and quantifying cell phenotypes," *Genome Biology*, vol. 7, no. 10, p. R100, 2006.

5

Level Set Methods in Segmentation of SDOCT Retinal Images

Padmasini N, Umamaheswari R, Mohamed Yacin Sikkandar, and Manavi D Sindal

CONTENTS

5.1 Introduction

Optical Coherence Tomography (OCT) is a powerful non-contact type imaging modality used to image various aspects of biological tissues, such as structural information, blood flow, elastic parameters, change of polarization states, and molecular content [1]. The latest technology using a spectral domain optical coherence tomography (SDOCT) scanner, helps to view fine details of the retina. This retinal image is used to diagnose systemic eye diseases such as diabetic retinopathy, macular edema, age related macular degeneration etc. In diabetic maculopathy the fluid filled macular edema region has to be assessed volumetrically. For this assessment it is essential to perform segmentation of fluid filled regions. Figure 5.1 shows a typical SDOCT scanner used for imaging the retina, and Figures 5.2 and 5.3 show a typical SDOCT retinal image of a normal and with fluid filled region.

SDOCT makes use of a low coherence interferometer to generate two- or three-dimensional imaging of biological samples by obtaining high-resolution cross-sectional backscattering profiles. The estimation of the depth at which specific backscatter originated is from its time of flight. In SDOCT, the source is broadband and continuous wave; the reference arm length is fixed at a position corresponding to the position of the sample and a spectrometer is used to analyze the interference pattern between the light returning from the reference arm and the sample, as shown in Figure 5.1. The typical OCT images obtained using Cirrus HD-OCT which is capable of 5-mm axial and 15-mm transverse resolution in tissue is shown in Figures 5.2 and 5.3. The axial resolution varies from 3 to 5 mm, and the size of the picture is 500-700 mm.

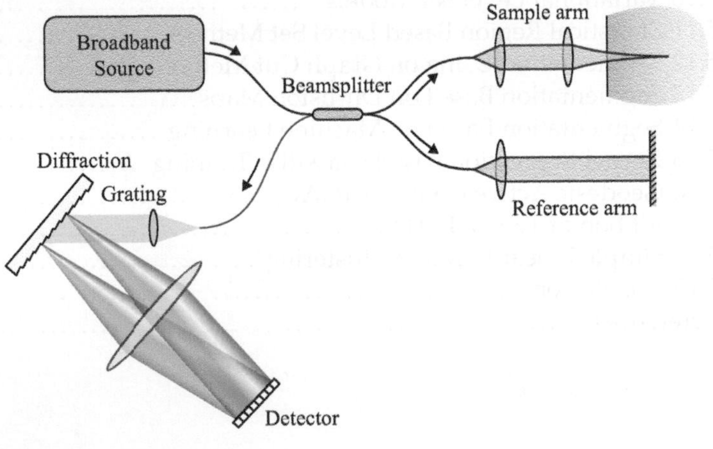

FIGURE 5.1
The principle of SDOCT.

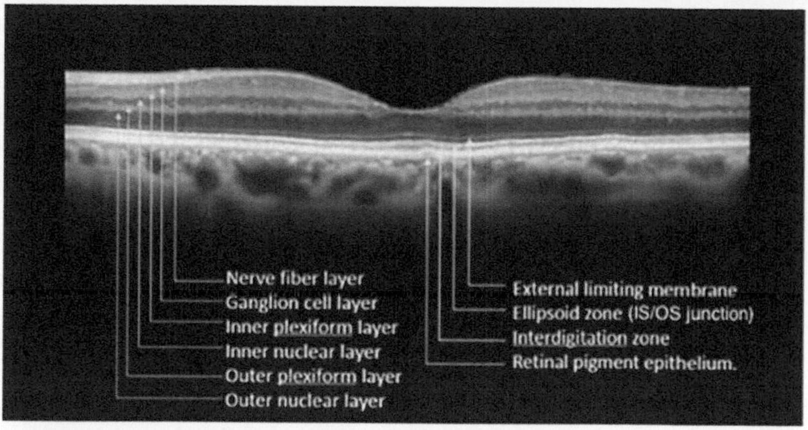

FIGURE 5.2
SDOCT normal image.

As shown in Figure 5.2, the retina is a ten layered structure, viz., Nerve fiber layer (NFL), Ganglion cell layer (GCL), Inner plexiform layer (IPL), inner nuclear layer (INL), outer plexiform layer (OPL), outer nuclear layer (ONL), External limiting membrane (ELM), Ellipsoid zone (previously referred to as the IS/OS junction), Interdigitation zone, and Retinal pigment epithelium (RPE). Automatic detection of diabetic maculopathy from SDOCT retinal images is extremely important in analyzing the stage of diabetic retinopathy. Diabetic maculopathy is the condition of fluid being accumulated in between the retinal layers. As shown in Figure 5.3, SDOCT images provide more details about the intraretinal fluid and subretinal fluid present in the macula scan images.

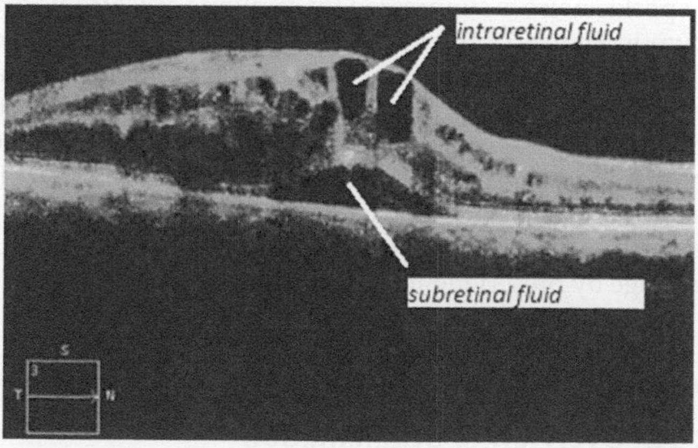

FIGURE 5.3
Diabetic maculopathy condition with intraretinal and subretinal fluid (Courtesy: Aravind Eye Hospital, Puducherry).

Even though, in the recent times there are some automatic algorithms proposed to segment retinal layers; the accuracy in edge detection is still challenging problem. There are some researchers who have developed different automatic algorithms for segmenting intraretinal fluid based on region based level set method. The features of the segmented region are analyzed volumetrically and based on their temporal characteristics, the severity of the disease can be estimated [2]. Segmentation, however, remains one of the most difficult and at the same time most commonly required steps in OCT image analysis. No typical segmentation method exists that can be expected to work equally well for all the tasks. One of the most challenging problems in OCT image segmentation is designing a system to work properly in clinical applications. There is no doubt that algorithms and research projects work on a limited number of images with some determinate abnormalities (or even on normal subjects) and such limitations make them more appropriate for the bench, not the bedside. Moreover, OCT images are inherently noisy, thus often requiring the utilization of 3D contextual information. Furthermore, the structure of the retina can drastically change during disease. The SDOCT scanner uses coherent wave pattern to acquire images and hence it produces the image with speckle noise. The speckle noise masks the low contrast lesions which interrupts the physician for effective diagnosis [3]. Speckle is a multiplicative, randomly distributed granular noise of a size of 1-2μm. It has a negative impact on the image [4]. Eq. (5.1) gives the general form of speckle noise,

$$g(n,m) = f(n,m) * u(n.m) + \partial(n,m) \tag{5.1}$$

where g(n,m) is the noisy image, u(n,m) is the multiplicative object, and δ(n,m) is the additive object of the speckles. The presence of speckle noise occurring in the OCT image degrades the quality of the image [5]. For effective elucidation of the image, speckle noise has to be reduced. In our work the speckle noise is suppressed by applying anisotropic diffusion filtering as shown in Figure 5.4 [6]. Diagnosing the retinal disorders can be carried out by performing segmentation of the region of interest in the processed image effectively. In this proposed work speckles are reduced by the fuzzy logic approach. The peak signal to noise ratio is calculated to be 10.67db in an average. To improve peak signal to noise ratio and for further effective removal of speckles, an anisotropic diffusion filter is used. The PSNR value is increased to about 64.5db in an average and, further it is found that this filter enhance the image by preserving its edges.

5.2 An Overview of Segmentation

In any image processing, the task of image segmentation is to find a collection of non-overlapping sub regions of a given image. In medical imaging

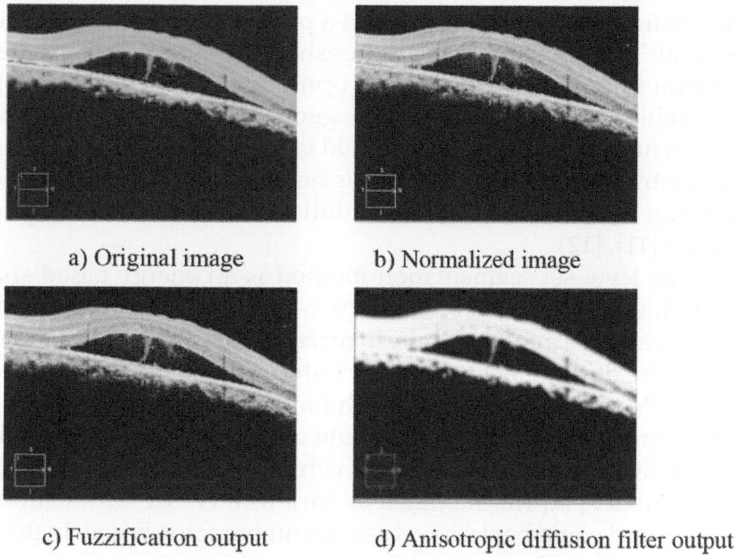

FIGURE 5.4
Output after filteration (Courtesy: Aravind Eye Hospital, Puducherry).

for example, one might want to segment the tumor region from a CT or MRI brain image. In airport screening, one might wish to segment certain "sensitive" shapes, such as guns. There are many other obvious applications. Image segmentation is the division of an image into different regions, each having certain properties. The first step of image analysis aims at either a description of an image or a classification of the image if a class label is meaningful. An example of the former is the description of an office scene. An example of the latter is the classification of the image of a cancerous cell. Image segmentation is a critical component of an image recognition system because errors in segmentation might propagate to feature extraction and classification. Many image segmentation techniques have been proposed to date as shown in Figure 5.5. These segmentation techniques can be categorized into three main classes, viz., (1) characteristic feature thresholding or clustering, (2) edge detection, and (3) region extraction [7]. Almost all image segmentation techniques proposed so far are ad hoc in nature. There are no general algorithms which will work for all images. One of the reasons that we do not have a general image understanding system is that a two-dimensional image can represent a potentially infinite number of possibilities. To build a general image understanding system would require the representation and storage of a vast amount of knowledge. [8] commented that an image segmentation problem is basically one of psychophysical perception, and therefore not susceptible to a purely analytical solution. Any mathematical algorithms must be supplemented by heuristics, usually involving semantics about the class of pictures under consideration. Quite often, one must go beyond simple heuristics, and the introduction of a priori knowledge about the picture is essential. The main limitations of thresholding based methods are that it is difficult (or impossible) to determine optimum threshold values [9], [10] and one is unable to take into account the geometric information of the objects to be segmented, which limit its potential to be generalizable to wider applications. In contrast, active contour models have demonstrated good performance in dealing with challenging segmentation problems, including vessel segmentation [11], [12].

The level set segmentation method is an energy based spatially guided technique. The level set method was first introduced by Osher and Sethian [13] to capture moving fronts. In recent years, there has been a growing interest in the development of active contour models based on level set methods. David Mumford and Jayant Shah have formulated an energy minimization problem that allows one to compute optimal piecewise-smooth or piecewise-constant approximations of a given initial image. This original Mumford Shah model [14] was modified as various level set formulations. Further, energy based could be classified as contour or region based. In the contour based method, it could be geometric or parametric active contours. Coupled Level sets, Distance regularized level sets, Pseudo level sets, and Geodesic active contours are some of the level set methods which are based on geometric active contours. Edge based contours were developed before region based contours came into the picture.

5.3 Level Set Methods

Level sets can be used for image segmentation by using image based features such as mean intensity, gradient, and edges in the governing differential equation. In a typical approach, a contour is initialized by a user and is then evolved until it fits the form of an anatomical structure in the image. Many different implementations and variants of this basic concept have been published in the literature. An overview of the field has been made by Sethian [15].

The role of a level set method for image processing often relates to PDE techniques involving one or more of the following features: 1) view of an image as a function sampled on a given grid with the grid values corresponding to the pixel intensity in suitable color space, 2) regularization of the solutions, 3) representation boundaries, and 4) development of numerics for the level set methods. Particularly in light of 3), it is not hard to seek an application of the level set method for segmentation. There are, however, efforts which combine different disciplines (mentioned above) to accomplish special tasks.

The paradigm of the level set is that it is a numerical method for tracking the evolution of contours and surfaces. Instead of manipulating the contour directly, the contour is embedded as the zero level set of a higher dimensional

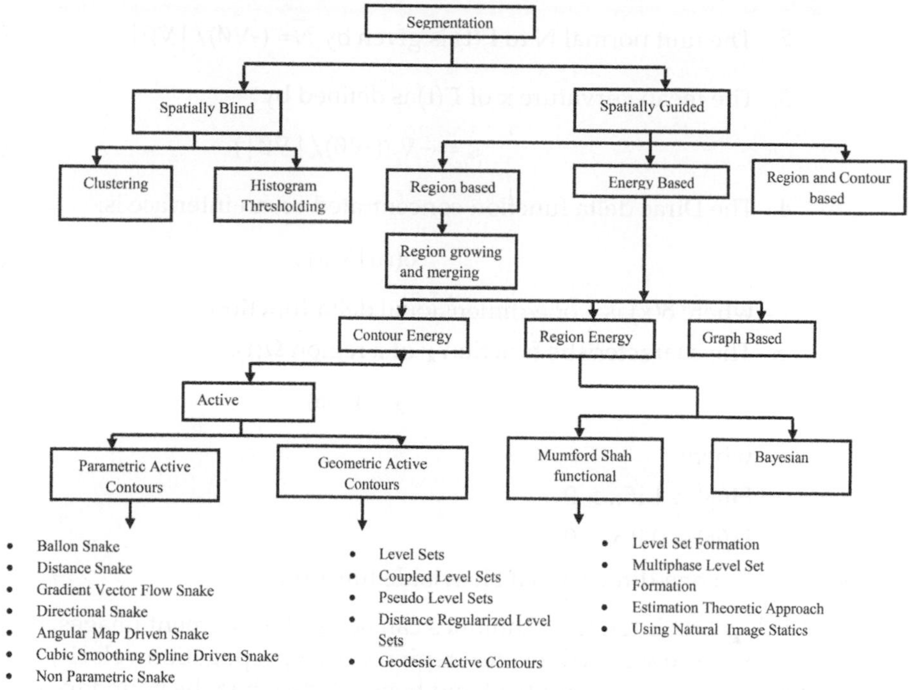

FIGURE 5.5
Segmentation Techniques.

function called the level set function, ψ(X,t). The level set function is then evolved under the control of a differential equation. At any time, the evolving contour can be obtained by extracting the zero level set Γ(X,t) = {ψ(X,t) = 0} from the output. The main advantages of using level sets is that arbitrarily complex shapes can be modeled and topological changes such as merging and splitting are handled implicitly.

There are two important considerations when analyzing the processing time for any particular level set segmentation task: the surface area of the evolving interface and the total distance that the surface must travel. Because the level set equations are usually solved only at pixels near the surface (fast marching methods are an exception), the time taken at each iteration depends on the number of points on the surface. This means that as the surface grows, the solver will slow down proportionally. Because the surface must evolve slowly to prevent numerical instabilities in the solution, the distance the surface must travel in the image dictates the total number of iterations required.

The key terms used in level set representation are as follows

1. The interface boundary Γ(t) is defined by: $\{x|\emptyset(x,t)=0\}$. (5.2)
   The region Ω(t) is bounded by Γ(t): $\{x|\emptyset(x,t)>0\}$ (5.3)
   and its exterior is defined by: $\{x|\emptyset(x,t)<0\}$ (5.4)

2. The unit normal N to $\Gamma(t)$ is given by $\vec{N} = (-\nabla\emptyset)/|\nabla\emptyset|$ (5.5)

3. The mean curvature κ of $\Gamma(t)$ is defined by

$$\kappa = -\nabla.((-\nabla\emptyset)/|\nabla\emptyset|) \tag{5.6}$$

4. The Dirac delta function concentrated on an interface is:

$$\delta(\phi)\,|\nabla\phi|, \tag{5.7}$$

   where $\delta(x)$ is a one-dimensional delta function.

5. The characteristic function χ of a region $\Omega(t)$:

$$\chi = H(\phi) \tag{5.8}$$

   where
   $H(\phi) \equiv 1$ if $x > 0$
   $H(\phi) \equiv 0$ if $x < 0$
   is a one-dimensional Heaviside function.

The level set interface techniques can be used to segment images; the central idea is to grow a seed inside a region with a propagation velocity which depends on the image gradient and hence stops when the boundary is reached. This strategy was proposed by [16].

5.4 Snakes-Active Contour Approach

Image segmentation methods using active contours are usually based on minimizing functionals which are so defined that curves close to the target boundaries have small values. To solve these functional minimization problems, a corresponding partial differential equation (PDE) is constructed as the Gateaux derivative gradient flow resulting in a curve evolution. The numerical methods to solve the curve evolution PDEs can be classified into three categories depending on the models to represent the active contours:

(1) Particle model: In this model, an active contour is approximated by a finite set of connected points [17]. The contour evolves as the points move. The local geometric properties essential to the curve evolution such as normal and curvature are approximated by using finite difference method on the adjacent points.

(2) Parametric model: In this model, an active contour is represented analytically in the parametric form $C(t) = (x(t), y(t))$ (such as B-splines in [18] whose shape is controlled by a few parameters and whose local geometric properties can be derived in close forms.

(3) Level set model: In this model, an active contour is embedded implicitly as a constant set in a function defined in a higher dimensional space.

The function is called embedding function and denoted as φ in contrast to the other two models where active contours are represented explicitly. The level set model has remarkable advantages which include

(1) the topological changes of the contours can be easily handled;
(2) the concept and numerical implementation can be easily adapted to solve any dimensional problems;
(3) the areas inside and outside an active contour can be easily determined.

Due to these advantages, since the level set method was first proposed for solving some specific PDEs in [19], a large amount of active contour models have been developed in the level set framework for the image segmentation purpose. Among these models, two of them, namely geodesic active contour model [20] and Chan-Vese model [21] stand out respectively as the paradigms for boundary based and region based segmentation methods.

The basic idea in active contour models (or snakes) is to evolve a curve, subject to constraints from a given image u_0, in order to detect objects in that image [22]. Ideally, we begin with a curve around the object to be detected, and the curve then moves normal to itself and stops at the boundary of the object. Since its invention this technique has been used both often and successfully. The classical snakes model involves an edge detector, which depends on the gradient of the image u_0, to stop the evolving curve at the boundary of the object. Let $u_0(x, y)$ map the square $0 \leq x, y \leq 1$ into R, where u_0 is the image and $C(I) : [0, 1] \rightarrow R2$ is the parameterized curve.

$$E(C) = -v_0 \int \nabla |I(c)|^2 ds + v_1 \int |C_s^2|\, ds + v_2 \int |C_{ss}^2| ds \tag{5.9}$$

The snake model is to minimize Eq. (5.9) where v_0,v_1,v_2 are positive parameters. The first two terms control the smoothness of the contour, while the third attracts the contour toward the object in the image (the external energy). They are called snakes because of the way the contours slither while minimizing their energy. Changes in high-level interpretation can exert forces on a snake as it continues its minimization. Even in the absence of such forces, snakes exhibit hysteresis when exposed to moving stimuli. Snakes do not try to solve the entire problem of finding salient image contours. They rely on other mechanisms to place them somewhere near the desired contour. However, even in cases where no satisfactory automatic starting mechanism exists, snakes can still be used for semiautomatic image interpretation. If an expert user pushes a snake close to an intended contour, its energy minimization will carry it the rest of the way. The minimization provides a 'power assist' for a person pointing to a contour feature. Snakes are an example of a more general technique of matching a deformable model to an image by means of energy minimization. [23], [24].

Though the snakes approach had an enormous impact in the segmentation community, it also suffers from several drawbacks outlined below as discussed by [25]:

1. The implementation of contour evolutions based on an explicit parameterization requires a delicate regridding (or reparameterization) process to avoid self-intersection and overlap of control or marker points.
2. The explicit representation by default does not allow the evolving contour to undergo topological changes such that the segmentation of several objects or multiply-connected objects is not straightforward. The segmentations obtained by a local optimization method are bound to depend on the initialization.
3. The snake algorithm is known to be quite sensitive to the initialization. For many realistic images, the segmentation algorithm tends to get stuck in undesired local minima—in particular in the presence of noise.
4. The snakes approach lacks a meaningful probabilistic interpretation. Extensions to other segmentation criteria—such as color, texture or motion—are not straight-forward.

Snake based methods [26] attempt to minimize the sum of internal and external energy of the current contour. These methods work well on those images with high contrast, high gradient and smooth boundaries between the layers; however, the performance is adversely affected by blood vessel shadows, other morphological features of the retina, or irregular layer shapes.

Zhu et al. [27] proposed a floating canvas method to segment 3D intraretinal layers. This method can produce relatively smooth layers; however, it is sensitive to any low gradients between layers [28]. Proposed an active contour method, which incorporates a circular shape prior information, to segment the intraretinal layers from 3D OCT image. This method can effectively overcome the effects of the blood vessel shadows and other morphological features of the retina; however, it cannot work well on those images with irregular layers.

Level set methods provide a non-parametric way to describe the interface. In contrast to parametric methods—such as snakes that provide an explicit parameterization of the interface—level sets embed the interface implicitly, which has some computational advantages (i.e., regarding propagation and topology of the interface). The level set function φ is defined in the same space as the input data (which is three-dimensional for volumetric OCT data) and maps an input coordinate x to a scalar. The interface is then defined as the curve C for which the level set is zero: $C = \{x \mid \varphi(x) = 0\}$. The level set is evolved according to the general level set equation

$$\varphi t = -F|\nabla\varphi| \tag{5.10}$$

Here, φt is the update step of the level set, F is some force that drives the level set and ∇φ is the gradient of the level set [29]. It is clear that Γ is the zero level set of the function φ. In the case that Γ is not closed, but divides the domain into two parts, then the function can be defined to be positive on one side of the curve and negative on the other side of the curve. The function φ is called a level set function for Γ. It is clear that φ satisfies the partial differential equation in Ω.:

$$|\nabla\varphi| = 1 \tag{5.11}$$

However, φ is not the only function that satisfies equation (5.11) in the distribution sense. In order to define a unique solution for the equation, the concept of viscosity solution need to introduced. The existence and uniqueness of viscosity solutions for linear and nonlinear partial differential equations constitutes an active field of research with rich literature [30]. One way to introduce the viscosity function is to add an extra time variables t. Let $\tilde{\emptyset}$ be any function such that Γ is the zero level set curve of $\tilde{\emptyset}$ and $\tilde{\emptyset}$ is positive inside Γ and negative outside Γ. Then the distance function φ is the steady state of the following time dependent equation

$$\frac{\partial d}{\partial t} + sign(d)(|\nabla d| - 1) = 0 \tag{5.12}$$

$d(x,0) = d_0 = \tilde{\emptyset}$, i.e. $d(x, t; \tilde{\emptyset}) \to \varphi(x)$ as $t \to \infty$. Moreover the steady state is unique. Once the level set function is defined, we can use it to represent general piecewise constant functions. For example, assuming that q(x) equals c1 inside Γ and equals c2 outside Γ, it is easy to see that q can be represented as:

$$q = c_1 H(\varphi) + c_2(1 - H(\varphi) \tag{5.13}$$

where the Heaviside function H(φ) is defined by:

$$H(\varphi) = \begin{cases} 1, \varphi > 0, \\ 0, \ \varphi \le 0 \end{cases}$$

In order to identify the function q, we just need to identify the level set function φ and the piecewise constant values c_i's. If the function q(x) has many pieces, then we need to use multiple level set functions. The ideas of Chan and Vese are followed [21], [31]. Assume that we have two closed curves Γ1 and Γ2, and we associate the two level set functions $\varphi_j, j = 1, 2$, with these curves. Then the domain Ω is divided into four parts:

$$\Omega 1 = \{x \in \Omega, \varphi 1(x) > 0, \varphi 2(x) > 0\} \tag{5.14}$$

$$\Omega 2 = \{x \in \Omega, \varphi 1(x) > 0, \varphi 2(x) < 0\} \tag{5.15}$$

$$\Omega 3 = \{x \in \Omega, \varphi 1(x) < 0, \varphi 2(x) > 0\} \tag{5.16}$$

$$\Omega 4 = \{x \in \Omega, \varphi 1(x) < 0, \varphi 2(x) < 0\} \tag{5.17}$$

Using the Heaviside function again, we can express q with possibly up to four pieces of constant values as:

$$q = c_1 H(\varphi 1)H(\varphi 2) + c_2 H(\varphi 1)(1 - H(\varphi 2) + c_3(1 - H(\varphi 1)H(\varphi 2) + c_4(1 - H(\varphi 1)(1 - H(\varphi 2)) \tag{5.18}$$

By generalizing, we see that n level set functions give the possibility of 2n regions.

For i = 1, 2, · · · , 2n, let $bin(i - 1) = (b_1^i, b_2^i, b_3^i, \ldots . b_n^i)$ be the binary representation of i-1, where $b_1^i = 0 \; or \; 1$. A piece wise constant function q with constant values c_i, i = 1,2,3.... 2^n could be represented as

$$q = \sum_{i=1}^{2^n} c_i \prod_{j=1}^{n} R_i(\emptyset_j) \tag{5.19}$$

where

$$R_i\,(\emptyset_j) = \begin{cases} H(\emptyset_j), & if\, b_j^i = 0; \\ 1 - H(\emptyset_j), & if\, b_j^i = 1; \end{cases} \tag{5.20}$$

5.5 Challenges in OCT Images

- Perturbation of 3D OCT images and image artefacts are produced by eye movements during the imaging. It is difficult to remove all the noise and at the same time keep the relevant image structures;
- Intraretinal layers segmentation can be difficult in images affected by disease;
- The leakages and irregular shapes of the optic nerve head can make it difficult to detect the intraretinal layers accurately in ONH images;
- The layer boundaries within the retina are not distinct because of immature imaging modalities. The appearance of the layers may be inhomogeneous and inconsistent because of the presence of blood vessels and blood vessel shadows inside the layers.

5.6 Level Set Methods for OCT Image Segmentation

5.6.1 Loosely Coupled Level Sets (LCLS)

The LCLS approach is based on a probabilistic framework, which performs segmentation of interfaces between retinal layers. Every interface C_i is represented by its own level set function φ_i, which is propagated according to:

$$\frac{\partial \varphi_i}{\partial t} = -\Delta t((p_r(^{l_i}/_{\mu}) - 0.5) + \alpha\kappa_i + \beta\zeta_i)|\nabla\emptyset_i| \tag{5.21}$$

where $p_r(^{l_i}/_{\mu})$ is the probability of a pixel belonging to layer l_r and μ the attenuation coefficient of that pixel, and κ_i and ζ_i are the geometric regularization terms. The weights of the terms are denoted by α and β, while Δt is the time step. The probabilistic term expresses the posterior probability of pixels along an interface belonging to the adjacent layer as:

$$p_r(^{l_i}/_{\mu}) = \frac{p_r(^{\mu}/l_i)p_r(l_i)}{\sum_{j\epsilon\{i,i+1\}} p_r(^{\mu}/l_j)p_r(l_j)} \tag{5.22}$$

where $p_r(^{l_i}/_{\mu})$ is the likelihood based on the available image data inside the set Ω_i containing all pixels assigned to l.

In the work by Jelena Novosel et al. [32], the retinal layer in OCT images is segmented by simultaneous detection of their interfaces. This is done by means of a level set approach based on Bayesian inference where the ordering of the layers is enforced via a novel level set coupling.

A quantitative comparison with manual annotations was used to estimate the method's accuracy, which showed very good agreement (mean absolute deviation (MAD) of 3.11- 8.58 μm). The large errors were mainly due to differences in handling the vessels. Based on repeated OCT images of the same eye acquired on consecutive days, the reproducibility of manual and automated segmentations, expressed by the MAD of the RNFL thickness, were 10.97 μm and 7.68 μm. For simultaneous detection of multiple interfaces between different layers, the force F is comprised of probabilities that are derived from the imaging data through Bayesian inference and constraints that enforce the predefined ordering. By using uncoupled level sets, detection of multiple interfaces becomes problematic as the level sets can cross each other. This may happen because the level sets are propagating independently of each other, each driven by its own image derived information. Coupling ensures proper ordering of the level sets, thereby preventing interfaces to cross. With current approaches of level set coupling either the complexity of the coupling increases with the number of the level sets or the coupling cannot be extended to layered structures [33]. Novosel et al. have reported that the RMS error for the three interfaces varied between 4.23-15.24 μm (1- 4 pixels). The larger errors were primarily due to differences in handling the vessels. The automatic segmentation included blood vessels in the RNFL, while manual annotations sometime differed. In addition, the blood vessels are not a part of the retinal layer tissue and segmentation in those areas is of limited interest. When excluding those areas from the accuracy evaluation, the RMS error for the three interfaces was 4.23-8.84 μm (1-2 pixels).

A locally-adaptive approach to segment the fluid and the interfaces between retinal layers in the B-scans of eyes affected by CSR is carried out by [34]. It is based on their previously developed loosely-coupled level sets (LCLS) method. In [35] retinal layers and fluids are segmented simultaneously and thus aid each other in retrieving the right segmentation. The approach operates on the attenuation coefficient, which is an optical property of tissue estimated from the OCT data [36] and thus invariant to some imaging artefacts. At each iteration of the optimization approach, the likelihoods are approximated by the histograms of the attenuation coefficients of layers that surround an interface. Instead of computing the normalized histogram of the complete layers, a window was set around a pixel of interest and normalized histograms were computed from values within the window. The local histograms still model the likelihoods, but only within a window of interest. This method could simultaneously segment fluid-associated pathologies and interfaces between retinal layers by utilizing local attenuation coefficient contrast of layers surrounding the interfaces and introducing auxiliary interfaces. Hence, the method can adapt to abrupt changes in attenuation coefficients within a layer and segment pathologies such as fluid pockets. An efficient adaptive multigrid level set method for front propagation purposes in three-dimensional medical image processing and segmentation is presented by [37]. It is able to deal with non sharp segment boundaries. A flexible, interactive modulation of the front speed depending on various boundary and regularization criteria ensure this goal. Efficiency is due to a graded underlying mesh implicitly defined via error or feature indicating values on the cells of the underlying hexahedral grid. A suitable saturation condition ensures an important regularity condition on the resulting adaptive grid. This simplifies the adaptive fast marching method on the compressed data significantly.

5.7 Bayesian Based Level Set Segmentation

In the work by Wang et al., segmentation of retinal vessels is carried out based on level set and region growing. The former is used for wide retinal vessel segmentation as it can converge to the wide vessels boundary, and the latter is used for thin retinal vessel segmentation as it can grow the object region with similar grayscale distribution. Zhao et al., propose a new retinal vessel segmentation method based on level set and region growing. Firstly, contrast-limited adaptive histogram equalization (CLAHE) is used to compensate for the effects of a non-uniform lighting, followed by a 2D Gabor wavelet to enhance the contrast of the retinal image. Then the retinal vessel segmentation is conducted in two parallel ways. The first way uses the anisotropic diffusion filter to smooth the retinal image and extract wide retinal vessels by the active contour model. The second way detects the thin vessels by the method of region growing directly. In the end, both the segmentation results are combined to obtain the final extracted retinal vessels [38].

5.8 Distance Regularized Level Set Evolution (DRLSE)

The level set evolution is derived as the gradient flow that minimizes an energy functional with a distance regularization term and an external energy that drives the motion of the zero level set toward desired locations. The distance regularization term is defined with a potential function such that the derived level set evolution has a unique forward-and-backward (FAB) diffusion effect, which is able to maintain a desired shape of the level set function, particularly a signed distance profile near the zero level set. This yields a new type of level set evolution called distance regularized level set evolution (DRLSE). This formulation has an intrinsic capability of maintaining regularity of the level set function, particularly the desirable signed distance property in a vicinity of the zero level set, which ensures accurate computation and stable level set evolution. DRLSE can be implemented by a simpler and more efficient numerical scheme than conventional level set methods. DRLSE also allows more flexible and efficient initialization than generating a signed distance function as the initial level set function. In the work by [39], DRLSE has been applied to an edge based active contour model for image segmentation, and provided a simple and efficient narrowband implementation of this model. This active contour model in DRLSE formulation allows the use of relatively large time steps to significantly reduce iteration numbers and computation time, while maintaining sufficient numerical accuracy in both full domain and narrowband implementations, due to the intrinsic distance regularization embedded in the level set evolution. The CV and DRLSE models are easy to formulate and optimize but the regularization term of the shortest smooth boundary length makes them not necessarily suitable for vessel segmentation problems [40]. A new level set based segmentation method is proposed to integrate both boundary and region information by [41]. Different from the hybrid model proposed in [42] that provides a statistical framework, the new model in this paper tries to solve the problem from more of a geometric perspective. The theory of the new model, its numerical solution, and some experimental results on 2D and 3D medical data are discussed.

Although the final result of a level set method is the zero level set of the level set function (LSF), it is necessary to maintain the LSF in good condition, so that the level set evolution is stable and the numerical computation is accurate. This requires that the LSF is smooth and not too steep or too flat (at least in a vicinity of its zero level set) during the level set evolution. This condition is well satisfied by signed distance functions for their unique property $|\nabla \emptyset| = 1$, which is referred to as the signed distance property. Wu, H., et al proposed a self-adaptive distance regularized level set evolution method for OD segmentation without the periodically re-initializing steps in the level set function execution to a signed distance function during the evolution. The proposed algorithm consists of two steps—in the first step, preprocessing of an image was performed using Fourier correlation coefficient filtering to obtain initial boundary as the beginning contour; while in the second step, an accurate boundary of an optic disc was formed using level set method [43].

Chen et al proposed a level set method based on the Selective Binary and Gaussian Filtering Regularized Level Set (SBGFRLS) method [44] and the Local Binary fitting (LBF) term proposed by Li et al. [45]. The active contour is driven by the Selective Binary and local fitting term in this work. Due to the local intensity term, the proposed model can avoid the numerical result trapped into the local minimum. The re-initialization method in this method is described in SBGFRLS model. This kind of re-initialization method simplified the computation during the evolution. Thus, the proposed method is called combined global and local information method (CGLI). The CGLI method takes the global force and the local force into consideration. Thus, the method has the ability to deal with intensity inhomogeneous retinal images and also can get subpixel accuracy and is robust to the position of the initial contour if the weight of the force is set appropriately [46].

In the work done by Chiu et al for segmentation of seven retinal layers in a SDOCT image, in order to determine the presence or absence of hyperreflectivity the image is first low-pass filtered with a Gaussian kernel and thresholded using Otsu's method to generate a binary mask. This step isolates the NFL-OPL and IS-RPE complexes. The fraction of bright pixels in the region above the cut off is then calculated for the binary image. If the fraction exceeds 0.025, then Chiu et al concluded that the segmented layer boundary is the IS-OS due to the presence of the NFL-OPL complex. Otherwise, they concluded that the vitreous-NFL layer boundary was segmented [47]. In the work by [48] on 3D retinal layer segmentation they had used an adaptive Otsu threshold for setting the intensity threshold [48]. In a similar manner Uji et al used Otsu's thresholding method for binarization with intensity thresholding used for automatic binarization-level decisions [49]. Active surfaces/contours are other popular methods that are widely used for the segmentation of 3D objects, implicitly in the form of a level set function or explicitly as a snake function. In recent years, the level set method has become popular due to its ability to handle complex geometries and topological changes. The level set is in fact a shape-driven tool which, using a properly defined speed function, can grow or shrink to take the shape of any complex object of interest. Unlike the traditional deformable models, the level set method does not depend on the parameterizations of the surface. In order to automatically segment the active area and inactive area in a displacement magnitude map, Wang et al used the classic automatic thresholding method for bi-modal images [50]. The central idea of the level set method, which was first introduced by Osher and Sethian, is the formulation of the correct equation of motion for front propagating with curvature-dependent speed. This equation is an initial-value Hamilton-Jacobi equation with right-hand-side that depends on curvature effects. The limit of the right-hand-side as the curvature effects go to zero is an eikonal equation with an associated entropy condition. By viewing the surface as a level set, topological complexities and changes in the moving front are handled naturally. With these equations as a basis, any number of numerical algorithms may be devised of arbitrary degree of accuracy using the technology developed for the solution of hyperbolic conservation laws. In particular, algorithms can be devised to have the correct limiting entropy-satisfying solution. In fact, some previous algorithms may be viewed as less sophisticated approximations to their equations of motion [51]. A basic idea in this field is to view a gray-scale image as a function $u_0(x, y)$ with u_0 taking on discrete values between 0 and 255, which we take as a continuum for the sake of this discussion. A standard operation on images is to convolve u0 with a Gaussian of equation (5.1).

$$J(x, y, \sigma) = \frac{1}{4\pi\sigma}\left(e^{-\frac{x^2+y^2}{4\sigma}}\right) \tag{5.23}$$

to obtain

$$u(x, y, \sigma) = \iint J(x - x', \ y - y', \sigma)u_o(x', y')dx'dy' = J * u_o \tag{5.24}$$

This has the same effect as solving the initial value problem for the heat equation $u_t = u_{xx} + u_{yy}$ $u(x, y, 0) = u_0(x, y)$ for $t > 0$ (ignoring boundary conditions) to obtain $u(x, y, \sigma)$ at $t = \sigma > 0$, i.e., the expression obtained in equation.

The subretinal fluid and intraretinal cysts are both detected using a level set segmentation method, due to the fact that the reflectance of cysts and subretinal fluid is significantly lower than the surrounding tissue in retina. Based on the difference between their position, shape, and size, these fluid regions can be classified as the intraretinal or the subretinal. Additionally, the variation in retinal thickness was calculated, normalized by the normal retina thickness range, and presented as a retinal thickness deviation map [52].

5.9 Geographic Atrophy

Geographic Atrophy (GA) segmentation was performed using a level set segmentation approach in SDOCT retinal images by [53]. The underlying principle of GA detection using the level set approach is to represent the GA

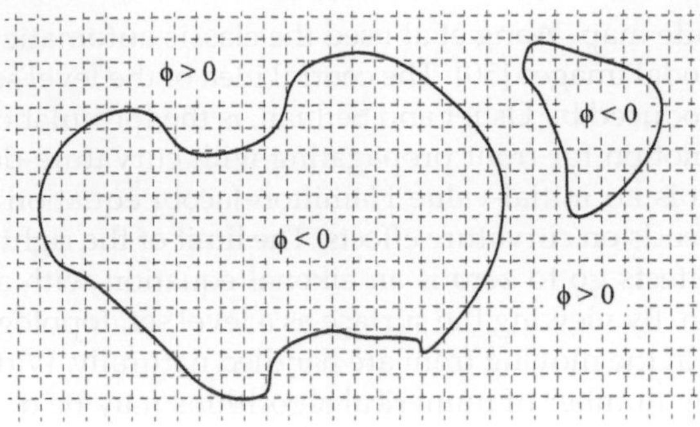

FIGURE 5.6
Two closed curves that are implicitly embedded by a single level set function defined on the grid.

contour C by the zero level set of a higher dimensional embedding function Ø, defined as the signed distance function (SDF) level set.

Figure 5.6 shows that inside the GA region the function has a value of Ø > 0; outside the GA region, the function has a value of Ø < 0. Thus on the GA contour, the function has a value of Ø = 0 and hence is called zero.

Fundamentally, rather than directly evolving the GA contour C, the algorithm evolves the level set function Ø. The level set evolution is governed by a partial differential equation (PDE) as shown below

$$\frac{d}{dt}\text{Ø}\alpha - \alpha P(x,y)|\nabla\text{Ø}| + \beta K(x,y)|\nabla\text{Ø}| \tag{5.25}$$

where P(x,y) represents a propagation speed term; K(x,y) represents a curvature term; and a and b are the heights reflecting the different influences of the propagation speed and curvature over the contour evolution. The evolving GA contour C was then obtained by extracting the zero level set.

5.10 Variational Level Set Models

Level set is an implicit deformable model, also called implicit active contours, that can model arbitrarily complex shapes and topological changes. This energy functional usually depends on the image data as well as the characteristic features used to identify the objects to be segmented. One of the primary and classical variational level set models was developed by Chan and Vese (CV model). Their method seeks the desired segmentation as the best piecewise constant approximation to a given image. In their proposed model for active contours to detect objects in a given image, they made use of curve evolution, Mumford–Shah functional for segmentation, and level sets. Their model could detect objects whose boundaries are not necessarily defined by gradient. They minimized the energy which is seen as a particular case of the minimal partition problem. In the level set formulation, the problem becomes a "mean-curvature flow" like evolving the active contour, which will stop on the desired boundary. However, the stopping term does not depend on the gradient of the image, as in the classical active contour models, but is instead related to a particular segmentation of the image. The initial curve can be anywhere in the image, and interior contours are automatically detected [54]. This type of variational level set model also known as the region based model, provides optimal segmentation by minimizing an energy functional. This energy functional usually depends on the image data as well as the characteristic features used to identify the objects to be segmented.

One of the primary and classical variational level set models was developed by Chan and Vese. Their method seeks the desired segmentation as the best piecewise constant approximation to a given image. They proposed to minimize the following energy functional:

$$\begin{aligned} E(c1, c2, \emptyset) &= \mu L(\emptyset) + E_{out}(c1, c2, \emptyset) \\ &= \mu \int \delta(\emptyset)|\nabla\emptyset| dxdy + \int (I - c1)^2\, H(\emptyset) dxdy \\ &\quad + \int (I - c2)^2 (1 - H(\emptyset)) dxdy \end{aligned} \tag{5.26}$$

Here, $\mu \geq 0$ is a fixed parameter, $\emptyset$ is the level set function, $L(\emptyset)$ is the length of the curve, c1 and c2 are the respective mean intensities inside and outside the contour, $H(\emptyset)$ and $\delta(\emptyset)$ are the 1D Heaviside and Dirac delta function, respectively; and I is the original image to be segmented. $L(\emptyset)$ denotes the internal energy which controls the smoothness of the curve and Eout(c1, c2, $\emptyset$) is the external energy which is driven by image features and forces the contour towards object boundaries. The Chan-Vese model assumes intensity homogeneity and seeks to partition an image into regions of constant mean intensity. This often leads to poor segmentation results in complicated images. Additionally, the Chan-Vese model is dependent on the placement of the initial contour, yielding different results for different initial locations of the contour. The segmentation of medical images generally faces challenges, including noise introduced during the acquisition process, missing or broken boundaries, and complex biological structures. In such cases, the introduction of prior information, such as an approximation of the shape, intensity, and other features of the tissue of interest could help the segmentation algorithm perform better. Recently, level set based approaches that integrate shape priors have been proposed using different shape models. These approaches either use specific shapes known a priori, or the shape parameters are obtained from available training data. Fourier descriptors are a highly effective and compact means of representing object shape and thus make an ideal candidate for use as a shape prior in the level set formulation. The work by Mohammad et al. (2015), has focussed on the description of shape priors using Fourier descriptors to simulate pathologies occurring in the human retina. The shape signatures are derived using the centroid distance function. They included a cost-function which serves as a weighting function to determine the similarity between the target curve and the derived curve. They have obtained the automated segmentation of pathologies visible in seven enface retinal images generated at different retinal depths. After segmentation, they measured the co-localization of pathologies in the inner retina and inter segmented layers to determine the effect of DR pathologies of the inner retina on the integrity of the photoreceptor cells [55]. Edge based level set models use an edge detector, which depends on the gradient of the image to stop the curve on the object boundaries. Region based models assume intensity homogeneity and are not as sensitive to the location of initial contours as they do not use the image gradient for segmentation.

A multi-resolution approach that used wavelets was proposed in [56]. Wavelets improve the convergence speed by using a coarse resolution for curve initialization. An edge based model that does not use initial contours was proposed by [57]. Their model derives the edge information and neighborhood distribution with two different localized region based operators. Shi et al. [48] added to the Chan-Vese model a restriction item that is a non-linear heat equation with a balanced diffusion rate to eliminate the re-initialization procedure. A new level set method which combines the average values of global regions and local boundary information to detect lung nodules in CT images was proposed by Wei Y et al [58]. A method which does not require solutions of partial differential equations—and is therefore fast,—was proposed by [59]. The method uses region information to guide the evolution of initial curves. A level set method with shape model was developed. After obtaining an initial segmentation using the Chan-Vese method, parameters of the pre-segmented region are calculated to establish shape models. The region then has improved segmentation on the object with the calculated shape.

To avoid level set function irregularities during curve evolution, re-initialization is employed by periodically replacing degraded level set function with a signed distance function. However, the re-initialization procedure raises serious problems as to when and how it should be performed. In addition, re-initialization is time-consuming and thereby largely increases calculation cost. An improved region based active contour model was proposed by Lei et al. [60]. In particular, their work highlighted the following three points: (a) the distance regularized level set evolution is introduced into active contour model to partition the difference image into changed and unchanged regions, respectively. The added distance regularization term makes the derived level set function have a unique forward and backward diffusion effect to maintain a desired shape of the level set function; (b) compared with the traditional Chan-Vese model, the proposed method eliminates the need of re-initialization procedure, which avoids numerical errors caused by the re-initialization procedure and greatly speeds up the curve evolution; (c) the proposed method exploits both region and edge gradient information for partitioning the difference image into changed and unchanged regions, which can detect the small holes and discontinuous boundary of the changed region.

5.11 Statistical Region Based Level Set Method

The statistical region based level set method was used by [61], where the contour is not evolved by fitting to local gradient information (as in the Snakes) but rather by fitting statistical models to intensity, color, texture, or motion within each of the separated regions. The respective cost functionals tend to have less local minima for most realistic images. As a consequence, the segmentation schemes are far less sensitive to noise and to varying initialization. To avoid the drawbacks faced with traditional statistical distances, the authors in [62] propose to use the Wasserstein distance. In their formulation, the distribution estimated from patches, but does not take into account the explicit dependence of the Wasserstein distance to the region. The Wasserstein distance originates from the theory of optimal transport [63]. It defines a natural metric between probability distributions, that takes into account the relative distance between the different modes. In the case of unimodal distributions, this distance reduces to the distance between the modes, thus enabling a precise discrimination of the features. This Wasserstein distance have found a wide range of applications such as the comparison of histogram features for image retrieval [64], [65] and color transfer [66]. Xie et al. implemented Radial Basis Function RBF level set method in a new region based active contour model. Its external force field is derived through statistical modeling of color pixels in multiscale and treats the color image in full 3D, without channel separation or decomposition, in order to simultaneously capture spatial and spectral interactions. It also has the potential to model multi-band data with more than three channels. Additionally, they showed that it is convenient for the proposed RBF based level set method to extend from the 2D image domain to 3D space; i.e., extension from active contours to active surfaces [67].

The common goal of region based level set approaches is to identify boundaries such that the color, texture, dynamic texture, or motion in each of the separated regions is optimally approximated by simple statistical models. Given a set of features or measurements f(x) at each image location, minimization of the respective cost functionals leads to an estimation of a boundary C. Depending on the chosen segmentation criterion, the features f may be the pixel colors, the local structure tensors or the spatio-temporal intensity gradients, while the parameter vectors $\{\theta i\}$ model distributions of intensity, color, texture, or motion. Region based active contour models employ the image statistical information inside and outside the contour to construct the constraints derived from the image data to control the whole evolution process. Compared with the edge based models, region based models have the following advantages in terms of the initial contour localization and the boundary antileakage and antinoise capability. First, region based models have more freedom for the initialization of the contour and the exterior and interior contours can be detected simultaneously. Second, they are significantly less sensitive to noise and can efficiently segment the images with weak edges or even without edges. One of the most popular region based models is the C-V model, which has been widely applied to binary phase segmentation [68] with the assumption that images only have two regions and each region is completely homogeneous. However, the C-V model fails to segment the images with intensity inhomogeneity.

Energy minimization leads to a gradient descent evolution of the embedding function interlaced with an update of the parameter vectors {θi} modeling the statistical distributions in the separated regions. These region based approaches are quite robust to noise and to varying initialization, making them well-suited for local optimization methods such as the level set method.

5.12 Segmentation Using on Graph Cut Method

The authors of [69] performed the pre-processing step using a bias correction operation around the ONH and the segmentation step includes kernel graph cuts and continuous max-flow algorithms. The method proved to be flexible, accurate, robust, and fast, leading to successful segmentation results of the three main retinal layers boundaries used to assess and monitor retinal diseases.

An effective segmentation algorithm was designed by [70] which is capable of segmenting total retina and retinal pigment epithelium (RPE) drusen complex (RPEDC). The algorithm segments all drusen types, including soft drusen, cuticular drusen, and subretinal drusenoid deposits. Their work of automated segmentation included downsampling the image, separation of layers, and flattening by convex hull followed by the active graph search method to find the shortest path.

Convex hull or convex envelope of a set X of points in the Euclidean plane or in a Euclidean space (or, more generally, in an affine space over the reals) is the smallest convex set that contains X. For instance, when X is a bounded subset of the plane, the convex hull may be visualized as the shape enclosed by a rubber band stretched around X [71]. Formally, the convex hull may be defined as the intersection of all convex sets containing X or as the set of all convex combinations of points in X. With the latter definition, convex hulls may be extended from Euclidean spaces to arbitrary real vector spaces; they may also be generalized further, to oriented matroids [72], the algorithmic problem of finding the convex hull of a finite set of points in the plane or other low dimensional Euclidean spaces is one of the fundamental problems of computational geometry.

In the work done by Yazdanpanah et al. (2011) [28], they used Active Contours without Edge with Shape constraint and contextual Weights (ACWOE–SW). ACWOE–SW detects the six interfaces of the five retinal layers properly, highlighting the performance of this method on the images with intensity inhomogeneity. Even very thin layers such as INL and OPL, which are difficult to distinguish visually, are segmented by this active contour approach.

Layer segmentation of thick retinal layers, such as the IPL and the outer nuclear layer (ONL) in OCT tomograms, is fairly straightforward when the images are acquired in healthy retinas that are characterized with well defined, parallel layers. However, diseased retinas contain a variety of morphological features such as macular holes, detachments, drusen, etc. that vary in size, shape, and image contrast and interrupt the regular layered structure of the retina. To test the capability of the proposed algorithm to properly segment retinal layers in diseased retinas, the authors have tested the code on OCT images acquired from rat retinas with drug-induced photoreceptor degeneration [73].

In SDOCT images, retinal layers are primarily horizontal structures distinguishable by a change in pixel intensity in the vertical direction. Weights can therefore be calculated solely based on intensity gradients as follows:

$$W_{ab} = 2 - g_a + g_b + W_{min} \tag{5.27}$$

W_{ab} is the weight assigned to the edge connecting nodes a and b, g_a is the vertical gradient of the image at node a, g_b is the vertical gradient of the image at node b, W_{min} is the minimum weight in the graph, a small positive number added for system stabilization. Eq. (5.27) assigns low weight values to node pairs with large vertical gradients. In our implementation, g_a and g_b are normalized to values between 0 and 1, and $W_{min} = 1 \times 10{-}5$. These weights are further adjusted to account for the directionality of the gradient. To segment the vitreous-NFL layer boundary, for example, it is known that the boundary exhibits a darker layer above a brighter layer [74]. In contrast, the NFL-GCL layer boundary has a light-to-dark layer change. As a result, edge maps such as [1;-1] and [-1;1] can be utilized when calculating the gradient to extract the appropriate layers. Finally, for automatic endpoint initialization the end columns are duplicated and added to either [47].

Several potentially blinding eye diseases, such as age-related macular degeneration and glaucoma, cause structural changes in the retina and the choroid. Successful quantitative evaluation of these changes requires a segmentation based determination of the thicknesses of tissue layers. For glaucoma patients, one of the most important layers that could be identified is the Ganglion cell layer. Thus, it is of paramount importance that imaging devices used for detecting glaucoma-related structural changes in the retina be able to identify this layer and measure its thickness. The results of the present study indicate that the Cirrus GCA segmentation algorithm allows identification of macular intraretinal layers and measurement of GCIPL thickness parameters with excellent reproducibility.

In the recent work by [75], which employed geodesic distance method (GDM), they could detect variations in both the directions by making use of both horizontal and vertical gradient information. GDM can highlight weak and low contrast boundaries. They were able to segment complex retinal structures with large curvatures and other irregularities caused by pathologies.

5.13 Segmentation Based on Diffusion Maps

In the work done by [76] in 2013, diffusion maps were used to construct input data points. They aggregated a group of pixels/voxels together to form a node. They had selected 10 × 10 × 10 pixel cubes as graph nodes of the first diffusion map and very thin horizontal cubic boxes (15 × 1 pixels) are used as graph nodes of the second diffusion map. A distance function is defined by matrices with a size of N × N, where N is the number of input points (nodes of the graph). To form the geometric distance, each element of the matrix is calculated as the Euclidean distance $\|X_{(i)} - X_{(j)}\|_2$. In the next step they calculated the eigen-functions of the symmetric matrix. Preceding this k-means clustering is applied on diffusion coordinates and the algorithm is iterated many times to select the clustering result for minimization of distortion. The corresponding input data points with respect to the clustered diffusion coordinates are recovered and then the graph partitioning is replaced with an image segmentation task.

5.14 Segmentation Based on Machine Learning

A supervised method, based on Extreme Learning Machine (ELM) [77], [78] is also used to segment retinal vessel. In this work a set of 39-D discriminative feature vectors, consisting of local features, morphological features phase congruency, Hessian and divergence of vector fields are extracted for each pixel of the fundus image. Then, a matrix is constructed for pixel of the training set based on the feature vector and the manual labels and acts as the input of the ELM classifier. The output of classifier is the binary retinal vascular segmentation. Finally, they implemented an optimization processing to remove the region less than 30 pixels which is isolated from the retinal vasculature. They claim that their proposed method is much faster than the other methods in segmenting the retinal vessels and have stated that the average accuracy, sensitivity, and specificity are 0.9607, 0.7140 and 0.9868 respectively. ELMs are feed forward neural network for classification or regression with a single layer of hidden nodes, where the weights connecting inputs to hidden nodes are randomly assigned and never updated. The weights between hidden nodes and outputs are learned in a single step, which essentially amounts to learning a linear model. The name "extreme learning machine" (ELM) was given to such models by [79]. According to their creators, these models are able to produce good generalization performance and learn thousands of times faster than networks trained using back propagation.

5.15 Kernel Regression Based Classifier Training

In the work by [80] Kernel regression (KR) based segmentation is used to identify fluid filled regions and seven retinal layers on spectral domain optical coherence tomography images of eyes with diabetic macular edema (DME). Classification based graph theory and dynamic programming (GTDP) segmentation includes embedded denoising which is advantageous for reducing the noise present within the classification feature vectors. While many different denoising methods may be also used to reduce the noise, the exciting properties of KR include its direct estimation of the denoised first and second order derivatives ($\beta 1$ and $\beta 2$), as well as the generation of locally weighted kernels which can be used directly as features or reused for non-linear feature denoising. A limitation of KR is the dependence of parameter values on the image noise level. Thus, in order to optimally denoise images of varying scan types, future versions of the algorithm should adapt the KR parameter values based on the estimated noise level.

Pattern recognition based techniques perform layer segmentation by using boundary classifier, which is used to classify each voxel either as a layer boundary or a non boundary. The classifier is trained through a learning process by using reference layer boundaries. Fuller et al. [81] designed multi-resolution hierarchical support vector machines (SVMs) to segment OCT retinal layer. However, the performance of this algorithm is not good enough. It has 6 pixels of line difference and 8% of the thickness difference. Lang et al. [82] trained a random forest classifier to segment retinal layers from macular images. However, the performance of the pattern recognition based techniques are highly dependent on training sets.

Graph based methods find the global minimum cut of the segmentation graph, which is constructed with a regional term and a boundary term. Garvin [83] proposed a 3D graph search method by constructing a geometric graph with edge and regional information. Five intraretinal layers were successfully segmented. This method was extended in [80], which combined graph theory and dynamic programming to segment the intraretinal layers.

Eight retinal layer boundaries were located. Although these methods provide good segmentation accuracy, they cannot segment all layer boundaries simultaneously and the processing speed is relatively slow. [84] proposed a parallel graph search method to overcome these limitations. Kafieh et al., [85] proposed coarse grained diffusion maps relying on regional image texture without requiring edge based image information. Ten layers were segmented accurately. However, this method has high computational complexity and cannot work well for abnormal images.

5.16 Geodesic Active Contours (GAC)

The geodesic active contour is a boundary based segmentation model whose basic idea is to find a minimum length curve measured in a Riemannian space induced from the image. Let Γ be a closed curve in $\Omega \subset R2$. Associated with Γ, we define a φ as a signed distance function by:

$$\emptyset(x) = \begin{cases} distance\ (x, \Gamma),\ \mathrm{x} \in \text{interior of } \Gamma \\ -distance\ (x, \Gamma),\ \mathrm{x} \in \text{exterior of } \Gamma \end{cases} \tag{5.28}$$

The major step in variational method based image segmentation was the Geodesic active contour proposed simultaneously by Caselles et al. (1995; 1997) [86], [87] and Yezzi et al. [88], and Kichenassamy et al. [89]. In this work, it is shown that a special case of the Snakes model can be interpreted as finding geodesics (locally shortestpaths) in a space with a metric derived by image content is formalism provides an analogue between segmentation using active contours and minimal distance (geodesic) computations. The GAC model requires careful good initialization [90]. Formally, the energy to be minimized has the following form:

$$E_{GAC}[C(s)] = \int_0^{L(C)} g(|\nabla I C(s)|) ds \tag{5.29}$$

where L(C) is the length of C. We can note that choosing g = 1 gives the length of the curve C(s), so minimizing Eq. (5.29) gives a minimal curve where the length of the curve is weighted by the function $g(|\nabla I|)$. The procedure for finding an optimal solution is to evolve the curve in the steepest direction (gradient) of the energy which is given by the first variation of E_{GAC} [91]

$$\frac{\partial E_{GAC}}{\partial C} = (\kappa g + \nabla g.n)n \tag{5.30}$$

where κ is the curvature and n is the outward curve normal. To find a minimum solution to Eq. (5.30) above, the curve C can then be evolved in the negative direction of Eq. (5.31)

$$\frac{\partial C}{\partial t} = -\frac{\partial E_{GAC}}{\partial C} = -((\kappa g + \nabla g.n)n) \tag{5.31}$$

To avoid the problems with parametric curves (e.g. difficult handling of topology changes), it is practical to perform this curve evolution using an implicit (level set) representation. Eq. (5.31) specifies what we need: Here, the motion of C corresponds to $d\alpha/dt$ which is combined with $n = \nabla\phi/|\nabla\phi|$, gives Eq. (5.32):

$$\frac{\partial \emptyset}{\partial t} = (\kappa g + \nabla g.n)|\nabla \emptyset| \tag{5.32}$$

which corresponds to the gradient of the energy E_{GAC} with respect to the curve represented as the zero level set of ϕ. Comparing Eq. (5.32) with the geometrically motivated active contour we see that the "balloon term" has been replaced by a term involving the gradient g. The effect of this is an "advection" (transportation) of the curve by the gradient of g, which pulls the curve to stationary points of g (i.e. edges), we could generally expect a more robust convergence behavior than with Eq. (5.29). Moreover, being derived from an energy formulation, the geodesic active contour model enjoys a more rigorous mathematical framework. In the derivation of the curve evolution above they included the notion of gradient of the energy. However, the standard derivations in literature have generally lacked a proper definition of gradient by omitting the definition of an inner product on the "manifold of curves". This inner product has been investigated in work by Yezzi and Mennucci [92] and Solem and Overgaard [93]. They had proposed to use a Sobolev-type inner product which tends to avoid local optima solutions of the energy. Although the model works well with finding the blood vessels, it does crucially depend on the choice of the seeds placed for the initialization of the level set. To overcome this disadvantage an Infinite Perimeter Active Contour (IPAC) Model was proposed for the segmentation of objects with irregular boundaries [94].

$$F^{IPAC}(\Gamma, C_1, C_2 = L^2(\gamma - \Gamma) + \lambda_1 \int_{inside\,(\Gamma)} |\mu_0(x) - c_1|^2\,dx$$
$$+ \lambda_2 \int_{outside\,(\Gamma)} |\mu_0(x) - c_2|^2\,dx \tag{5.33}$$

where is L^2 the 2D Lebesgue measure of the -neighborhood of the edge set and λ_1 and λ_2 and are fitting term parameters.

5.17 Ribbon of Twins (ROT)

The Ribbon of Twins is an active contour based model to segment retinal vessels [95]. Each ROT contains four linked active contours, $v_c(s,t) = (x_c(s,t), y_c(s,t))$, $c \in \{-2, -1, 1, 2\}$, where x and y are coordinate functions of the parameter $s \in [0, 1]$, and t is time. There are two contours inside the vessel, that move outwards toward the internal side of the edges (v±1) and are linked together to maintain vessel width consistency (the "ribbon"); and two located outside the edges and moving towards internal contours (v±2), so that each edge is sandwiched within a "twin" of external and internal contours. The energy of the four contours are defined as

$$E_c(t) = \int_0^1 \left(E_c^{int}(v_c(s,t)) + E_c^{pho}(v_c(s,t)) + E_c^{rot}(v_c(s,t))\right)ds \tag{5.34}$$

where E_c^{int}, E_c^{pho}, E_c^{rot} are the internal, photometric and ROT model energy functions respectively. The combination of the twin convergence criteria, with an "escape procedure" to deal with photometric distractions, and the edge direction criterion, makes the ROT very effective at locating vessels even in noisy and difficult situations, while also being able to detect the absence of the vessel. Segmentation based on gradient descent with momentum was proposed by Lathen et al. [96].

Because of the intensity inhomogeneity of the difference image due to the hemorrhages, exudates and neovascularisation, it is difficult to use one single Gaussian to model the blood vessels and one single Gaussian to model the background. Therefore, a Gaussian mixture model is used to accurately estimate blood vessels. Automatic Choroidal Layer Segmentation Using Markov Random Field and Level Set Method was carried out by Chuang Wang et al. [97]. The region based term, incorporating the neighbouring pixel information with the single pixel log-likelihood function by using the Markov Random Field, is modeled into the level set method; The Gaussian Mixture Model is constructed and updated at each level set iteration, instead of learned offline from a fixed training set; and Finally, the Gaussian Vector Field method is used to estimate more comprehensive narrowband around the zero level set to increase the speed of the segmentation. The energy functional of this segmentation model is formulated as:

$$E(\varphi) = E_M(\varphi) + E_E(\varphi) + E_R(\varphi) \tag{5.35}$$

The first term E_M is a region based term, which the Markov Random Field method is used to incorporate the neighbouring pixels with the single pixel likelihood function to smooth and tighten the choroidal boundary and to avoid leakages from the boundary. The second term E_E incorporates the edge information to direct the initial contour to the boundary. Although the edge between the choroid and sclera is indistinct or even invisible at some locations, the edge information is still important in guiding the contour to the desired boundary. Therefore, they incorporated the edge based information to assist the segmentation. The Geodesic Active Contour model (GAC), based edge term has its regularization effect. However for this particular problem the edge information of the data is not clear and the shapes are irregular so the distance regularization term is necessary to smooth the boundary and avoid small contours.The last term E_R is a distance regularisation term, which keeps the choroidal layer boundary smooth.

5.18 Simple Linear Iterative Clustering

In this work by [98] Superpixel segmentation is designed to generate a coherent grouping of pixels that contain similar grayscale and spatial information. In this the authors have proposed an boundary segmentation framework for retinal OCT images and volumes. This SLIC (Simple Linear Iterative Clustering) algorithm is used to segment internal layer boundaries, since it produces super pixels at a low computational cost while achieving accurate segmentation. The SLIC superpixels, and the modified active contour, segment the remaining boundaries in a sequential order. This proposed adaptive-curve detection method searches the retinal region with boundary evolution. The SLIC superpixels, and the modified active contour, segment the remaining boundaries in a sequential order. By combining superpixels and active contour methods, cell layers can be reliably segmented from low contrast B-scans containing strong speckle noise. In low contrast regions, the super pixels can group local pixels according to contrast in A-scans. Also, the active contour balances contour shape and gradient information to reduce the influence of blood vessels and their shadows.

5.19 Conclusion

As glaucoma and diabetic retinopathy are more prevalent among the Indian population, retinal image analysis is crucial at the current time. The various level set segmentation techniques and their application to OCT retinal image analysis have been discussed in detail in this chapter. Manual image analysis is a time consuming task, but automated segmentation methods can help medical professionals to reduce diagnosis time. Level set methods have been the focus for the past two decades because of their promising results. The major advantages of the method include its robustness to noisy conditions, its ability in extracting curved objects with complex topology, and its neat numerical framework. Despite their success, these methods have to address the following limitations. First and foremost is the need for computation time to be reduced for viability in clinical application and the next is the robustness to variation in image quality needs to be studied.

References

1. Abramoff, M. D., Garvin, M. K., & Sonka, M. (2010). Retinal imaging and image analysis. *IEEE Reviews in Biomedical Engineering*, 3, 169–208.

2. Padmasini, N., Umamaheswari, R., & Sikkandar, M. Y. (2018). State-of-the-Art of Level-Set Methods in Segmentation and Registration of Spectral Domain Optical Coherence Tomographic Retinal Images. In *Soft Computing Based Medical Image Analysis*. Chapter: 10 Publisher: Academic Press pp. 163 –181.
3. Tsantis, S., Dimitropoulos, N., Ioannidou, M., Cavouras, D., & Nikiforidis, G. (2007). Inter-scale wavelet analysis for speckle reduction in thyroid ultrasound images. *Computerized Medical Imaging and Graphics, 31*(3), 117–127.
4. Hitesh H. Vandra & Pandya, H.N. (2010). Comparative analysis on Speckle noise reduction techniques on computed tomographic images. *Oriental Journal of Computer Science & Technology*, 3(2), 261–264.
5. Schmitt, J. M., Xiang, S. H., & Yung, K. M. (1999). Speckle in optical coherence tomography. *Journal of Biomedical Optics*, 4(1), 95–105.
6. Padmasini, N., Abbirame, K. S., Yacin, S. M., & Umamaheswari, R. (2014, November). Speckle noise reduction in spectral domain optical coherence tomography retinal images using anisotropic diffusion filtering. *2014 IEEE International Conference* In *Science Engineering and Management Research (ICSEMR)*, (pp. 1–5).
7. Fu, K. S., & Mui, J. K. (1981). A survey on image segmentation. *Pattern Recognition*, 13(1), 3–16.
8. Pavlidis, T. (2012). *Algorithms for graphics and image processing*, Springer Science & Business Media.
9. Bankhead, P., McGowan, J., & Curtis, T. (2009). "Fast retinal vessel detection and measurement using wavelets and edge location refinement", *PLoS ONE*, 7, p. e32435.
10. Rossant, F., Badellino, M., Chavillon, A., Bloch, I., & Paques, M. (2011). A morphological approach for vessel segmentation in eye fundus images, with quantitative evaluation. *J. Med. Imag. Health. Inf.*, 1, 42–49.
11. Al-Diri, B., Hunter, A., & Steel, D. (2009, September). An active contour model for segmenting and measuring retinal vessels. *IEEE Trans. Med. Imag.*, 28(9), 1488–1497.
12. B. Dizdaroglu et al. (2012). Level sets for retinal vasculature segmentation using seeds from ridges and edges from phase maps, in *Proc. IEEE Int. Workshop Mach. Learn. Signal Process*, 1–6.
13. Osher S., & Sethian, J.A. (1988). Fronts propagating with curvature-dependent speed: algorithms based on Hamilton–Jacobi formulation. *Journal of Computational Physics*, 79(1):12–49.
14. Mumford, D., & Shah, J. (1989), Optimal approximations by piecewise smooth functions and associated variational problems. Communications on pure and applied mathematics, 42(5), 577–685.
15. Sethian, J.A. *Level set methods and fast marching methods*, Cambridge University Press, 1996.
16. Malladi, R., & Sethian, J. A. (1995). Image processing via level set curvature flow. *Proceedings of the National Academy of Sciences*, 92(15), 7046–7050.
17. Kass, M., Witkin, A., & Terzopoulos, D. (1988). Snakes: Active contour models. *International Journal of Computer Vision*, 1:321–331.
18. Precioso, F., Barlaud, M., Blu, T., & Unser, M. (2005). Robust real-time segmentation of images and videos using a smooth-spline snake-based algorithm. *IEEE Transactions on Image Processing*, 14(7):910–924.

19. Osher, S., & Sethian, J.A. (1988). Fronts propagating with curvature-dependent speed: algorithms based on Hamilton-Jacobi formulations. *Journal of Computational Physics*, 79(1):12–49.
20. Caselles, V., Kimmel, R., & Sapiro, G. (1997). Geodesic Active Contours. *International Journal of Computer Vision*, 22(1):61–79.
21. Chan, T. F., & Vese, L.A. (2001). Active contours without edges. IEEE Transactions on Image Processing, 10(2):266–277.
22. Kass, M., Witkin, A., & Terzopoulos, D. (1988). Snakes: active contour models. *Int. J. Comput. Vis.*, 1 (4), 321–331.
23. Osher, S., & Fedkiw, R. (2006). Level set methods and dynamic implicit surfaces (Vol. 153). Springer Science & Business Media.
24. Li, C., Xu, C., Gui, C., & Fox, M. D. (2005, June). Level set evolution without re-initialization: a new variational formulation. In *Computer Vision and Pattern Recognition*, 2005. CVPR 2005. IEEE Computer Society Conference ,Vol. 1, pp. 430–436.
25. Cremers, D., Rousson, M., & Deriche, R. (2007). A review of statistical approaches to level set segmentation: integrating color, texture, motion and shape. *International Journal of Computer Vision*, 72(2), 195–215.
26. Kass, M., Witkin, A., & Terzopoulos, D. (1987, June), Snakes: Active contour models. In *Proc. 1st Int. Conf. on Computer Vision* (Vol. 259, p. 268).
27. Zhu, C., Zou, B., Zhao, R., Cui, J., Duan, X., Chen, Z., & Liang, Y. (2017). Retinal vessel segmentation in colour fundus images using Extreme Learning Machine. Computerized Medical Imaging and Graphics, 55, 68–77.
28. Yazdanpanah, A., Hamarneh, G., Smith, B.R., & Sarunic, M.V. (2011). Segmentation of intra-retinal layers from optical coherence tomography images using an active contour approach. *IEEE Trans. Med. Imaging*, 30(2), 484–496.
29. Vermeer, K. A., Van der Schoot, J., Lemij, H. G., & De Boer, J. F. (2011). Automated segmentation by pixel classification of retinal layers in ophthalmic OCT images. *Biomedical optics express*, 2(6), 1743–1756.
30. Crandall, M.G., Ishii, H., & Lions, P.-L. (1992). User's guide to viscosity solutions of second order partial differential equations. *Bull. Amer. Math. Soc.* (N.S.), 27(1):1–67.
31. Luminita A.V. & Chan, T.F. (2002). A new multiphase level set framework for image segmentation via the Mumford and Shah model. *International Journal of Computer Vision*, 50(3):271–293.
32. Novosel, J., Vermeer, K. A., Thepass, G., Lemij, H. G., & Van Vliet, L. J. (2013, April). Loosely coupled level sets for retinal layer segmentation in optical coherence tomography. In *Biomedical Imaging (ISBI), 2013 IEEE 10th International Symposium on* (pp. 1010–1013). IEEE.
33. Mitiche, A., & Ayed, I. B. (2010). *Variational and level set methods in image segmentation* (Vol. 5). Springer Science & Business Media.
34. Novosel, J., Wang, Z., de Jong, H., van Velthoven, M., Vermeer, K. A., & van Vliet, L. J. (2016, April). Locally-adaptive loosely-coupled level sets for retinal layer and fluid segmentation in subjects with central serous retinopathy. In *Biomedical Imaging (ISBI), 2016 IEEE 13th International Symposium on* (pp. 702–705). IEEE.
35. Novosel, J. et al. (2015). Loosely coupled level sets for simultaneous 3d retinal layer segmentation in optical coherence tomography. *Med. Image Anal.*, 26, 146–158.
36. Vermeer, K.A. et al. (2014). Depth-resolved model-based reconstruction of attenuation coefficients in optical coherence tomography. *Biomed. Opt. Express*, 322–337.

37. Droske, M., Meyer, B., Rumpf, M., & Schaller, C. (2001, June). An adaptive level set method for medical image segmentation. In *Biennial International Conference on Information Processing in Medical Imaging* (pp. 416–422). Springer, Berlin, Heidelberg.
38. Zhao, Y. Q., Wang, X. H., Wang, X. F., & Shih, F. Y. (2014). Retinal vessels segmentation based on level set and region growing. *Pattern Recognition*, 47(7), 2437–2446.
39. Chunming Li (Li, C., Xu, C., Gui, C., & Fox, M. D. (2010). Distance regularized level set evolution and its application to image segmentation. *IEEE transactions on image processing*, 19(12), 3243–3254.
40. Zhao, Y., Rada, L., Chen, K., Harding, S. P., & Zheng, Y. (2015). Automated vessel segmentation using infinite perimeter active contour model with hybrid region information with application to retinal images. *IEEE Transactions on Medical Imaging*, 34(9), 1797–1807.
41. Zhang, Y., Matuszewski, B. J., Shark, L. K., & Moore, C. J. (2008, July). Medical image segmentation using new hybrid level-set method. In *BioMedical Visualization, 2008. MEDIVIS'08. Fifth International Conference* (pp. 71–76). IEEE.
42. Paragios, N., & Deriche, R. (2000, June). Coupled geodesic active regions for image segmentation: A level set approach. In *European Conference on Computer Vision* (pp. 224–240). Springer, Berlin, Heidelberg.
43. Wu, H., Geng, X., Zhang, X., Qiu, M., Jiang, K., Tang, L., & Dong, J. (2014). A self-adaptive distance regularized level set evolution method for optical disk segmentation. *Bio-medical Materials and Engineering*, 24(6), 3199–3206.
44. K. Zhang, L. Zhang, H. Song, and W. Zhou. (2010). Active contours with selective local or global segmentation: a new formulation and level set method. *Image and Vision Computing*, 28(4), 668–676.
45. Li, C., Kao, C.-Y., Gore, J.C., & Ding, Z. (2007). Implicit active contours driven by local binary fitting energy. In Proceedings of the IEEE Computer Society Conference on Computer Vision and Pattern Recognition (CVPR '07), Minneapolis, Minn, USA, June 2007.
46. Chen, G., Chen, M., Li, J., & Zhang, E. (2017). Retina image vessel segmentation using a hybrid CGLI level set method. *BioMed Research International*, 2017.
47. Chiu, S.J., Lokhnygina,Y., Dubis, A.M., Dubra, A., Carroll, J., Izatt, J.A., & Farsiu, S. (2013). Automatic cone photoreceptor segmentation using graph theory and dynamic programming. *Biomed. Opt. Express*, 4 (2013) 924–937.
48. Shi, F., Chen, X., Zhao, H., Zhu,W., Xiang, D., Gao, E., & Chen, H. (2015). Automated 3-D retinal layer segmentation of macular optical coherence tomography images with serous pigment epithelial detachments. *IEEE Trans. Med. Imaging*, 34 (2), 441–452.
49. Uji, A., Murakami, T., Unoki, N., Ogino, K., Horii, T., Yoshitake, S., & Yoshimura, N. (2014). Parallelism for quantitative image analysis of photoreceptor–retinal pigment epithelium complex alterations in diabetic macular edema parallelism in DME. *Invest. Ophthalmol. Vis. Sci.*, 55 (5), 3361–3367.
50. Wang,B., Zhang, Q., Lu, R., Zhi, Y. & Yao, X. (2014). Functional optical coherence tomography reveals transient phototropic change of photoreceptor outer segments. *Opt. Lett.*, 39 (24), 6923–6926.
51. Peng, D., Merriman, B., Osher, S., Zhao, H., & Kang, M. (1999). A PDE-based fast local level set method. *Journal of Computational Physics*, 155(2), 410–438.
52. Jia, Y., Bailey, S. T., Wilson, D. J., Tan, O., Klein, M. L., Flaxel, C. J., & Fujimoto, J. G. (2014). Quantitative optical coherence tomography angiography of choroida

neovascularization in age-related macular degeneration. *Ophthalmology*, 121(7), 1435–1444.
53. Hu, Z., Medioni, G.G., Hernandez, M., Hariri, A., Wu, X., & Sadda, S.R. (2013). Segmentation of the geographic atrophy in spectral-domain optical coherence tomography and fundus autofluorescence images geographic atrophy segmentation in SD-OCT and FAF images. *Invest. Ophthalmol. Vis. Sci.*, 54 (13), 8375–8383.
54. Chan, T. F., Sandberg, B. Y., & Vese, L. A. (2000). Active contours without edges for vector-valued images. *Journal of Visual Communication and Image Representation*, 11(2), 130–141.
55. Mohammad, F., Ansari, R., Wanek, J., Francis, A., & Shahidi, M. (2015). Feasibility of level-set analysis of enface OCT retinal images in diabetic retinopathy, *Biomed. Opt. Express*, 6(5), 1904–1918.
56. Al-Qunaieer, F. S., Tizhoosh, H. R., & Rahnamayan, S. (2011). Multi-resolution level set image segmentation using wavelets, *18th IEEE International Conference in Image Processing (ICIP)* (pp. 269–272).
57. He, L., Peng, Z., Everding, B., Wang, X., Han, C. Y., Weiss, K. L., & Wee, W. G. (2008). A comparative study of deformable contour methods on medical image segmentation, *Image and Vision Computing*, 26(2), 141–163.
58. Wei, Y., Xu, X. H., Jia, T., & Zhao, D. Z. (2006, October). An optimal level sets method for lung nodules detection in ct images. In *Intelligent Systems Design and Applications, 2006. ISDA'06. Sixth International Conference on* (Vol. 2, pp. 251–255). IEEE.
59. Pan, S., & Dawant, B.M. (2001). Automatic 3D segmentation of the liver from abdominal CT images: a level-set approach. In *Medical Imaging 2001, International Society for Optics and Photonics*, 2001, pp. 128–138.
60. Lei, Y., Shi, J., & Wu, J. (2017). Region-driven distance regularized level set evolution for change detection in remote sensing images. *Multimedia Tools and Applications*, 76(23), 24707–24722.
61. Rousson, M., & Deriche, R. (2002, December), A variational framework for active and adaptative segmentation of vector valued images. In *Motion and Video Computing, 2002. proceedings. workshop on* (pp. 56–61). IEEE.
62. K. Ni, X. Bresson, T. Chan, and S. Esedoglu. Local histogram based segmentation using the wasserstein distance August 2009, *International Journal of Computer Vision*, 84, 97–111.
63. Villani, C. (2003). Topics in optimal transportation (No. 58). American Mathematical Society.
64. Rabin, J., Delon, J., & Gousseau, Y. (2009). A statistical approach to the matching of local features. *SIAM Journal on Imaging Sciences*, 2(3), 931–958.
65. Delon, J. (2004). Midway image equalization. *Journal of Mathematical Imaging and Vision*, 21(2), 119–134.
66. Rabin, J., Peyré, G., Delon, J., & Bernot, M. (2011, May). Wasserstein barycenter and its application to texture mixing. In International *Conference on Scale Space and Variational Methods in Computer Vision* (pp. 435–446). Springer, Berlin, Heidelberg.
67. Xie, X., & Mirmehdi, M. (2011). Radial basis function based level set interpolation and evolution for deformable modelling. *Image and Vision Computing*, *29*(2-3), 167–177.
68. Li, C., Kao, C. Y., Gore, J. C., & Ding, Z. (2007). Implicit active contours driven by local binary fitting energy. Presented at the Comput. Vis. Pattern Recog.

69. Kaba, D., Wang, Y., Wang, C., Liu, X., Zhu, H., Salazar-Gonzalez, A.G., & Li, Y. (2015). Retina layer segmentation using kernel graph cuts and continuous maxflow, *Opt. Express*, 23 (6), 7366–7384.
70. Farsiu, S., Chiu, S. J., O'Connell, R. V., Folgar, F. A., Yuan, E., Izatt, J. A., & Toth, C. A. (2014). Quantitative classification of eyes with and without intermediate age-related macular degeneration using optical coherence tomography. *Ophthalmology*, 121(1), 162–172.
71. A.M. Andrew, Another efficient algorithm for convex hulls in two dimensions, *Inf. Process. Lett.*, 9 (5), (1979) 216–219.
72. Brown, K.Q. (1979). Voronoi diagrams from convex hulls, *Inf. Process. Lett.*, 9(5), 223–228, https://doi.org/10.1016/0020-0190(79)90074-7.
73. Mishra, A., Wong, A., Bizheva, K., & Clausi, D. A. (2009). Intra-retinal layer segmentation in optical coherence tomography images. *Optics Express*, 17(26), 23719–23728.
74. M.K. Garvin, M.D. Abramoff, X. Wu, S.R. Russell, T.L. Burns, & Sonka, M. (2009). Automated 3-D intraretinal layer segmentation of macular spectral domain optical coherence tomography images, *IEEE Trans. Med. Imaging*, 28 (9),1436–1447.
75. Duan, J., Tench, C., Gottlob, I., Proudlock, F., & Bai, L. (2016). Automated segmentation of retinal layers from optical coherent tomography images using geodesic distance. arXiv preprint arXiv:1609.02214.
76. Kafieh, R., Rabbani, H., Abramoff, M. D., & Sonka, M. (2013). Intra-retinal layer segmentation of 3D optical coherence tomography using coarse grained diffusion map. *Medical Image Analysis*, 17(8), 907–928.
77. G.B. Huang, Q.Y. Zhu, & Siew, C.K. (2006). Extreme learning machine: theory and applications. *Neurocomputing*, 70 (1), 489–501.
78. Shanmugam, V., & Banu, R. D. W. (2013, January). Retinal blood vessel segmentation using an extreme learning machine approach. In *Point-of-Care Healthcare Technologies (PHT), 2013 IEEE* (pp. 318–321). IEEE.
79. Yılmaz Kaya, L. K., & Tekin, R. (2013). A computer vision system for the automatic identification of butterfly species via gabor-filter-based texture features and extreme learning machine: GF+ ELM. *Tem Journal*, 13.
80. Chiu, S. J., Allingham, M. J., Mettu, P. S., Cousins, S. W., Izatt, J. A., & Farsiu, S. (2015). Kernel regression based segmentation of optical coherence tomography images with diabetic macular edema. *Biomedical Optics Express*, 6(4), 1172–1194.
81. Fuller, A., Zawadzki, R., Choi, S., Wiley, D., Werner, J., & Hamann, B. (2007). Segmentation of three-dimensional retinal image data. *IEEE Transactions on Visualization and Computer Graphics*, 13(6), 1719–1726.
82. Lang, A., Carass, A., Hauser, M., Sotirchos, E. S., Calabresi, P. A., Ying, H. S., & Prince, J. L. (2013). Retinal layer segmentation of macular OCT images using boundary classification. *Biomedical Optics Express*, 4(7), 1133–1152.
83. Garvin, M. K., Abràmoff, M. D., Kardon, R., Russell, S. R., Wu, X., & Sonka, M. (2008). Intraretinal layer segmentation of macular optical coherence tomography images using optimal 3-D graph search. *IEEE Transactions on Medical Imaging*, 27(10), 1495–1505.
84. Quellec, G., Lee, K., Dolejsi, M., Garvin, M. K., Abramoff, M. D., & Sonka, M. (2010). Three-dimensional analysis of retinal layer texture: identification of fluid-filled regions in SD-OCT of the macula. *IEEE Transactions on Medical Imaging*, 29(6), 1321–1330.

85. Kafieh, R., Rabbani, H., Hajizadeh, F., Abramoff, M. D., & Sonka, M. (2015). Thickness mapping of eleven retinal layers segmented using the diffusion maps method in normal eyes. *Journal of Ophthalmology*.
86. Caselles, V., Kimmel, R., & Sapiro, G. (1997). Geodesic active contours. In *Computer Vision, 1995. Proceedings. 5th International Conference on*, (pp. 694–699).
87. Caselles, V., Kimmel, R., & Sapiro, G. (1997, February). Geodesic active contours. *International Journal of Computer Vision*, 22(1):61–79.
88. Yezzi, A., Kichenassamy, S., Kumar, A., Olver, P., & Tannenbaum, A. (1997). A geometric snake model for segmentation of medical imagery. *IEEE Transactions on Medical Imaging*, 16(2), 199–209.
89. Kichenassamy, S., Kumar, A., Olver, P., Tannenbaum, A., & Yezzi, A. (1996). Conformal curvature flows: from phase transitions to active vision. *Archive for Rational Mechanics and Analysis*, 134(3), 275–301.
90. Läthén, G., Jonasson, J., & Borga, M. (2010). Blood vessel segmentationusing multi-scale quadrature filtering, *Pattern Recogn. Lett.*, 31, 762–767.
91. Kumar, A., Yezzi, A., Kichenassamy, S., Olver, P., & Tannenbaum, A. (1995, December). Active contours for visual tracking: a geometric gradient based approach. In *Decision and Control, 1995., Proceedings of the 34th IEEE Conference on* (Vol. 4, pp. 4041–4046). IEEE.
92. Yezzi, A. & Mennucci, A. (2005). Conformal metrics and true "gradient ž flows" for curves. *International Conference on Computer Vision*, 1, 913–919.
93. Solem, J. E., & Overgaard, N. C. (2005, April). A geometric formulation of gradient descent for variational problems with moving surfaces. In *International Conference on Scale-Space Theories in Computer Vision* (pp. 419–430). Springer, Berlin, Heidelberg.
94. M. Barchiesi, S. H. Kang, T. M. Le, M. Morini, and M. Ponsiglione, (2010). A variational model for infinite perimeter segmentations based on Lipschitz level set functions: Denoising while keeping finely oscillatory boundaries. *Multiscale Model. Sim.*, 8, 1715–1741.
95. Al-Diri, B., & Hunter, A. (2005). A ribbon of twins for extracting vessel boundaries, eprints.lincoln.ac.uk.
96. Lathen, G., Andersson, T., Lenz, R., & Borga, M. (2009, June). Momentum based optimization methods for level set segmentation. In *International Conference on Scale Space and Variational Methods in Computer Vision* (pp. 124–136). Springer, Berlin, Heidelberg.
97. Wang, C., Wang, Y. X., & Li, Y. (2017), Automatic choroidal layer segmentation using Markov random field and level set method. *IEEE journal of Biomedical and Health Informatics*, 21(6), 1694–1702.
98. Bai, F., Gibson, S. J., Marques, M. J., & Podoleanu, A. (2018, March). Superpixel guided active contour segmentation of retinal layers in OCT volumes. In *2nd Canterbury Conference on OCT with Emphasis on Broadband Optical Sources* (Vol. 10591, p. 1059106). International Society for Optics and Photonics.

6

Numerical Techniques for Level Set Models: an Image Segmentation Perspective

Elisabetta Carlini, Maurizio Falcone, and Roberto Ferretti

CONTENTS

6.1 Introduction

The level set (LS) method, proposed in the late 80s, has proven a very successful technique for the analysis of front propagation problems and has permitted the treatment of many different physical and conceptual models within the same theoretical framework. The major asset of LS methods is their capability to handle the onset of singularities and topological changes in the front.

This review is focused on Finite Difference (FD) and Semi-Lagrangian (SL) numerical techniques for LS models and will introduce the most basic concepts of LS methods. For a more extensive introduction, we refer the reader to the books by Sethian [22] and Osher–Fedkiw [20].

In the basic version of the LS method (as first proposed in [21]), the unknown evolution of a $(d-1)$-dimensional interface in a d-dimensional space is tracked via a "representation" function $u : \mathbb{R}^d \times [0,T] \to \mathbb{R}$, the position of the interface Γ_t at time t being given by the zero-level set of $u(\cdot, t)$, i.e.,

$$\Gamma_t = \{x : u(x,t) = 0\}.$$

Throughout the paper, for simplicity, we will mostly take $d = 2$ and assume that, for any $t \in [0,T]$, the curve Γ_t is closed (although it will not be assumed to be simple, nor connected), and denote by Ω_t the set enclosed, so that $\Gamma_t = \partial\Omega_t$. The initial position of the front $\Gamma_0 = \partial\Omega_0$ is described by an initial function u_0, which must satisfy

$$\begin{cases} u_0(x) < 0, & \text{for } x \in \mathbb{R}^2 \backslash \overline{\Omega}_0 \\ u_0(x) = 0 & \text{for } x \in \partial\Omega_0 \\ u_0(x) > 0 & \text{for } x \in \Omega_0. \end{cases} \tag{6.1}$$

After describing Γ_0 as the zero-level set of u_0, our plan is to describe the front Γ_t at a generic time t as the zero-level set of the solution of a Cauchy problem, having u_0 as its initial condition.

In the simplest situation, we assume that each point of Γ_0 evolves in the normal direction with velocity $c(x)$, and that the front is shrinking (a suitable change of sign would produce an expansion). A generic point $P \in \Gamma_t$ will be represented as $P = (x_1(s,t), x_2(s,t))$, where s refers to the parametric representation of Γ_t (see Figure 6.1). Since the velocity V at every point has magnitude $c(P)$ and is directed in the normal direction η, we can write

$$V(P) = (\dot{x}_1(s,t), \dot{x}_2(s,t)) = c(P)\eta(P) \tag{6.2}$$

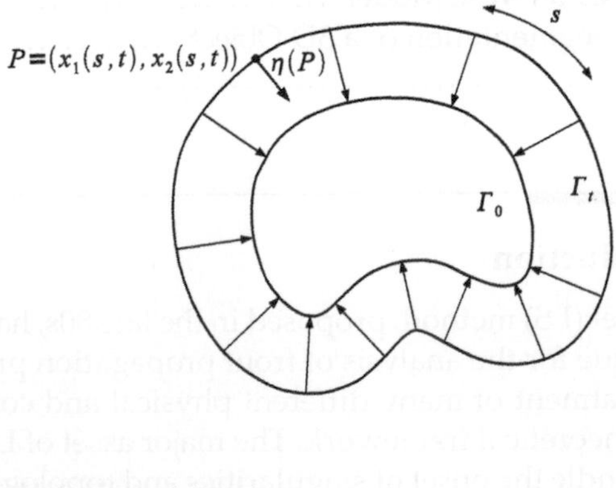

FIGURE 6.1
Propagation of a front in the normal direction.

Considering the total derivative of $u(x_1(s,t), x_2(s,t))$, and taking into account that this derivative vanishes on a level set of constant value, we have:

$$\begin{aligned}
0 &= \frac{d}{dt}u(x_1(s,t), x_2(s,t), t) \\
&= u_t(x_1(s,t), x_2(s,t)) + Du(x_1(s,t), x_2(s,t)) \cdot (\dot{x}_1, \dot{x}_2) \\
&= u_t(P) + c(P)Du(P) \cdot \eta(P) \\
&= u_t(P) + c(P)|Du(P)|,
\end{aligned}$$

where Du denotes the gradient of u, $|\cdot|$ denotes the Euclidean norm, and the normal direction to a level set of u (computed at P) has been written in terms of u as $\eta(P) = Du(P)/|Du(P)|$. In conclusion, solving the equation

$$\begin{cases} u_t + c(x)|Du| = 0 & (x,t) \in \mathbb{R}^2 \times (0,T] \\ u(x) = u_0(x) & x \in \mathbb{R}^2, \end{cases} \tag{6.3}$$

and looking at the zero-level set of the solution $u(x,t)$ we can recover the front Γ_t. Note that the choice of the zero level is arbitrary, and in fact all level sets of u are moving according to the same law.

If more general forms of the velocity are considered, then the model equation corresponding to the LS method (see, e.g., [21] for details) becomes

$$\begin{cases} u_t + c(x, Du, D^2u)|Du| = 0 & (x,t) \in \mathbb{R}^2 \times (0,T] \\ u(x) = u_0(x) & x \in \mathbb{R}^2. \end{cases} \tag{6.4}$$

In this form, the model can describe isotropic and anisotropic front propagation, Mean Curvature Motion (MCM) and other situations with velocity depending on some geometrical properties of the front. This includes the basic cases:

$c(x,t)$	isotropic motion with space-time varying velocity
$c(x,t,\eta)$	anisotropic motion, i.e., speed depending on the normal direction
$c(x,t,k)$	curvature-dependent motion

with $k = k(x,t)$ denoting the mean curvature of the front at (x,t). Among further extensions of the model, we quote the case in which the velocity is obtained by convolution (nonlocal velocity).

Analytical study of these equations has received in the last decades a great impulse from the notion of *viscosity solution*, which allows strong nonlinearities and degeneracy of the equation, as well as singularities and low smoothness of the solution. We will not enter into the theoretical details here, but an extensive overview of the related literature can be found in [14].

6.2 Basic Level Set Models and Related Numerical Techniques

We will consider in this review two basic situations in level set models: the first describes propagation of an interface with given (possibly variable) speed, and the second is curvature-driven propagation. The two cases lead respectively to a first-order and a second-order nonlinear PDE. Although the focus of this chapter is on image segmentation, we will point out the possible relevance of both models in other fields of image processing.

An explicit numerical approximation for (6.4) is in the form

$$\begin{cases} U^{n+1} = S_\Delta(U^n), & n \geq 0, \\ u_j^0 = u_0(x_j), \end{cases} \tag{6.5}$$

in which we denote by $U^n = (u_1^n, \ldots, u_N)^t$ the vector collecting all the node values $u_j^n \approx u(x_j, t_n)$ of the numerical solution at the j-th node x_j and at the n-th time step $t_n = n\Delta t$. In what follows, it can be convenient to denote by $\mathcal{I}$ the set of indices $\{1, \ldots, N\}$ of the nodes. In practice (and this is the rule when treating biomedical images), the numerical grid is typically structured and orthogonal with a constant space discretization step Δx, and the index j should be understood as a multi-index: for example, in two dimensions we set $j = (j_1, j_2)$, $\mathcal{I} = \{1, \ldots, N_1\} \times \{1, \ldots, N_2\}$, $N = N_1 N_2$ and (up to a translation) $x_j = j\Delta x$.

We point out that convergence of numerical schemes for the two models under consideration, as well as for other models satisfying a *comparison principle* (see [1], [14]) follows from the Barles–Souganidis theorem [3], under the assumption that the scheme is consistent, L^∞ stable and monotone. We refer the interested reader to [14] for an extensive discussion of the theory. Here we simply remark that consistency requires the scheme to be a "small perturbation" of the exact equation, and may take a slightly different form in the various theoretical settings. Monotonicity requires that

$$S_\Delta(V) \geq S_\Delta(W) \tag{6.6}$$

whenever $V \geq W$ elementwise. In all the schemes considered here, this property also implies L^∞ stability.

6.2.1 Eikonal Equation

This is the basic level set model, and its simplest version results from using $c(x) \equiv 1$ in the construction of the previous section, thus leading to the first order hyperbolic equation

$$\begin{cases} u_t + |Du| = 0 & (x,t) \in \mathbb{R}^2 \times [0, T] \\ u(x) = u_0(x) & x \in \mathbb{R}^2, \end{cases} \tag{6.7}$$

under which a given level set moves with constant speed in the normal direction, and describes the locus of points with increasing, constant distance from its initial position.

The well-posedness of this equation can be proved, for example, in the space of bounded and Lipschitz continuous functions. Existence, in particular, follows from the Hopf–Lax representation formula for the solution $u(x,t)$, which, in the case of (6.7), takes the form (see [14]):

$$u(x,t) = \min_{a \in B(0,1)} u_0(x - at), \tag{6.8}$$

where $B(0,1)$ denotes the unit ball of $\mathbb{R}^2$:

$$B(0,1) = \{x \in \mathbb{R}^2 : |x| \leq 1\}.$$

The representation formula (6.8) might be seen as a generalization of the classical formula of characteristics for the linear advection equation. We also point out that, in addition to level set models, the eikonal equation also appears in other image processing problems, in particular in the so-called *Shape-from-Shading* (see [12] for an in-depth presentation).

We show below the basic ingredients for the numerical approximation, in the case of Finite Difference and Semi-Lagrangian schemes, respectively.

6.2.1.1 FD Schemes

This is the most popular class of methods, which stem, in their elementary version, from finite difference schemes developed in the 60s for conservation laws. Most of the theory is constructed (see the seminal paper [11]) on the slightly more general case of a Hamilton–Jacobi equation of the form

$$u_t + H(x, Du) = 0 \tag{6.9}$$

where $H : \mathbb{R}^d \times \mathbb{R}^d \to \mathbb{R}$ is a continuous Hamiltonian, and in particular, for the case under consideration,

$$H(x, Du) = c(x)|Du|. \tag{6.10}$$

Typical FD schemes for (6.9) are set in the so-called *differenced form*, which in the simplest two-dimensional case has the structure

$$\begin{aligned} u_j^{n+1} &= S_\Delta\left(u^n_{j_1 \pm 1, j_2}, u_j^n, u^n_{j_1, j_2 \pm 1}\right)_j \\ &= u_j^n - \Delta t\, G\left(x_j, \frac{u^n_{j_1+1,j_2} - u_j^n}{\Delta x}, \frac{u_j^n - u^n_{j_1-1,j_2}}{\Delta x}, \frac{u^n_{j_1,j_2+1} - u_j^n}{\Delta x}, \frac{u_j^n - u^n_{j_1,j_2-1}}{\Delta x}\right), \end{aligned} \tag{6.11}$$

that is, in which the j-th component of the scheme S_Δ depends only on the values at x_j and at its first neighbours, and the dependence on the neighbours appears only via the partial incremental ratios. The function G is termed as *numerical Hamiltonian,* and is clearly the key ingrediant of a specific scheme.

Given the general form (6.9) with a Hamiltonian function $H(x, u_{x_1}, u_{x_2})$, consistency for schemes in differenced form can be recast as the condition

$$G(x, a, a, b, b) = H(x, a, b),$$

whereas monotonicity requires the numerical Hamiltonian G to be nondecreasing w.r.t. right incremental ratios (i.e., its second and fourth argument) and nonincreasing w.r.t. left incremental ratios (i.e., its third and fifth argument).

We provide a couple of examples of schemes in this class.

- 2D Lax-Friedrichs scheme
  This classical scheme [11] corresponds to a numerical Hamiltonian of the form

$$G^{LF}(x, a^+, a^-, b^+, b^-) := H\left(x, \frac{a^+ + a^-}{2}, \frac{b^+ + b^-}{2}\right) - \theta\frac{\Delta x}{\Delta t}((a^+ - a^-) + (b^+ - b^-)),$$

  with $0 < \theta < 1/4$. In particular, for the Hamiltonian (6.10), we would obtain the scheme

$$u_j^{n+1} = u_j^n - \Delta t\left[c(x_j)\left(\left(\frac{u^n_{j_1+1,j_2} - u^n_{j_1-1,j_2}}{2\Delta x}\right)^2 + \left(\frac{u^n_{j_1,j_2+1} - u^n_{j_1,j_2-1}}{2\Delta x}\right)^2\right)^{1/2} - \theta\frac{\Delta x}{\Delta t}\left(\frac{u^n_{j_1+1,j_2} - 2u^n_j + u^n_{j_1-1,j_2}}{\Delta x} + \frac{u^n_{j_1,j_2+1} - 2u^n_j + u^n_{j_1,j_2-1}}{\Delta x}\right)\right].$$

  The Lax–Friedrichs scheme is monotone and stable under a linear refinement law $\Delta t \sim C\Delta x$, for a sufficiently small constant C depending on the initial condition u_0. We refer to [11] for a complete study of stability.

- Osher–Sethian scheme
  This scheme has been proposed in [21], and, although especially suited for level set models, it is applicable in general to all Hamiltonians in the form

$$H(x, u_{x_1}, u_{x_2}) = f\left(x, u_{x_1}^2, u_{x_2}^2\right).$$

  In this case, and assuming for example that f is nondecreasing w.r.t. both $u_{x_1}^2$ and $u_{x_2}^2$ (as it would be the case in (6.10) for a positive speed $c(x)$), the numerical Hamiltonian is defined (see [21]) as

$$G^{OS}(x, a^+, a^-, b^+, b^-) := f\left(x, \bar{a}^2, \bar{b}^2\right),$$

with $\bar{a}^2$ and $\bar{b}^2$ given by

$$\bar{a}^2 = \begin{cases} \min(a^+,0)^2 + \max(a^-,0)^2 & \text{if } f(x,\cdot,u_{x_2}^2) \text{ is increasing} \\ \max(a^+,0)^2 + \min(a^-,0)^2 & \text{if } f(x,\cdot,u_{x_2}^2) \text{ is decreasing} \end{cases} \tag{6.12}$$

$$\bar{b}^2 = \begin{cases} \min(b^+,0)^2 + \max(b^-,0)^2 & \text{if } f(x,u_{x_1}^2,\cdot) \text{ is increasing} \\ \max(b^+,0)^2 + \min(b^-,0)^2 & \text{if } f(x,u_{x_1}^2,\cdot) \text{ is decreasing.} \end{cases} \tag{6.13}$$

In particular, for the eikonal case (6.10) under consideration, and if $c(x) > 0$, f is increasing w.r.t. both the second and the third argument, and we obtain the scheme

$$u_j^{n+1} = u_j^n - \Delta t\left[c(x_j)\left(\bar{a}_j^2 + \bar{b}_j^2\right)^{1/2}\right],$$

where

$$\bar{a}_j^2 = \min\left(\frac{u_{j_1+1,j_2}^n - u_j^n}{\Delta x}, 0\right)^2 + \max\left(\frac{u_j^n - u_{j_1-1,j_2}^n}{\Delta x}, 0\right)^2$$

$$\bar{b}_j^2 = \min\left(\frac{u_{j_1,j_2+1}^n - u_j^n}{\Delta x}, 0\right)^2 + \max\left(\frac{u_j^n - u_{j_1,j_2-1}^n}{\Delta x}, 0\right)^2,$$

while the opposite choice of $\bar{a}^2$ and $\bar{b}^2$ would be required for $c(x) < 0$ – the result is a purely upwind scheme. Stability conditions require again a linear $\Delta t/\Delta x$ relationship.

Last, we remark that monotone schemes can be at most first-order accurate. To overcome this limitation, the basic blocks of differenced schemes have been used to build *high order schemes*, which provide a more accurate and efficient approximation. We refer to [23] for an extensive review on this topic.

6.2.1.2 SL Schemes

Representation formulae like (6.8) are typically the base for the semi-Lagrangian treatment of advection terms. A SL scheme for (6.7) is obtained by discretizing the representation formula (6.8) rather than (6.7) itself. In a first stage, a time discretization step Δt is fixed, and the representation formula is written on a single time step, from $t_n = n\Delta t$ to $t_{n+1} = (n+1)\Delta t$, as

$$u(x, t_{n+1}) = \min_{a \in B(0,1)} u(x - a\Delta t, t_n). \tag{6.14}$$

Next, for $j \in \mathcal{I}$, (6.14) is computed at each node x_j:

$$u(x_j, t_{n+1}) = \min_{a \in B(0,1)} u(x_j - a\Delta t, t_n).$$

Last, since the numerical solution is represented via the values $u_j^n \approx u(x_j, t_{n+1})$, the exact computation of $u(x_j - a\Delta t, t_n)$ at the right-hand side is replaced by

$$\Pi[u^n](x_j - a\Delta t). \tag{6.15}$$

The notation in (6.15) stands for a given space reconstruction Π (e.g., an interpolation) based on the values $\{u_j^n\}_{j\in\mathcal{I}}$ and computed at the point $x_j - a\Delta t$. The scheme takes therefore the form

$$\begin{cases} u_j^{n+1} = \min\limits_{a\in B(0,1)} \Pi[u^n](x_j - a\Delta t) & j \in \mathcal{I}, n \geq 0 \\ u_j^0 = u_0(x_j) & j \in \mathcal{I}. \end{cases} \tag{6.16}$$

The basic ingredients for a specific implementation of (6.16) are therefore an interpolation operator Π and an optimization method to recover the minimum among all the values. A complete review of the various recipes is beyond the scope of this chapter, but a detailed overview can be found in [14]. The scheme is monotone as long as the space interpolation Π is monotone itself, and no stability restriction on the relationship $\Delta t/\Delta x$ is required.

Note that, in the case of the more general form (6.3), and as long as $c(x) > 0$, the scheme (6.16) is changed accordingly as

$$u_j^{n+1} = \min_{a\in B(0,1)} \Pi[u^n](x_j - ac(x_j)\Delta t), \tag{6.17}$$

whereas, if $c(x) < 0$, the min should be changed into a max. High-order versions may be constructed by increasing the order of the interpolation.

6.2.2 Mean Curvature Motion

A second typical level set model describes the Motion by Mean Curvature (MCM) and takes the form:

$$\begin{cases} u_t(x,t) - \operatorname{div}\left(\frac{Du(x,t)}{|Du(x,t)|}\right)|Du(x,t)| = 0 & (x,t) \in \mathbb{R}^2 \times (0,T], \\ u(x,0) = u_0(x) & x \in \mathbb{R}^2, \end{cases} \tag{6.18}$$

where the term in divergence form represents precisely the mean curvature of level sets, so that

$$c(x,t,k(x,t)) = -k(x,t) = -\operatorname{div}\left(\frac{Du(x,t)}{|Du(x,t)|}\right).$$

Equation (6.18) is known to have a unique continuous viscosity solution (see [10,13]).

In image processing, (6.18) provides a model in which an interface is not only shrunk, but regularized at the same time, this being a key feature in the segmentation of noisy images. In addition, MCM equation plays a role in the denoising of images. In this case, $\{u(x,t)\}_{t\geq 0}$ represents a family of successive restored versions of the initial noisy image u_0. The variable t is called *scale variable* and, as t increases, we expect $u(x,t)$ to be smoothed, and the noise removed. The model was introduced by Alvarez, Lions and Morel in [2], and the connection between scale space analysis and PDEs has been since studied in [1], proving in particular that the MCM operator satisfies most of the relevant properties in multi-scale analysis, as monotonicity, invariance under grey scale change, and translation invariance.

The term $\operatorname{div}(\frac{Du(x,t)}{|Du(x,t)|})|Du(x,t)|$ represents a degenerate diffusion term, which diffuses in the direction orthogonal to the gradient Du. In fact, denoting by $\sigma(Du) = (\frac{Du}{|Du|})^{\perp}$ the unit vector orthogonal to Du, (6.18) might be rewritten as:

$$u_t = \sigma(Du)^{\top} D^2 u \, \sigma(Du),$$

where $D^2 u$ is the Hessian matrix of u.

We review the main ideas behind FD and SL numerical techniques, for the case of the Mean Curvature Motion.

6.2.2.1 FD Schemes

Once the schemes in differenced form (6.11) have been introduced, it becomes natural to use this general structure, replacing the fixed propagation speed $c(x)$ with a speed depending on the solution, in particular the Mean Curvature. For example, we start by rewriting the Osher–Sethian scheme as

$$u_j^{n+1} = u_j^n - \Delta t \, G^{OS}\left(x_j, \frac{u^n_{j_1+1,j_2} - u^n_j}{\Delta x}, \frac{u^n_j - u^n_{j_1-1,j_2}}{\Delta x}, \frac{u^n_{j_1,j_2+1} - u^n_j}{\Delta x}, \frac{u^n_j - u^n_{j_1,j_2-1}}{\Delta x}\right) \tag{6.19}$$

where

$$G^{OS}(x_j, a^+, a^-, b^+, b^-) = c(x_j)\left(\bar{a}_j^2 + \bar{b}_j^2\right)^{1/2} \tag{6.20}$$

In (6.20), we use as speed term $c(x) = -k(x)$, where k is the mean curvature of a generic level set of u, which can be computed as

$$k(x) = \operatorname{div}\left(\frac{Du(x)}{|Du(x)|}\right) = \frac{u_{x_1x_1}{u_{x_2}}^2 - 2u_{x_2}u_{x_1}u_{x_1x_2} + u_{x_2x_2}u_{x_1}^2}{\left({u_{x_1}}^2 + {u_{x_2}}^2\right)^{3/2}}, \tag{6.21}$$

and $\bar{a}_j^2, \bar{b}_j^2$ are obtained via (6.12)–(6.13) according to the sign of $k(x)$. Last, we obtain the final form of the scheme for (6.18) by replacing the continuos expression (6.21) by its discrete approximation based on centered finite differences and computed at the node x_j (see [22] for more details). This scheme gives a first order approximation, whereas a second order scheme for the same equation can be obtained using more sophisticated approximations of the derivatives and of the nonlinear terms as proposed in [21].

In this case, stability of the scheme requires a parabolic-type CFL condition of the form $\Delta t \sim \Delta x^2$, which results from approximating a diffusion operator in explicit form, and forces the use of very small time steps.

6.2.2.2 SL Schemes

As in the case of the eikonal equation, the construction of a semi-Lagrangian scheme for equation (6.18) stems from a suitable representation formula for the solution. In this case, the formula has a stochastic character. The interested reader can find in [4] the details, along with the relevant literature, whereas we limit ourselves here to a mere presentation of the scheme.

Let again u_j^n denote the numerical approximation of $u(x_j, t_n)$. We denote by $D_j u^n$ the central finite difference approximation of the space gradient on the numerical solution at the n-th step, so that

$$D_j u^n = \frac{1}{2\Delta x}\begin{pmatrix} u^n_{j_1+1,j_2} - u^n_{j_1-1,j_2} \\ u^n_{j_1,j_2+1} - u^n_{j_1,j_2-1} \end{pmatrix}, \tag{6.22}$$

and we define $\sigma_j^n = \sigma(D_j u^n)$, i.e., the unit normal vector computed on the approximate gradient.

Now, we can write the SL scheme for (6.18) as:

$$\begin{cases} u_j^{n+1} = \dfrac{1}{2}\left(\Pi[u^n](x_j + \sigma_j^n\sqrt{\Delta t}) + \Pi[u^n](x_j - \sigma_j^n\sqrt{\Delta t})\right) \\ u_j^0 = u_0(x_j). \end{cases} \tag{6.23}$$

Note that the average at the right-hand side of (6.23) is computed at the extreme points of a segment of length $2\sqrt{\Delta t}$, orthogonal to the approximate gradient. This is precisely what generates the correct (degenerate) diffusion in the scheme. Note also that the vector σ is not defined at nodes where the approximate gradient D_j^n vanishes. Although this is a very unlikely occurrence in image analysis, the scheme can be defined so as to overcome this problem. Roughly speaking, two main techniques have been proposed (see [4,5]):

- the scheme (6.23) is only applied when the discrete gradient is above a given threshold (depending on Δx), say, $|D_j^n| \geq C\Delta x^s$, with C and s suitable positive constants. When D_j^n is under the threshold, the scheme switches to isotropic diffusion (heat equation);
- rather than computing the approximate gradient, the correct direction of diffusion is detected via a minmax operator (as first proposed in [17]), obtaining the scheme

$$u_j^{n+1} = \min_{a\in S^1}\max\left\{\Pi[u^n]\left(x_j + a\sqrt{2\Delta t}\right), \Pi[u^n]\left(x_j - a\sqrt{2\Delta t}\right)\right\}, \tag{6.24}$$

in which S^1 denotes the unit circle, i.e., $S^1 = \{x \in \mathbb{R}^2 : |x| = 1\}$.

Finally, we remark that, despite being explicit, the scheme remains stable under hyperbolic type (i.e., linear) $\Delta t/\Delta x$ relationships.

6.3 Active Contours Models for Segmentation

The so-called *active contours* models are segmentation strategies in which a curve (the "active contour" or "snake") evolves according to the gradient of a suitable energy functional towards a regime position, which solves the segmentation problem in the chosen energy. They were first introduced in [16] using closed parametric curves, and then reformulated, starting with [7], in terms of level set models. We discuss in this section some level set models of this kind, built with the basic blocks shown above, aimed at image segmentation. Depending on the criterion used to stop the evolution of the interface (and ultimately of the underlying energy functional), we can single out two subclasses, respectively making and not making use of the information from the gradient of the initial image. In what follows, we will denote by $I_0(x)$ the image to be segmented.

6.3.1 Active Contours Models Using the Image Gradient

The basic idea underlying this class of models is to start from an initial position of the interface enclosing the object to be extracted from the image background, and use a model which shrinks the level sets (clearly, the opposite choice could also be implemented). The key feature of the model is to stop the propagation of the front once an edge is detected, so that the speed of propagation $c(x, Du, D^2u)$ should ideally vanish when the gradient of $I_0(x)$ is large. In order to identify regions with large gradients, a positive edge-detection function is defined. This function has the property of decreasing at the increase of $|DI_0(x)|$, and having for example a zero limit for $|DI_0(x)| \to \infty$. In practice, since the initial image $I_0(x)$ might be noisy, its gradient is regularized via a Gaussian convolution kernel G_σ with unit mass and a proper scale parameter σ, that is

$$G_\sigma(x) = \sigma^{-1/2} e^{-\frac{|x|^2}{4\sigma}}.$$

Two typical edge-detection functions have been proposed in the literature. The first one [18] is of the form

$$g_1(x) = 1 - \frac{|G_\sigma * DI_0(x)| - m}{M - m},$$

in which M and m denote the maximum and minimum norm for the regularized gradient of I. Here, $g_1(x) = 0$ at points at which $|DI_0(x)| = M$. A second form is

$$g_2(x) = \frac{1}{1 + |G_\sigma * DI_0(x)|^p} \qquad p \geq 1,$$

and satisfies the asymptotic condition $g_2(x) \to 0$ as $|DI_0(x)| \to \infty$, with a decay rate depending on p. This latter form has been independently proposed in [7] for $p = 2$ and in [18] for $p = 1$.

Edge-detection functions as such are used in level set models to modulate the speed of propagation. A first-order level set model [18] uses g_1 in an eikonal equation as

$$\begin{cases} u_t + g_1(x)|Du| = 0 & (x,t) \in \mathbb{R}^2 \times [0, +\infty) \\ u(x) = u_0(x) & x \in \mathbb{R}^2. \end{cases} \tag{6.25}$$

According to (6.1), positive values of g_1 correspond to a shrinking curve, so that u_0 should be chosen so as to enclose the object with its zero-level set. Then, the evolution of the interface converges to the set where g_1 vanishes.

On the other hand, a regularizing curvature term could be used to smooth out the active contour in case of noisy images. Such a model evolves according to a linear combination of eikonal and curvature operators, and uses the edge detecting function g_2, thus taking the form (see [7], [18]):

$$\begin{cases} u_t - g_2(x)|Du| \left(1 + \varepsilon \operatorname{div}\left(\frac{Du(x,t)}{|Du(x,t)|}\right)\right) = 0 & (x,t) \in \mathbb{R}^2 \times [0, +\infty) \\ u(x) = u_0(x) & x \in \mathbb{R}^2. \end{cases} \tag{6.26}$$

In (6.26), the eikonal term keeps the front evolving also at zero-curvature points. The term $g_2(x)$ modulates the speed of evolution, and stops the front on edges at which $DI_0(x) \to \infty$. The sign of the first-order part is chosen so as to force expansion, in contrast to the curvature term which tends to shrink the interface.

Last, we mention a third model, termed as *level set geodesic flow* [8], which tries to circumvent the problem occurring in the model (6.26) whenever the edges of the image are not ideal, i.e., if they do not satisfy an infinite gradient condition. In this model, the eikonal term is replaced by a transport term driven by $-Dg_2(x)$, which pushes the interface towards the minima of the edge-detection function. The resulting level set equation reads

$$\begin{cases} u_t - \varepsilon g_2(x)|Du| \operatorname{div}\left(\frac{Du(x,t)}{|Du(x,t)|}\right) - Dg_2(x) \cdot Du = 0 & (x,t) \in \mathbb{R}^2 \times [0, +\infty) \\ u(x) = u_0(x) & x \in \mathbb{R}^2. \end{cases} \tag{6.27}$$

In this case, the interface is expected to reach a stationary state in a wider range of conditions, and may converge to local minima of the energy, e.g. when the initial position of the interface is close to an edge of the image. We note that a similar model has been proposed [26] for the reconstruction of a surface from an unorganized set of points.

6.3.2 Chan–Vese Model

A second model for image segmentation stems from the Mumford–Shah theory [19], and could be formulated as follows: given an observed image

$I_0 : \Omega \to [0,1]$, find a decomposition made of open sets $\Omega = \cup_i \Omega_i \cup C$ with $C = \cup_i \partial\Omega_i$, such that I_0 varies smoothly within each Ω_i and is allowed to have discontinuities across the boundaries of Ω_i (i.e., along C).

A simplified model can be obtained by assuming the segmented image I to be a piecewise constant functions, i.e., $I \equiv c_i$ inside each Ω_i. In particular, for the special case of isolating an object from the background, we can set $i \in \{1,2\}$ and the functional to be minimized is

$$E^{MS}(c_1, c_2, C) = \lambda_1 \int_{\Omega_1} (I_0 - c_1)^2 dx + \lambda_2 \int_{\Omega_2} (I_0 - c_2)^2 dx + \mu |C|, \tag{6.28}$$

where $|C|$ denotes the length of C and plays the role of a regularizing term, $\lambda_1, \lambda_2, \mu$ are constants to be suitably tuned, and the c_i ($i = 1, 2$) denote the mean values of I_0 in the sets Ω_i.

In order to reformulate this problem in terms of a LS method, the curve C is defined as the zero-level set of the function $u(x,t)$ and, denoting by $H(\cdot)$ the usual Heaviside function, (6.28) becomes (see [24])

$$E^{CV}(c_1, c_2, u) = \lambda_1 \int_{\Omega} (I_0 - c_1)^2 H(u) dx + \lambda_2 \int_{\Omega} (I_0 - c_2)^2 (1 - H(u)) dx + \mu \int_{\Omega} |DH(u)| dx, \tag{6.29}$$

where the integral averages c_1 and c_2 are defined in terms of u as:

$$c_1 = \frac{\int_{\Omega} I_0(x) H(u) dx}{\int_{\Omega} H(u) dx}, \quad c_2 = \frac{\int_{\Omega} I_0(x)(1 - H(u)) dx}{\int_{\Omega} (1 - H(u)) dx}.$$

Denoting now by H_ε and δ_ε two C^1 regular approximations of the Heaviside function H and of the delta function so that $H'_\varepsilon = \delta_\varepsilon$, we can write the Euler–Lagrange equation corresponding to the corresponding regularized energy E^{CV}_ε. The evolution of u along the gradient of E^{CV}_ε gives

$$\frac{\partial u}{\partial t} = \delta_\varepsilon(u) \left[\mu \operatorname{div}\left(\frac{Du}{|Du|} \right) - \lambda_1 (I_0 - c_1)^2 + \lambda_2 (I_0 - c_2)^2 \right]. \tag{6.30}$$

The solution of (6.30) converges, for $t \to \infty$, to a regime solution witch minimizes the functional (6.28).

A standard rescaling can be made, as in Zhao et al. [25], by replacing $\delta_\varepsilon(u)$ by $|Du|$. This does not affect the steady-state solution, but helps remove stiffness near the zero level sets of u. Finally, we end up with the nonlinear evolution equation:

$$\frac{\partial u}{\partial t} - |Du| \left[\mu \operatorname{div}\left(\frac{Du}{|Du|} \right) - \lambda_1 (I_0 - c_1)^2 + \lambda_2 (I_0 - c_2)^2 \right] = 0, \tag{6.31}$$

wich is solved for $t \to \infty$. Note that, due to the definition of c_1 and c_2, (6.31) is a nonlocal equation.

In a slightly more general version, the functional E^{CV} contains also a term $\nu \int_\Omega H(u)dx$ penalizing (with a coefficient ν) the area enclosed by the curve C. The corresponding level set model reads then

$$\frac{\partial u}{\partial t} - |Du| \left[\mu \operatorname{div} \left(\frac{Du}{|Du|} \right) - \nu - \lambda_1 (I_0 - c_1)^2 + \lambda_2 (I_0 - c_2)^2 \right] = 0.$$

6.4 Numerical Simulations

In this section, we show some numerical tests where an X-ray image is segmented, and compare three active contour models on the same image. We have used SL schemes to compute the approximate solution. In our last test we consider the segmentation of a 3D object starting from a synthetic tomographic image.

6.4.1 Active Contour Model Using Image Gradient

We first consider model (6.25). Since, in a real image, an edge does not necessarily correspond to an infinite gradient, it might be necessary to subtract a positive constant k to the speed $g_1(x)$, so that the evolution of the front would stop when approaching an intermediate value between m and M for the norm of the regularized gradient.

To implement the method we use scheme (6.17) with speed

$$c(x) = g_1(x) - k$$

and $k \in (m, M)$. The initial contour, i.e., the zero level set of the initial condition, should be located outside of the region to be segmented. In this region the speed is positive, and then the contour would shrink. We set $\sigma = 5 \cdot 10^{-4}$ and $\Delta t = 2\Delta x$.

Figure 6.2 shows the image to be segmented together with the zero-level contour of numerical solutions, at the initial iteration (top left), at iteration $n = 65$ with $k = 0.6$ (top right) and at iteration $n = 112$ and $k = 0.7$ (bottom left). Although simple, the method depends critically on the choice of the parameters (in particular, on the constant k), and the result is not completely robust and accurate. In addition, the method requires a stopping criterion, since, depending on the image under consideration, the evolution might not converge to an equilibrium.

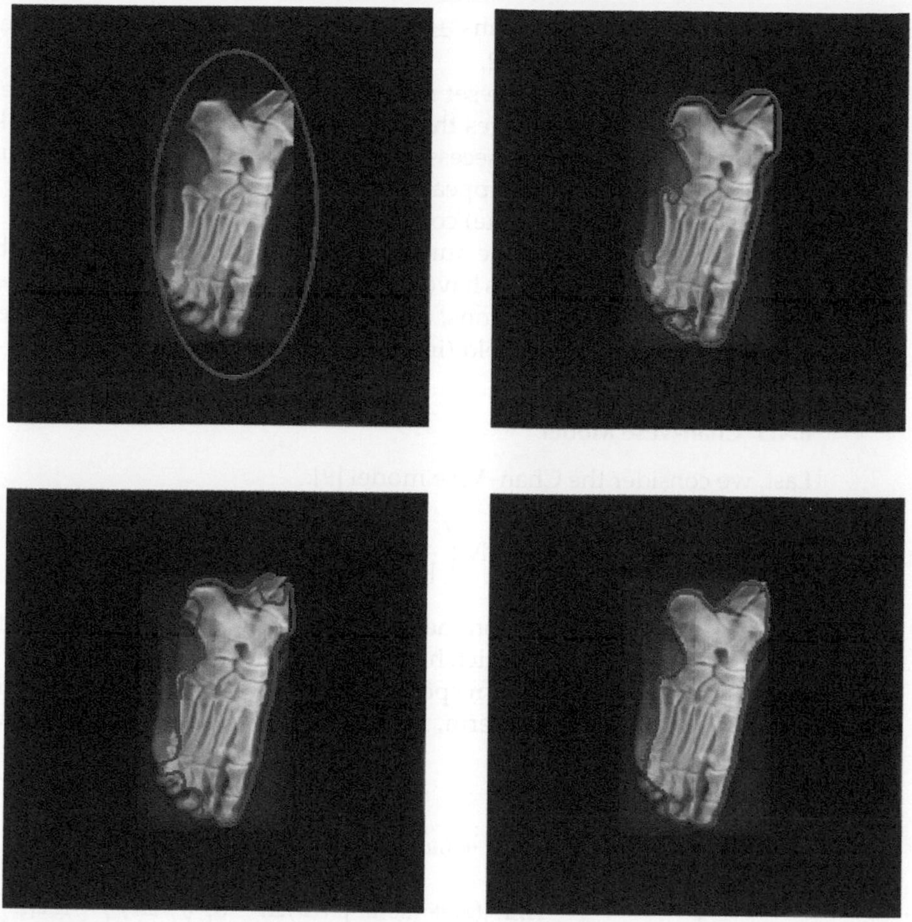

FIGURE 6.2
Zero-level contour of the numerical solution of (6.25): Initial condition (top left), iteration $n = 112$ with speed $g_1(x) - 0.7$ (top right), iteration $n = 65$ with speed $g_1(x) - 0.6$ (bottom left). Zero-level contour of the numerical solution of (6.32) at iteration $n = 175$ (bottom right).

6.4.2 Level Set Geodesic Model

Next, we consider the geodesic model (6.27), and the following SL scheme to approximate its solution:

$$u_j^{n+1} = \frac{1}{2}\Pi[u_j^n]\left(x_j + D_j g_2 \Delta t + \sigma_j^n \sqrt{\varepsilon g_2(x_j)\Delta t}\right) + \frac{1}{2}\Pi[u_j^n]\left(x_j + D_j g_2 \Delta t - \sigma_j^n \sqrt{\varepsilon g_2(x_j)\Delta t}\right). \tag{6.32}$$

In (6.32), $D_j g_2$ stands for the centered difference approximation of the gradient defined in (6.22) and computed on g_2, and the related displacement $D_j g_2 \Delta t$ implements the advection term in (6.27). On the other hand, the average computed with the two terms $\pm\sigma_j^n\sqrt{\varepsilon g_2(x_j)\Delta t}$ treats the curvature term, as already shown in Section 6.2.

In the numerical test, we set $\varepsilon = 0.3$ and $\Delta t = \Delta x/4$. The presence of the mean curvature term enlarges the stencil of the scheme, and this makes the use of smaller time steps necessary to maintain accuracy. The solution is smoother, although it also appear more robust, and in particular the model (and, accordingly, the scheme) converges to a steady state solution.

In Figure 6.2, we show the numerical solution at iteration $n = 175$ (bottom right), in which the iterations have been stopped when the difference between two successive approximations, measured in the discrete 1-norm, becomes smaller than a given threshold (in our case, $5 \cdot 10^{-3}$).

6.4.3 Chan-Vese Model

Last, we consider the Chan–Vese model [9]:

$$u_t = \left(\mu \operatorname{div}\left(\frac{Du}{|Du|}\right) - \nu + c[u(t)]\right)|Du| \tag{6.33}$$

where $c[u(t)]$ denotes the nonlinear speed which corresponds to the term in square brackets in (6.31), which has a nonlocal dependence on u via c_1 and c_2.

Using the techniques of respectively (6.23) for the mean curvature term and (6.16) for the eikonal term, we derive the following approximation of (6.33):

$$u_j^{n+1} = \begin{cases} \max\limits_{a\in B(0,1)} \left\{ \frac{1}{2}\Pi[u_j^n](x_j + (ac[u^n] - \nu)\Delta t + \sigma_j^n\sqrt{\mu\Delta t}) \right. \\ \qquad \left. + \frac{1}{2}\Pi[u_j^n](x_j + (ac[u^n] + \nu)\Delta t - \sigma_j^n\sqrt{\mu\Delta t}) \right\} & \text{if } c[u^n] \geq 0, \\ \min\limits_{a\in B(0,1)} \left\{ \frac{1}{2}\Pi[u_j^n](x_j + (ac[u^n] - \nu)\Delta t + \sigma_j^n\sqrt{\mu\Delta t}) \right. \\ \qquad \left. + \frac{1}{2}\Pi[u_j^n](x_j + (ac[u^n] + \nu)\Delta t - \sigma_j^n\sqrt{\mu\Delta t}) \right\} & \text{if } c[u^n] < 0. \end{cases} \tag{6.34}$$

We set $\Delta t = \Delta x$ and $\lambda = \lambda_1 = \lambda_2 = 20$ and we vary the parameters μ and ν. In Figure 6.3, we show the zero-level contour of the initial condition (top left), which can be located in any place of the image. We show the zero-level set of the numerical solution computed by setting respectively $\mu = 0$ and $\nu = 0$ (top right), $\mu = 0.05$ and $\nu = 0$ (bottom left), $\mu = 0.01$ and $\nu = 0.5$ (bottom right).

In Figure 6.4, we show the initial condition u^0 and the solution u^n of (6.34) at iteration $n = 60$ with $\mu = 0.01$, $\nu = 0.5$ and $\lambda = 20$. Although the choice of the parameters has a clear influence on the detection of details, the model shows no critical dependence on this choice.

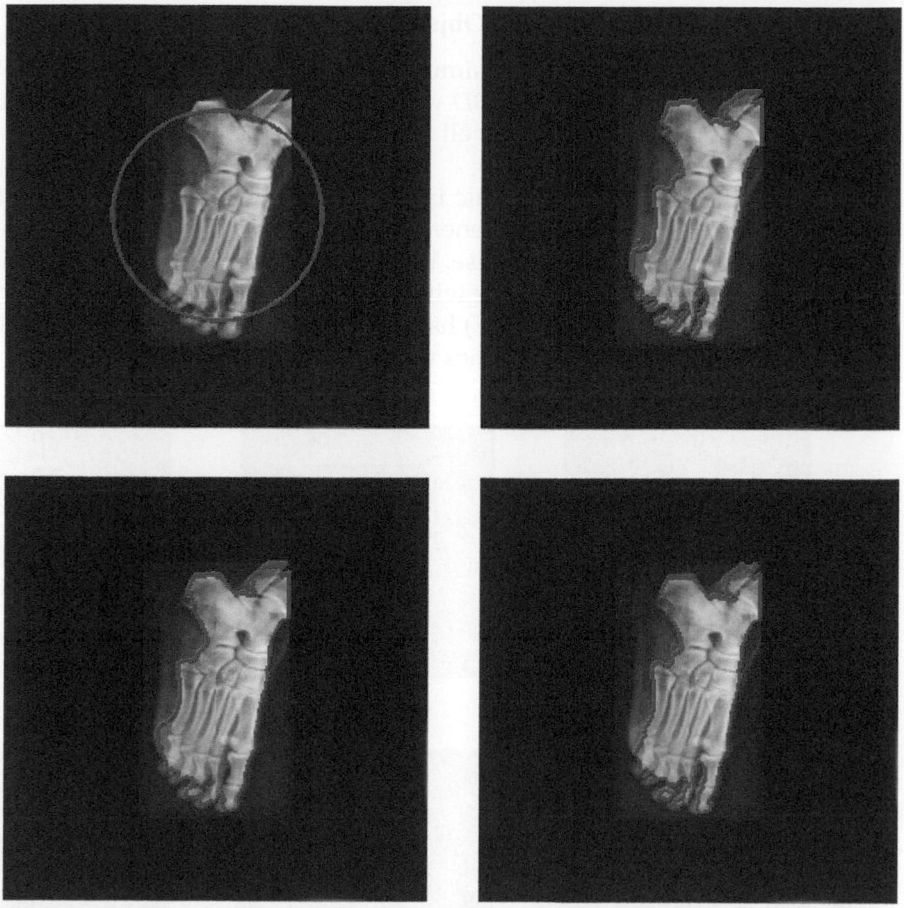

FIGURE 6.3
Chan–Vese model. zero-level contour of the numerical solution of (6.34). Initial Condition, iteration 62 with $\mu = 0, \nu = 0, \lambda = 20$, iteration 45 with $\mu = 0.05, \nu = 0, \lambda = 20$, iteration 60 with $\mu = 0.01, \nu = 0.5, \lambda = 20$.

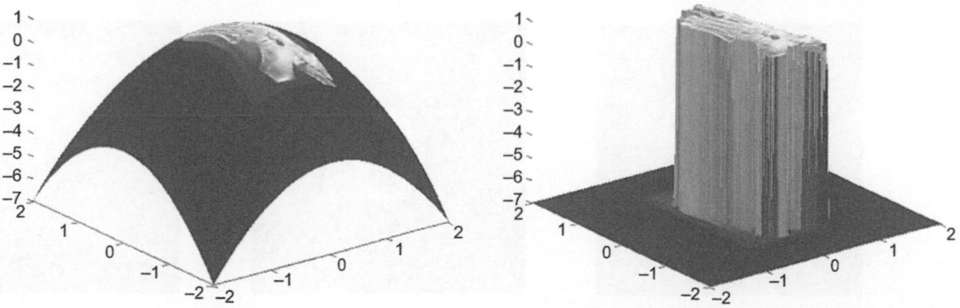

FIGURE 6.4
Chan-Vese model. Numerical solution of (6.34). Initial Condition and u^n at iteration $n = 60$ with $\mu = 0.01, \nu = 0.5, \lambda = 20$.

6.4.4 Segmentation of a 3D Object

We conclude by showing a simulation where a three-dimensional object is segmented by applying the 3D version of scheme (6.32). For a complete description of the scheme, as well as for its extension to the 3D case, we refer the readers to [6].

The synthetic tomographic image, representing a simplified 3D Shepp-Logan phantom, has been generated by running the tomobox Matlab tools [15] and adding Gaussian noise. We show in Figure 6.5 nine slices of the noisy synthetic tomographic image with size $81 \times 81 \times 81$, with an added noise of variance 0.1. The model (6.27) has been applied by setting $\varepsilon = \sigma = 0.01$. The scheme has been run four times with four different initial conditions, chosen

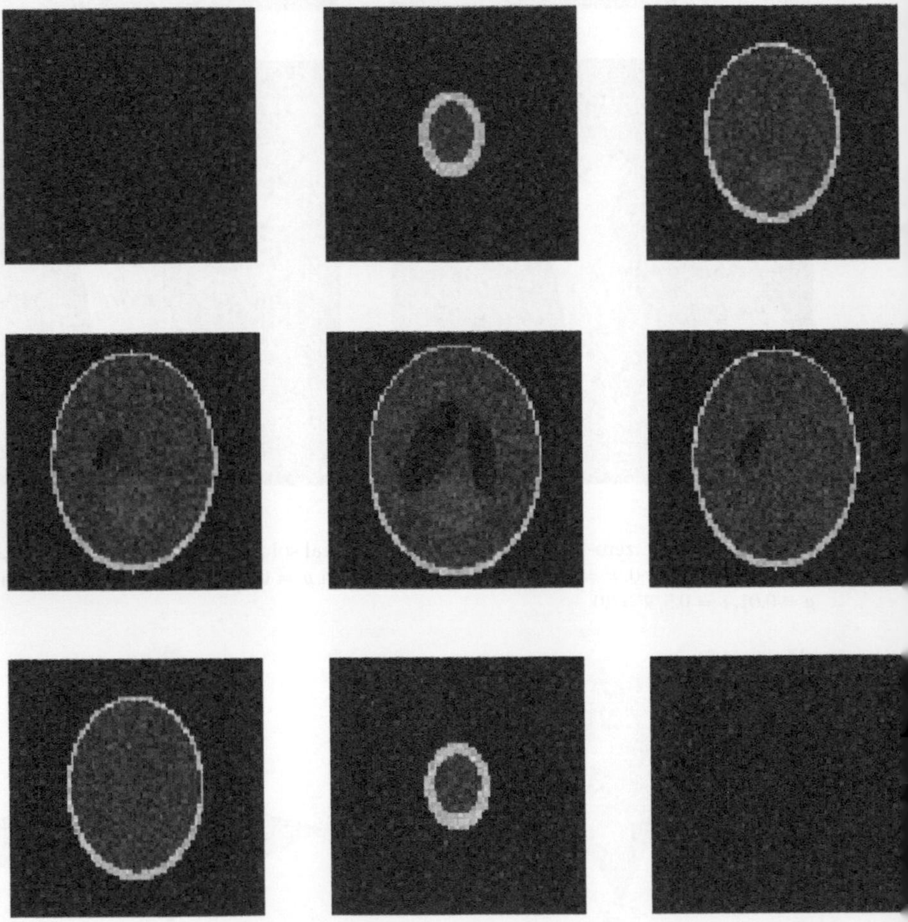

FIGURE 6.5
Shepp-Logan phantom with noise: slices corresponding to vertical levels at the distance of 1[illegible] pixels, from level 1 to level 81.

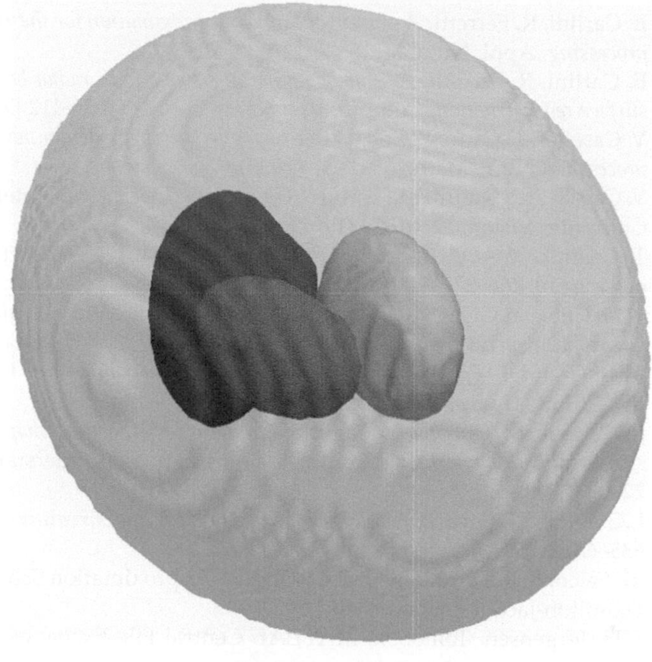

FIGURE 6.6
3D view of the segmented Shepp-Logan phantom.

so as to let the method converge to four different equilibrium surfaces, which correspond to the external surface of the phantom and three of the homogeneous subsets (which can be easily located on the 2D slices). The result of the segmentation is represented in Figure 6.6. The iterative method has been run with $\Delta t = \Delta x = 0.05$ and stopped when the difference between two successive approximations, measured in the discrete 1-norm, becomes smaller than the threshold of 10^{-2}.

References

1. L. Alvarez, F. Guichard, P. L. Lions, J. M. Morel, *Axioms and Fundamental Equations of Image Processing*, Arch. for Rational Mechanics, *Arch. for Rational Mechanics*, 123, 199–257 (1993).
2. L. Alvarez, P. L. Lions, J. M. Morel, *Image selective smoothing and edge detection by nonlinear diffusion*, SIAM J. Num. Anal., 29, 845–866 (1992).
3. G. Barles, P.E. Souganidis, *Convergence of approximation schemes for fully nonlinear second-order equations* , Asymp. Anal., 4, 271–283 (1991).
4. E. Carlini, M. Falcone, R. Ferretti, *Convergence of a large time-step scheme for mean curvature motion*, Interfaces and free boundaries, 12, 409–441 (2010).

5. E. Carlini, R. Ferretti, *A semi-Lagrangian approximation for the AMSS model of image processing*, Appl. Num. Math., 73, 16-32 (2013).
6. E. Carlini, R. Ferretti, *A semi-Lagrangian scheme with radial basis approximation for surface reconstruction*, Comput. Vis. Sci. 18 , no. 2-3, 103–112 (2017).
7. V. Caselles, F. Catté, T. Coll, F. Dibos, *A geometric model for active contours in image processing*, Num. Math., 66, 1–31 (1993).
8. V. Caselles, R. Kimmel, G. Sapiro, *Geodesic active contours*, International Journal of Computer Vision, 22, 61–79 (1997).
9. T. Chan, L. Vese, *Active contours without edges*, IEEE Transactions on Image Processing, 10, 266–277 (2001).
10. Y. G. Chen, Y. Giga, S. Goto, *Uniqueness and existence of viscosity solutions of generalized mean curvature flow equation*, J. Diff. Geom, 33, 749–786 (1991).
11. M.G. Crandall, P.L. Lions, *Two approximations of solutions of Hamilton–Jacobi equations*, Math. Comp., 43, 1–19, (1984).
12. J.D. Durou, M. Falcone, M. Sagona, *Numerical Methods for Shape from Shading: a new survey with benchmarks*, Computer Vision and Image Understanding, Elsevier, 109, 22–43 (2008).
13. L.C. Evans, J. Spruck, *Motion of level sets by mean curvature*, I. J. Diff. Geom, 33, 635–681 (1991).
14. M. Falcone, R. Ferretti, Semi-Lagrangian Approximation Schemes for Linear and Hamilton-Jacobi Equations, SIAM, 2013.
15. J. H. Jørgensen. Tomobox, MATLAB Central File Exchange, Retrieved Aug 17 2010.
16. M. Kass, A. Witkin, D. Terzopoulos. *Snakes: active contour models*, Internationa Journal of Computer Vision, 1, 321–331 (1988).
17. R. Kohn, S. Serfaty, *A deterministic-control-based approach to motion by curvature* Comm. Pure Appl. Math., 59, 344–407 (2006).
18. R. Malladi, J.A. Sethian, B.C. Vemuri, *A topology independent shape modeling scheme* in Proc. SPIE Conf. Geometric Methods Computer Vision II, vol. 2031, 246–258 (1993).
19. D. Mumford, J. Shah, *Optimal Approximations by Piecewise Smooth Functions and Associated Variational Problems*, Comm. on Pure and Appl. Math., 42, 577–685 (1989).
20. S. J. Osher, R. P. Fedkiw, Level Set Methods and Dynamic Implicit Surfaces, Applied Mathematical Sciences, 153, Springer-Verlag, New York, (2003).
21. S. J. Osher, J. A. Sethian, *Front propagating with curvature-dependent speed: algorithm based on Hamilton–Jacobi formulation*. J. of Comp. Physics, 79, 12–49 (1988).
22. J. A. Sethian, Level Set Methods and Fast Marching Methods: Evolving Interface in Computational Geometry, Fluid Mechanics, Computer Vision, and Material Science, Cambridge University Press, Cambridge Monograph on Applied and Computational Mathematics, (1999).
23. C.-W. Shu, *High order numerical methods for time dependent Hamilton-Jacobi equations* in Mathematics and Computation in Imaging Science and Information Processing S.S. Goh, A. Ron and Z. Shen, eds, Lecture Notes Series, Institute for Mathematica Sciences, National University of Singapore, vol. 11, World Scientific Press, Singapore, 47–91 (2007).

24. L. Vese, T. Chan, *A multiphase level set framework for image segmentation using the Mumford and Shah model*, Int. J. of Comp. Vision., 50, 271–293 (2002).
25. H. Zhao, T. Chan, B. Merriman, S. J. Osher, *A Variational Level Set Approach to Multiphase Motion*, J. of Comp. Physics, 127, 179–195 (1996).
26. H. Zhao, S. J. Osher, B. Merriman, M. Kang, *Implicit and nonparametric shape reconstruction from unorganized points using variational level set method*, Comput. Vis. Image Underst., 80, 295–319 (2000).

7

Level Set Methods for Cardiac Segmentation in MSCT Images

Ruben Medina, Sebastian Bautista, Villie Morocho, and Alexandra La Cruz

CONTENTS

7.1 Introduction

Early identification of myocardial muscle dysfunction by quantitative analysis allows a reliable diagnosis of cardiovascular diseases. The above analysis is based on the estimation of various clinical parameters including ventricular volumes, ejection fraction, thickening of the myocardium and myocardial mass. For the evaluation of such parameters it is generally required the proper delineation of endocardial and epicardial contours of cardiac cavities [1]. Quantification of cardiac function is usually performed using X-Rays 2-D contrast ventriculographic images, 2-D or 3-D echocardiographic images, 4-D MRI images, 4-D Multi–Slice CT (MSCT) or PET/SPECT images. Multi-Slice CT is a medical imaging modality that enables acquisition of 3-D or 4-D cardiac images including more than 20 3-D images per cardiac cycle. A key task to achieve cardiac quantification is accurate detection of the left ventricle in the MSCT images, which can be performed by means of a segmentation process. The segmentation is based on grouping of pixels/voxels in an image for representing a shape, where the procedure used for attaining this organization is based on proximity and similarity between attributes of an image [2, 3]. The segmentation of cardiac images is a difficult task because of several problems such as: 1) complexity and variability of the heart movement; 2) the low contrast exhibiting by the objects in these images; 3) contamination with noise; and 4) presence of artifacts that may arise during the acquisition and / or reconstruction of the images [4].

Several algorithms for cardiac segmentation have been proposed. Simpler segmentation techniques, such as region growing, have been widely reported. Approaches based on region growing techniques are used in interactive multi-object segmentation techniques coupled with a connectivity approach aiming at obtaining coherent shapes representing the cardiac cavities [5]. They have also been combined with landmark detection using Support Vector Machines for useful seed detection as proposed by Bravo et al. [6]. In [7] a 3-D region growing algorithm is validated. However, the region growing algorithm corresponds to a commercial implementation of Siemens and no details are reported about the type of region growing implemented. The validation is performed indirectly by measuring the volume and the ejection fraction rather than performing comparison of the actual 3-D shapes obtained. Additionally, authors acknowledge the fact that the algorithm exclude papillary muscles from the left ventricle lumen. They also perform the manual segmentation excluding the papillary muscles. This has the consequence of attaining better accuracy measures when the evaluation is performed using the Dice similarity. Otherwise, exclusion of papillary muscles from the left ventricle lumen has an important impact in left ventricle mass calculation as shown in [8] where they report that excluding papillary muscles from the left ventricle lumen can increase the left ventricle mass up to 30%.

Some other approaches correspond to the atlas based segmentation techniques where prior information is gathered during the training phase. An atlas can be constructed by manual segmentation of each heart cavity, and statistical techniques could combine either the surface of the cavities as well as the gray level information within the shape. During the segmentation process, several landmarks defining the location of the heart in the database could be estimated, and based on this information the heart model is positioned and adapted in space using affine transformations. And finally, the accurate segmentation is attained by deformable adaptation. These type of approaches have been proposed by Ecabert [9], Zhang et al. [10] and Van Assen et al. [11].

Also, registration based segmentation technique is proposed by Kirisli et al. [12], where a non-rigid registration technique is used for deforming a multi–atlas representing the four cardiac cavities. The approach is a fully automatic method for segmentation of cardiac cavities in multi-slice CT images. Machine learning techniques have also been used for cardiac cavities segmentation such as Zheng et al. [13] where a two stages method is proposed. The first stage performs anatomical structure localization, and in the second stage the boundary delineation is attained. Both stages use marginal space learning techniques for performing an accurate four chamber segmentation with a low computational cost.

Other approaches are based on level set contour deformation techniques. In Lynch et al. [14] a cardiac motion model based on the volume is used in a level set framework for performing the 4-D segmentation in MRI data. A user–guided 3-D active contour segmentation approach based on level set has been developed by Yushkevich et al. [15] as an open–software platform known as ITK–SNAP. This platform was initially conceived for neuroimaging modalities but their application can be extended to cardiac images. A deformable contour based approach has been used by Heiberg et al. [16] for developing a software platform that is freely available for non–commercial research. A level set approach for left ventricle segmentation in echocardiographic images has been proposed by Dydenko et al. [17] where a prior shape for the left ventricle is registered to the image, and a level set approach is used for performing the contour deformation that allows the recovering of the ventricle shape.

Accurate and advanced cardiac segmentation techniques have been proposed. In [10] Zhang et al., an advanced model based segmentation method is presented where a combination of active shape models and active appearance model is used for segmenting left and right ventricles. Even when the method is highly accurate, the main limitation is the computational cost. The time necessary for performing the segmentation for a full cardiac cycle is 15-30 min. A multi-atlas segmentation method with registration refinement is proposed in [18]. The method took about 5 minutes and attained an accuracy 0.92 for the Dice similarity.

Level set techniques have been used for cardiac segmentation and most of the applications use global energy minimization methods such as the Geodesic Active Contours by Caselles et al. [19] and region competition by Zhu and Yuille [20]. Other techniques use local energy minimization for coping with gray level variations, such as the Lankton and Tannenbaum [21] algorithms. However, they are seldom used for segmentation of medical images.

This paper reports the results of a research project aimed at 2-D and 3-D segmentation of left ventricle images in multi-slice computerized tomography. The contributions of this research are:

- Comparison of the performance of level set global minimization approaches against local minimization approaches when the segmentation of 2-D Multi-slice CT images is performed. Nine algorithms were compared: the Caselles algorithm, the algorithm proposed by Chan and Vese [22], the algorithm proposed by Lankton and Tannenbaum [21], the algorithm proposed by Bernard [23], a region growing algorithm [24], the algorithm proposed by Shi et al. [25]. The fast marching algorithm, the Chunming Li algorithm and the implementation of the sparse field method proposed by Lankton. The implementation of the algorithms tested is available online as the CREASEG software [26], as functions of the Matlab software (Caselles and Chan Vese) or software distributions provided by the authors proposing such algorithms.
- Extension to 3-D segmentation of the left ventricle external wall is performed using a custom designed software platform oriented to research.

The remainder of the paper is organized as follows: in section 7.2, the level set algorithms compared in this research, are briefly presented. Section 7.3 describes the numerical implementation behind level set algorithms. The method is presented in section 7.4. In section 7.5 the results are reported and finally in section 7.6 the conclusions and future work are presented.

7.2 Level Set Algorithms

7.2.1 Level Set Formulation

The level set method enables deformation of a contour in 2-D or a surface in 3-D by manipulating a higher dimensional function. This technique was proposed by Osher and Sethian [27] and it has been applied in image processing, computer graphics and physical simulation. In the level set formulation a curve is defined as the zeros of a Lipschitz continuous function ϕ. In consequence the set of points $\{(x,y) \in \mathbb{R}^2 : \phi(x,y) = 0\}$ describe the current location of the curve. If we consider a parameterized curve $\gamma(s,t)$ with a velocity field describing the dynamics of the curve denoted as $\partial\gamma/\partial t$. Then if $\phi(\gamma(s,t),t) = 0$ for $t \geq 0$ the following equation is satisfied along γ [28].

$$\phi_t + \frac{\partial \gamma}{\partial t} \cdot \nabla\phi(\gamma,t) = 0 \qquad (7.1)$$

It can be shown that the evolution of the level set is given by:

$$\frac{\partial \phi}{\partial t} = -|\nabla\phi| \cdot F \qquad (7.2)$$

where F is the velocity term that control the curve evolution. This is the propagation velocity of a point in the curve moving in the normal direction with respect to the curve. Given a particular initialization of the level set curve, it is possible to guide the level set to different features or shapes within the image by manipulating the term F. Velocity functional F could include a term based on image features and a second term that is based on the contour curvature. One of the advantages of using this method is the fact that topological changes of the shape such as merging or splitting are implicitly handled. Several algorithms for level set based segmentation have been proposed. They are constructed by deriving the velocity functional from an energy functional adapted to the segmentation application. Several level set segmentation algorithms are presented in the following sections.

7.2.2 Fast Marching Algorithm

The Fast Marching Method is an algorithm useful for monotonically advancing fronts using a computational efficient method as proposed by Sethian [29]. This approach can be used for segmentation by synthesizing an external speed term that is applied to the front for stopping it near the objects contours as explained in [30]. The Fast Marching algorithm is constructed based on the level set approach presented in section 7.2.1.

Let us consider in Eq. 7.2, the special case of a surface (a contour representing the zero level set) moving at a velocity $F(x,y) > 0$ and $T(x,y)$ the time at which the surface crosses a point (x,y). Such time function satisfies the following identity:

$$|\nabla T| \cdot F = 1 \qquad (7.3)$$

where it is evident that the gradient of the time of surface arrival is inversely proportional to the speed F. A possible solution for approximating the position of the moving contour is following an iterative procedure by approximating the derivatives in Eq. 7.1. Considering the following difference operator notation:

$$D_{ij}^{+x}\phi = \frac{(\phi_{i+1,j} - \phi_{i,j})}{\Delta x} \tag{7.4}$$

The solution for the arrival time in the 2-D domain consists in solving the following equation:

$$\left[max(D_{i,j}^{-x}T,0)^2 + min(D_{i,j}^{+x}T,0)^2 + max(D_{i,j}^{-y}T,0)^2 + min(D_{i,j}^{+y}T,0)^2\right]^{1/2} = 1/F_{i,j} \tag{7.5}$$

where D^- and D^+ are backward and forward difference operators. The procedure consists in solving this quadratic equation at each grid point and iterating until convergence. The algorithm is based on the fact that Eq. 7.5 has an *up-wind* difference structure where the information propagates from smaller values of T to larger values. The algorithm is implemented using narrow band techniques or the sparse field method (see section 7.3). The algorithm is detailed in [29,30].

Using the fast marching method for image segmentation requires defining a special image based speed function $F(x,y) = k_I(x,y) > 0$ that could control the outward propagation of the initial curve, such that the surface could evolve for approaching the object boundaries. A feasible speed function could be defined as:

$$F(x,y) = k_I(x,y) = e^{-\alpha|\nabla G_\alpha * I(x,y)|}, \quad \alpha > 0 \tag{7.6}$$

This function has values close to zero at high image gradient points that are usually located on the object contour. Other type of speed function that could be used is the expression in Eq. 7.30.

It is also possible to consider additional constraints such as a definition for the speed corresponding to $F = 1 - \epsilon\mathcal{K}$ ($\epsilon > 0$) with $\mathcal{K}$ representing the curvature for the surface ϕ. Variation of parameter ϵ enables the evolution of the surface for attaining a smooth contour. In general, one of the outputs of this type of algorithms is the evolved level set that can be post-processed with a threshold for obtaining the final segmentation [31].

7.2.3 Caselles Algorithm

The Caselles algorithm [19] is a contour based method, where the velocity term is calculated based on the image gradient as an energy function expressed as:

$$E(C) = \int_0^1 g(I(C(q)))|C'(q)|dq \tag{7.7}$$

where

$$g(I) = \frac{1}{1 + |\nabla(G * I)|^2} \tag{7.8}$$

The image intensity is denoted as I, while G is a Gaussian filter of variance 1 and C is a parametric curve where the parameter is a signed distance function $q = \phi(\mathbf{x})$. Minimization of Eq. 7.7 is attained by searching the gradient descent using the steepest-descent method. According to this method the initial contour $C(0) = C_0$ is deformed according to the evolution expression in Eq. 7.9.

$$\frac{\partial C(t)}{\partial t} = g(I)\mathcal{K}\vec{\mathcal{N}} - (\nabla g \cdot \vec{\mathcal{N}})\vec{\mathcal{N}} \tag{7.9}$$

where $\mathcal{K}$ is the curvature and $\vec{\mathcal{N}}$ is the unit inward normal. The curve C is the level set $\{(\mathbf{x}) \in \mathbb{R}^2 : \phi(\mathbf{x}) = 0\}$. Therefore, the solution of this minimization problem is equivalent to searching the steady state solution of the following evolution equation.

$$\frac{\partial \phi}{\partial t}(\mathbf{x}) = g(I(\mathbf{x}))|\nabla\phi(\mathbf{x})|(c + \mathcal{K}) + \nabla g(I(\mathbf{x}))\nabla\phi(\mathbf{x}) \tag{7.10}$$

where $\mathcal{K}$ is the curvature of the evolving contour and c is a constant that acts as a balloon force that pushes the contour either inward or outward [19]. The term $(c + \mathcal{K})$ is equivalent to the internal force in the classical energy based snake model [32]. The external image force is given by the stopping function in Eq. 7.8. This function allows to stop the curve when it arrives to the actual object contour. The Caselles algorithm is contour based and the narrow band implementation is efficient from the computational point of view. The limitations of this algorithm are related to the fact that the stopping term is not efficient; thus, the contour can leak to outside areas of the target object. Moreover, when the front is propagated further than the target boundary, it cannot return to the actual contour location.

7.2.4 Chan Vese Algorithm

The Chan Vese algorithm is an area based segmentation where minimization of the energy function allows the recovering of boundaries between regions with different intensities. This algorithm is a particular case of the Mumford-Shah model [33]. The model is not based on the gradient of the image for stopping the evolution process. The model can detect objects in the image with very smooth or discontinue boundaries. According to the Chan Vese algorithm, the energy function is defined in Eq. 7.11.

$$E(C) = \int_{inside(C)} |I(\mathbf{x}) - v|^2 dxdy + \int_{outside(C)} |I(\mathbf{x}) - u|^2 dxdy \tag{7.11}$$

where v is the average of pixels inside the contour C where $\phi \geq 0$ and u is the average of pixels outside the contour C where $\phi < 0$. In this active contour model, the previous energy function is minimized and a regularization term is included. The evolution of the contour is given by Eq. 7.12.

$$\frac{\partial \phi}{\partial t}(\mathbf{x}) = \delta(\phi(\mathbf{x}))((I(\mathbf{x}) - v)^2 - (I(\mathbf{x}) - u)^2) + \lambda\delta(\phi(\mathbf{x}))\mathcal{K} \tag{7.12}$$

where δ is the Dirac function and u and v are updated at each iteration. ϕ is a signed distance function that is re–initialized at each iteration and λ is a regularization parameter weighting the curvature term.

Details concerning the energy function can be found in Chan and Vese [22]. This is a region–based algorithm that performs the segmentation of the image by attaining two homogeneous regions. However, as the evolution is based only on a narrow region of the level set, the algorithm is sensible to initialization. The main parameter for this algorithm is the curvature term λ that acts as a regularization term. Another limitation is the fact that when the average of pixels inside the object is almost similar to the average of pixels outside the object, the segmentation is poor. In such a case, rather than the pixels intensities $I(\mathbf{x})$, it is necessary to consider other features such as the curvature, the orientation or any other feature.

7.2.5 Lankton Algorithm

The Lankton algorithm is a local region-based algorithm that is useful for performing the segmentation of objects with heterogeneous intensities. The work described in [21] reports three contributions: firstly, a framework for localizing any region-based energy is described. Secondly, a way for localizing active contours able to interact with one another is reported. Thirdly, the effect of the localization radius on segmentation results is analyzed. The segmentation approach can be adapted for using different types of energies such as the Yezzi or Chan Vese energies. The optimization is performed in a neighborhood that can be a circle or square with the size defined by a parameter known as radius term. Additionally in this algorithm there is also a regularization term denoted as λ.

$$\frac{\partial \phi}{\partial t}(\mathbf{x}) = \delta(\phi(\mathbf{x})) \int_{\Omega} B(\mathbf{x}, \mathbf{y}) \cdot \nabla_{\phi} F(I(\mathbf{y}), \phi(\mathbf{y})) d\mathbf{y} + \lambda\delta(\phi(\mathbf{x}))\mathcal{K} \tag{7.13}$$

where $B(x, y)$ represents the local neighborhood and $\nabla_{\phi} F(I(\mathbf{y}), \phi(\mathbf{y}))$ is the gradient of $F(.)$. The function, F is a generic internal energy measure representing the local adherence to a given model along the contour. This generic function can handle three specific types of energies: the uniform modeling energy that uses a constant intensity model and it is also known as the Chan Vese energy [22]. The mean separation energy is another global region-based energy using mean intensities and it is known as the Yezzi energy [34]. A third type is the histogram separation energy. This is a more complex energy that compares the full histograms of the foreground and background. Minimization of this energy works by separating intensity histograms of the region inside and outside of the curve. This type of energy allows interior and exterior regions to be heterogeneous as long as their intensity profiles are different. A measure of this energy is based on the Bhattacharyya coefficient [35]. The flow equation for the global version is capable of segmenting objects with nonuniform intensities as long as the intensity profile for the object and background is separable. In the localized version, the algorithm is capable of separating locally nonhomogeneous regions. The authors of the Lankton algorithm also show how to extend the localized segmentation method for performing simultaneous segmentation of multiple foreground objects. In this case, it is necessary to use several level sets where evolution of each one incorporates two competing components: *advance* and *retreat*. The *advance* component a is always positive and tries to move the curve outwards along its normal. In contrast, the *retreat* component r is negative and tries to move the curve inward along its normal. The curve evolution is governed by the relative magnitudes of a and r. Concerning the implementation, it improves the computational efficiency by calculating values of ϕ in a narrow band around the zero level set. They reinitialize ϕ every few iterations using the fast marching technique [36]. Analysis of the choice of radius parameter shows that when the proposed energy is evaluated with a very small radius, the F becomes an edge detector based on statistics of pixels centered in the local neighborhood. In contrast, if the radius grows in a manner that tends to include the entire image, the local statistics will be similar to the global statistics and the behavior will be similar to a global region-based algorithm. One limitation of the algorithm is the fact that the sensitivity to initialization is greater than global region-based methods. Additionally, the execution time for this algorithm tends to be slower than the global algorithms counterparts. A more detailed presentation of this algorithm can be found in Lankton and Tannenbaum [21].

7.2.6 Bernard Algorithm

The algorithm of Bernard [23] is based on using as a level set implicit function $\phi(.)$ a B–spline basis. The algorithm exploits the separable property of B–spline basis functions for attaining an efficient implementation. The algorithm is a region–based method that computes the level set evolution on the whole image. This fact means that new contours could appear far from the initialization. The segmentation functional is described in [37]. This functional is similar to the Chan Vese functional [22]. If Ω is an open subset in $\mathcal{R}^2$

$$E(C) = v_{in}\int_{\Omega} g_{in}(\mathbf{x}, \phi(\mathbf{x}))H(\phi(\mathbf{x}))d\mathbf{x} + v_{out}\int_{\Omega} g_{out}(\mathbf{x}, \phi(\mathbf{x}))(1 - H(\phi(\mathbf{x})))d\mathbf{x}$$

$$+ v_c\int_{\Omega} g_c(\mathbf{x}, \phi(\mathbf{x}))\delta(\phi(\mathbf{x}))|\nabla\phi(\mathbf{x})|d\mathbf{x} \tag{7.14}$$

where v_{in}, v_{out} and v_c are positive escalars. In particular, the Chan Vese functional in this case is expressed as:

$$E(C) = \int_{\Omega} |I(\mathbf{x}) - v|^2 H(\phi(\mathbf{x}))d\mathbf{x} + \int_{\Omega} |I(\mathbf{x}) - u|^2 (1 - H(\phi(\mathbf{x})))dx + v_c \int_{\Omega} \delta(\phi(\mathbf{x}))|\nabla\phi(\mathbf{x})|dx \quad (7.15)$$

However, the level set implicit function is given by:

$$\phi(\mathbf{x}) = \sum_{k \in Z^d} c[\mathbf{k}]\beta^n\left(\frac{\mathbf{x}}{h} - \mathbf{k}\right) \quad (7.16)$$

where $\beta^n(\cdot)$ is the uniform symetric d-dimensional B–spline of degree n. The coefficients of the B–spline representation are in $c\,[k]$. The knots of the B–spline are located in a grid with regular spacing represented by h. This level set function is separable and it can be built as the product of d 1-D B–splines as shown in Eq. 7.17.

$$\beta^n(\mathbf{x}) = \prod_{j=1}^{d} \beta^n(x_j) \quad (7.17)$$

The level set evolution is estimated using a gradient descent algorithm on the B–spline coefficients. This allows the estimation of the iterative variation of B–spline coefficients as:

$$\mathbf{c}^{i+1} = \mathbf{c}^i - \lambda\nabla_c E(\mathbf{c}^i) \quad (7.18)$$

where λ is the iteration step and ∇_c is the gradient of the energy with respect to B–spline coefficients. This energy gradient can be estimated as the convolution of the feature image and the down-sampled B-spline using a factor h as detailed in [23].

The algorithm has a main parameter that represents a scale parameter denoted by h, which controls the smoothness of the evolving contour. Values for this parameter should be lower than 4. Minimization of Eq. 7.15 is performed by using the gradient descent algorithm where at each step the candidate update $\mathbf{c}^{i+1}$ and its associated energy are estimated. If this update decreases the energy, the step is considered successful and the coefficients $\mathbf{c}^{i+1}$ are accepted. The step size λ is multiplied by a factor $\alpha_f \geq 1$. If not, a more conservative update is performed by dividing the step size by a factor $\alpha'_f \geq 1$. Normally, in the CREASEG implementation the factors controlling the step size are fixed as $\alpha_f = 1$ and $\alpha'_f = 1.5$; however, this parameter could be modified for certain applications. The implementation works in this case with $v_{in} = 1$, $v_{out} = 1$ and $v_c = 0$. The regularization term is zero and the smoothness of the final shape is controlled with the scale of the B-spline. This procedure allows reducing the computation time. Authors show that increasing the scale of the B-spline is more efficient at reducing the effect of noise than considering the curvature regularization term. The Bernard method has as an advantage the fact of simplifying the mathematical derivations. The proposed cost function depends of a finite number of parameters and its gradient is calculated exactly without using finite difference approximations. The discretization scheme is natural and incorporated within the B-spline model. In this way, all calculations are accurate including the derivative calculations. Additionally, the level set evolution is implemented as a sequence of 1-D convolutions that enable a smoothing filter operation where the amount of smoothing is controlled explicitly with the scale and degree of the B-spline basis.

7.2.7 Shi Algorithm

The algorithm proposed by Shi et al. [25] is an approximation for the level set curve evolution that should be suitable for real-time implementation. According to this method, the level set is defined over a regular grid D of size $M_1 \times M_2 \times \ldots \times M_K$. The coordinates of a point in the grid are denoted as $\mathbf{x} = (x_1, x_2, x_3, \ldots, x_K)$. The object region Ω includes a set of grid points enclosed by contour C and the set of points belonging to the background is denoted $D \backslash \Omega$.

The band of points located at the boundary between the object and the background is decomposed in two list of points. L_{in} with neighboring points inside the contour and L_{out} with neighboring points belonging to the background region.

The algorithm does not solve explicitly the Partial Differential Equations (PDEs) but they achieved the curve evolution by decomposing the evolution process in two cycles: the first cycle for the data dependent term and the second cycle for the smoothness regularization term. The curve is represented by an integer value level set function denoted by $\hat{\phi}$. This function takes the integer values $\{-3, -1, 1, 3\}$ that describes a narrow band around the evolving contour. The speed function is also represented by an integer array denoted by $\hat{F}$ with values $\{+\ 1, 0, -1\}$ representing the sign of the evolution speed F. The evolution is attained by a switching procedure between elements of two linked lists representing the interior or exterior of the shape. Two basic procedures are defined for this algorithm: the procedure *switch_in()* moves the boundary outwards by one pixel. The procedure *switch_out()* moves the boundary inwards by one pixel. At each iteration the speed term is calculated for points included in lists L_{out} and L_{in} and the sign is stored in the array $\hat{F}$. The next step consists in scanning both lists sequentially for evolving the curve. When scanning the list L_{out}, the *switch_in()* procedure is applied if $\hat{F} > 0$, moving the curve outwards by one grid point and moving the point to L_{in}. The moved points must be deleted from list L_{out} and the set of neighbor pixels must be updated. Then, the list L_{in} is scanned and the procedure *switch_out()* is applied if $\hat{F} \leq 0$. The moved points must be deleted from list L_{in} and the set of neighbor pixels must be updated. After scanning both lists, the stopping condition is checked. The curve evolution stops when $\hat{F}(\mathbf{x}) \leq 0\ \forall \mathbf{x} \in L_{out}$ or $\hat{F}(\mathbf{x}) \geq 0\ \forall \mathbf{x} \in L_{in}$ or the maximum number of iterations is attained.

During the second cycle corresponding to the smoothness regularization, the curve is evolved according to a smoothing speed $\hat{F}_{int}$ derived from a Gaussian filtering process. A binary indication function of the region Ω is defined as $\chi_\Omega(\mathbf{x})$ from the level set $\hat{\phi}$. The indication function is then processed with a Gaussian filter and the result is binarized using a threshold of 1/2 such that points in L_{out} have a value +1, points in L_{in} have a value of -1 and the rest of points have a value of zero. Once $\hat{F}_{int}$ is calculated, the curve is evolved using the same procedure of the first cycle.

The algorithm could work with edge based data dependent term such as Caselles or region-based data dependent term. In the CREASEG implementation the data dependent term is a region-based Chan Vese speed function.

7.2.8 Chunming Li Algorithm

An additional algorithm incorporated in the CREASEG software is the algorithm of Chunming Li [38]. This is a localized region-based algorithm where the evolution of the level set takes place on the whole domain of the image. Unfortunately, for left ventricle segmentation in MSCT images, the gray level values within the ventricle could be similar to other regions within the same image and the Li method could fail to detect the left ventricle shape. Instead, the algorithm could obtain an over-segmented image. A careful selection of algorithm parameters could reduce the possibility of obtaining new contours far from the left ventricle shape; however, this could happens in some images. Discussion of this limitation is presented in [38]. The algorithm is based in the introduction of a kernel function $\mathbf{K} : \mathcal{R}^n \rightarrow [0, +\infty)$

$$\mathbf{K}(-\mathbf{u}) = \mathbf{K}(\mathbf{u}) \tag{7.19}$$

$$\mathbf{K}(\mathbf{u}) \geq \mathbf{K}(\mathbf{v}) \quad \textit{if}\ |\mathbf{u}| < |\mathbf{v}| \quad \textit{and} \quad \lim_{|\mathbf{u}|\rightarrow\infty} K(\mathbf{u}) = 0 \tag{7.20}$$

$$\int \mathbf{K}(\mathbf{x})d\mathbf{x} = 1 \tag{7.21}$$

A closed contour C is defined in the image domain denoted by D. This contour separates the domain D into two regions: $D_1 = outside(C)$ and $D_2 = inside(C)$. For each pair of points $\mathbf{x}$ and $\mathbf{y}$ it is possible to define the local intensity fitting energy expressed in Eq. 7.22.

$$\varepsilon_{\mathbf{x}}^{Fit}(C, f_1(\mathbf{x}), f_2(\mathbf{x})) = \sum_{i=1}^{2} \lambda_i \int_{D_i} \mathbf{K}(\mathbf{x}-\mathbf{y})|I(\mathbf{y}) - f_i(\mathbf{x})|^2 d\mathbf{y} \tag{7.22}$$

where λ_1 and λ_2 are positive constants and $f_1(\mathbf{x})$, $f_2(\mathbf{x})$ are values approximating the image intensities in D_1 and D_2. $I(\mathbf{y})$ represents the intensity in a local region around $\mathbf{x}$ whose size is controlled by a Gaussian kernel function $\mathbf{K}_\sigma(\mathbf{u})$. For obtaining the object boundary C, it is necessary to minimize $\varepsilon_{\mathbf{x}}^{Fit}$ for all $\mathbf{x}$ in the domain D. This leads to minimizing the energy functional in Eq. 7.23,

$$\varepsilon(C, f_1(\mathbf{x}), f_2(\mathbf{x})) = \int \varepsilon_{\mathbf{x}}^{Fit}(C, f_1(\mathbf{x}), f_2(\mathbf{x}))d\mathbf{x} + \nu|C| \tag{7.23}$$

where ν is a constant penalizing the length of the contour $|C|$.

The standard level set formulation enables obtaining the evolution equation using gradient descent techniques as shown in Eq. 7.24,

$$\frac{\partial\phi}{\partial t} = -\delta_\varepsilon(\phi)(\lambda_1 e_1 - \lambda_2 e_2) + \nu\delta_\varepsilon(\phi) div\left(\frac{\nabla\phi}{|\nabla\phi|}\right) + \mu\left(\nabla^2\phi - div\left(\frac{\nabla\phi}{|\nabla\phi|}\right)\right) \tag{7.24}$$

where δ_ε is a smoothed Dirac delta function. The functions e_1 and e_2 are defined as:

$$e_i(\mathbf{x}) = \int \mathbf{K}_\sigma(\mathbf{y} - \mathbf{x})|I(\mathbf{x}) - f_i(\mathbf{y})|^2 d\mathbf{y}, \quad i = 1, 2 \tag{7.25}$$

f_1, f_2 are given by:

$$f_i(\mathbf{x}) = \frac{\mathbf{K}_\sigma(\mathbf{x}) * \left[\mathbf{M}_i^\varepsilon(\phi(\mathbf{x}))I(\mathbf{x})\right]}{\mathbf{K}_\sigma(\mathbf{x}) * \mathbf{M}_i^\varepsilon(\phi(\mathbf{x}))}, \quad i = 1, 2 \tag{7.26}$$

and $\mathbf{M}_1^\varepsilon(\phi) = H_\varepsilon(\phi)$, $\mathbf{M}_2^\varepsilon(\phi) = 1 - H_\varepsilon(\phi)$ and $H_\varepsilon(\phi)$ is an approximated smoothed Heaviside function.

The first term in Eq. 7.24 is the data fitting term that is responsible for driving the contour towards the object boundaries. The second term, known as arc length term, has a length shortening effect on the contour defined by the level set. The third term is the level set regularization term. This algorithm depends heavily on regularization techniques for keeping the regularity of the level set and avoiding degradation rather than using re-initialization of the level set [22].

In a second contribution, Li et al. [39] propose a modification of this algorithm that is more robust and does not require reinitialization. In this case, rather than using a region–based active contour algorithm where the region information is extracted using a Gaussian kernel, the authors propose to perform the minimization of an energy functional with a distance regularization term and an external energy. The distance regularization term is defined with a potential function that maintains the desired shape of the level set function. The algorithm is known as Distance Regularized Level Set Evolution (DRLSE). In this algorithm the energy functional is defined as:

$$\varepsilon(\phi) = \mu\mathcal{R}_p(\phi) + \varepsilon_{ext}(\phi) \tag{7.27}$$

where $\mu > 0$ is a weighting constant, the level set regularization term is denoted $\mathcal{R}_p(\phi)$ and the second term $\varepsilon_{ext}(\phi)$ is the external energy estimated from the image to be segmented. The regularization term is defined as:

$$\mathcal{R}_p(\phi) = \int_D p(|\nabla\phi|)d\mathbf{x} \tag{7.28}$$

where $p : [0, \infty) \rightarrow \mathbb{R}$ is a potential function aimed at maintaining the signed distance property $|\nabla\phi| = 1$ close to the zero level set, while keeping the level set function constant at locations far from the zero level set such that $|\nabla\phi| = 0$. The selected function $p(s)$ should have a minimum at $s = 1$ and $s = 0$. Such function is expressed as:

$$p(s) = \begin{cases} \frac{1}{(2\pi)^2}(1 - cos(2\pi s)), & \text{if } s \leq 1 \\ \frac{1}{2}(s-1)^2, & \text{if } s \geq 1. \end{cases} \tag{7.29}$$

This function is twice differentiable in $[0, \infty)$ and it has the specified minimum points.

The DRLSE formulation could be applied in several domains considering the appropriate definition for the external energy term ε_{ext}. In the case of image segmentation, there are several possible features for defining such external energy. The features could be region-based or edge-based image formation. In [39], the authors propose an active contour model using edge-based information. The method reported starts by defining an indicator function g in the image domain D as:

$$g = \frac{1}{1 + |\nabla G_\sigma * I|^2} \tag{7.30}$$

where G_σ is a Gaussian kernel with standard deviation σ. The convolution in Eq. 7.30 enables noise reduction and smoothing of the image. The energy function is defined as:

$$\varepsilon_\epsilon = \mu \int_D p(|\phi|)d\mathbf{x} + \lambda \int_D g\delta_\epsilon(\phi)|\nabla\phi|d\mathbf{x} + \alpha \int_D gH_\epsilon(\phi)d\mathbf{x} \tag{7.31}$$

The first term of the energy function is associated with the distance regularization energy $\mathcal{R}_p(\phi)$. The second term calculates the line integral of the function g along the zero level contour of ϕ. This line integral is equivalent to the Caselles energy for a parameterized contour C in their geodesic contour model formulation reported in [19]. The third term calculates a weighted area of the region $D_\phi^- = \{\mathbf{x} : \phi(\mathbf{x}) < 0\}$. This term increases the speed of motion of the zero level set during evolution when the initial contour is placed far away from the target object boundaries. When the initial contour is placed outside of the target object, the coefficient α should be positive and the zero level contour would shrink during the level set evolution. In contrast, when the initial contour is located inside the target object, the coefficient α should take negative values for attaining expansion of the contour. The edge indicator function in this term slow down the shrinking or expanding of the zero level set when it attains the target contour where the values taken by g are smaller.

In this method the Dirac delta and the Heaviside function are approximated by smoothed functions δ_ϵ and H_ϵ used in other methods [22].

$$\delta_\epsilon(\phi) = \begin{cases} \frac{1}{2\epsilon}\left[1 + cos\left(\frac{\pi\phi}{\epsilon}\right)\right], & \text{if } |\phi| \leq \epsilon \\ 0, & \text{if } |\phi| > \epsilon. \end{cases} \tag{7.32}$$

$$H_\epsilon(\phi) = \begin{cases} \frac{1}{2}\left(1 + \frac{\phi}{\epsilon} + \frac{1}{\pi} sin\left(\frac{\pi\phi}{\epsilon}\right)\right), & \text{if } |\phi| \leq \epsilon \\ 1, & \text{if } |\phi| > \epsilon \\ 0, & \text{if } |\phi| < -\epsilon. \end{cases} \tag{7.33}$$

where $H'_\epsilon = \delta_\epsilon$ and parameter ϵ is usually set as 1.5. Minimization of the energy function leads to the gradient flow equation in Eq. 7.34.

$$\frac{\partial\phi}{\partial t} = \mu div(d_p(|\nabla\phi|)\nabla\phi) + \lambda\delta_\epsilon(\phi)\, div\left(g\frac{\nabla\phi}{|\nabla\phi|}\right) + \alpha g\delta_\epsilon(\phi) \tag{7.34}$$

This level set evolution equation is implemented using a narrow band approach that restrict the computation to a narrow band around the zero level set. The DRLSE narrow band formulation does not require reinitialization due to the distance regularization effect. The iteration procedure is limited to updating of the level set function according to Eq. 7.35.

$$\phi_{i,j}^{k+1} = \phi_{i,j}^{k} + \Delta t L\left(\phi_{i,j}^{k}\right) \tag{7.35}$$

where the partial derivative is approximated by the forward difference. For the case, $\Delta x = \Delta y = h$ the time step should be $\mu\Delta t < (h/4)$.

7.2.9 Whitaker Algorithm

The Whitaker contribution reported in [40] presents a Maximum A Posteriori (MAP) approach to 3-D surface reconstruction from range data using the level set algorithm. Additionally, a novel computational technique for level set evolution, known as sparse field algorithm is presented. This type of algorithm has been implemented in open source libraries oriented to 3-D image processing such as ITK [41,42] and ITK-SNAP [15] where a software platform oriented to 3-D image segmentation is proposed.

The evolution equation for the 3-D surface S reconstruction solving the MAP model is expressed as:

$$\frac{\partial S}{\partial t} = -g(S)\vec{\mathcal{N}} + \rho(S) \tag{7.36}$$

where,

$$g(\mathbf{x}) = \sum_j c^j(\mathbf{x})D^j(\mathbf{x})\omega(D^i(\mathbf{x}))\gamma^j(\mathbf{x}) \tag{7.37}$$

represents the model for solving the MAP 3-D surface reconstruction, and $c(\mathbf{x})$ represents the confidence for any spatial point which is different from zero only in the space swept by the scanner. $D(\mathbf{x})$ represents the signed distance from the surface position to the range measurement sensor. $\gamma(\mathbf{x})$ is the Jacobian such that $\gamma(\mathbf{x})d\mathbf{x} = d\psi d\theta da$ representing the unit-volume relationship between scanner coordinates and Cartesian coordinates. The windowing function $\omega(\mathbf{x})$ control the depth of the region behind the range surface where the surface evolution takes place. The variable j counts the number of measurements associated to a particular range map. The term $\rho(S) = -\delta lnP(S)$ is the Euler-Lagrange of the prior. In this application the author proposes a prior that biases the solution toward smooth, continuous surfaces. In other words, given several surfaces near the given data, the algorithm should attain the surface with less area that in general tend to be the smoother surface. The probability distribution for this prior is given by:

$$P(S) = \left(\frac{\beta}{\pi}\right)^{\frac{1}{2}} \exp\left(-\beta \int_S \vec{\mathcal{N}} \cdot \vec{\mathcal{N}} d\mathbf{x}\right) \tag{7.38}$$

where, after orthonormal parameterization with r and s, the Euler Lagrange prior can be represented by the mean curvature of the surface as follow:

$$\rho(S(r,s,t)) = \beta\left(\frac{\partial^2 S}{\partial r^2} + \frac{\partial^2 S}{\partial s^2}\right) \tag{7.39}$$

The parameter β has the role of a regularization constant that control the probability distribution of the surfaces in the prior. A larger value of β enables obtaining smoother surfaces.

Solving the MAP problem expressed in Eq. 7.36 using the level set approach is performed through the following steps: 1) expressing the evolution equation for the problem using a parameterization described in terms of the differential structure of such model, 2) assuming the model is the level set of a function ϕ and 3) the geometry of the level set is expressed in terms of the differential structure of ϕ and the evolution equation of ϕ is derived.

The parametric deformable model for the surface is considered as $S(r,s,t)$, where $r, s \in \mathcal{U} \subset R$ is represented as:

$$S = \{\mathbf{x} \mid \phi(\mathbf{x}, t) = k\} \tag{7.40}$$

Using this definition, the evolution of the level set formulation combining the data term and the prior can be written [40] as:

$$\frac{\partial \phi}{\partial t} = g(\mathbf{x})|\nabla\phi| + \beta\left(\phi_x^2 + \phi_y^2 + \phi_z^2\right)^{-\frac{1}{2}}$$
$$\left[\left(\phi_y^2 + \phi_z^2\right)\phi_{xx} + \left(\phi_z^2 + \phi_x^2\right)\phi_{yy} + \left(\phi_x^2 + \phi_y^2\right)\phi_{zz} - \phi_p\right] \tag{7.41}$$
$$\phi_p = 2\phi_x\phi_y\phi_{xy} + 2\phi_y\phi_z\phi_{yz} + 2\phi_z\phi_x\phi_{zx} \tag{7.42}$$

In Whitaker et al. [43] they report an application of this algorithm for segmentation of 3-D images. The evolution equation for the level set is expressed as:

$$\frac{\partial \phi}{\partial t} = |\nabla\phi|\left[\alpha g(\mathbf{x}) + (1-\alpha)\nabla\cdot\frac{\nabla\phi}{|\nabla\phi|}\right], \tag{7.43}$$

where $\beta = 1-\alpha$ and the mean curvature is expressed as $\nabla\cdot\nabla\phi/|\nabla\phi|$. The data term $g(\mathbf{x})$ allows the model to expand or contract towards image features. The parameter $\alpha \in (0, 1]$ controls the smoothness of the contour obtained. In this application authors propose a simple data term aiming at real time visualization. The data term is expressed as:

$$g(\mathbf{x}) = \epsilon - |I(\mathbf{x}) - T|, \tag{7.44}$$

where T controls the brightness of the segmented region and ϵ sets the range of gray values around T that are considered inside the contour. In this way the model would expand to include voxels in the interval $T \pm \epsilon$ or it would contract to exclude voxels outside the given interval.

7.3 Numerical Implementation of Level Set Algorithms

Efficient implementations such as the method previously described of Shi [25] allows to reduce the computation time. Additionally, in a contribution of Adalstein and Sethian [33], they have proposed the *narrow band* method and later Whitaker has proposed the sparse field method [40].

The first term in Eq. 7.41 could attain an unstable or erroneous solution when simple forward finite differences are used. This equation is usually solved using the *up-wind* approach proposed by Osher and Sethian [27] for avoiding the instabilities and overshooting of simple forward finite differences. This approach uses one-side derivatives denoted as $d^{(+)}$ and $d^{(-)}$ that can be expressed as:

$$d^{(+)}\hat{\phi}_{x,y,z} = \frac{(\hat{\phi}_{x+h,y,z} - \hat{\phi}_{x,y,z})}{h} \tag{7.45}$$
$$d^{(-)}\hat{\phi}_{x,y,z} = \frac{(\hat{\phi}_{x,y,z} - \hat{\phi}_{x-h,y,z})}{h} \tag{7.46}$$

where h is the spacing within a regular rectilinear grid. The second term of Eq. 7.41 is solved using a finite forward difference approach with centralized differences and it does not require the *up-wind* method. Two efficient methods are described in the following paragraphs.

7.3.1 Narrow-Band Implementation

When dealing with applications where only a single level set $\phi(\mathbf{x}, t) = k$ is necessary. The evolution of ϕ is evaluated only in a neighborhood of this level set known as a *narrow-band*. The *narrow-band* approach calculates an embedding function around the level set using a signed distance transform. This distance transforms is calculated for a region width of only m points. The rest of points are set to a constant value indicating that they are outside of the *narrow-band*. The level set evolves in the band. The distance transform is re-calculated when the level set approaches the edge of the region and the process is repeated. Even when this method is useful for reducing the computational cost, it has several limitations such as the requirement of having a band with a large m ($m = 12$ in [33]) and using smoothing techniques for maintaining the stability of the contour at the boundaries of the band.

7.3.2 Sparse Field Algorithms

A more efficient computational solution approach is the sparse field method. According to this method, an implicit approximation to the distance transform is used at each time step in a neighborhood of the level set model. This method enables calculation of updates on a band of grid points that is only one point wide. The approximation to the level set function is denoted $\hat{\phi}$ and the set of grid points adjacent to $\hat{\phi}$ is the active set with elements known as *active points*. Deformation of the contour implies changing the values within this set. All derivatives up to the second order are estimated using nearest neighbor differences. In this way, only *active points* and their neighbors are relevant for the evolution of the approximated level set.

Active points must be adjacent to the estimated level set model $\hat{\phi}$ and this adjacency defines an implicit distance transform that is maintained by considering only a range of values for $\hat{\phi}$. When an *active point* is moved out of this *active range*, the point must be excluded from the *active set* and other grid points moving into the *active range* must be included within the *active set*. The neighborhoods of the *active set* are defined in layers: $L_N, \ldots, L_{+1}$ for the layers inside the object and $L_{-1}, \ldots, L_{-N}$ for the layers outside the object. The index represents a city-block distance from the nearest active point. For instance, with a city-block distance of 2 to the corners, five layers are required, two inside, two outside and the level set. They are denoted as $L_2, L_1, L_0, L_{-1}, L_{-2}$. The algorithm is implemented using linked-list data structures in combination with arrays for storing the values at each grid point and status. The status of each point is a label map that defines to which layer a point belongs. For the given example, it is required 5 labels plus an additional label for points outside the region. The label values are the set $\{-3, -2, -1, 0, 1, 2, 3\}$. A more detailed description of the algorithm can be found in [40]. An implementation of the sparse field algorithm of Whitaker is reported by Lankton in [44], including the open source software written in C and Matlab. The implemented algorithm works with a data term of the energy function of type Chan Vese [22].

7.4 Methods

7.4.1 Multi–Slice CT Image Dataset

A dataset of 307 axial slices extracted from 10, 3-D MSCT images was considered for this research. Each slice has a size of 512 × 512. The set is extracted from the region of interest where the left ventricle is located and from different locations along the left ventricle. The set includes contrast variations, low and high contrasted images, presence of papillary muscles and connection with the left atrium. Segmentation for this set is challenging due to the mentioned imperfections of the image dataset. The image dataset was subdivided in 20 images for training and 287 images for validation and comparison. The segmentation algorithms were also tested using a 3-D MSCT cardiac image in diastole.

An additional experiment concerning the 3-D segmentation of the external wall of the left ventricle was performed using the 3-D MSCT images in diastole for 14 patients. For this experiment all processing chores were implemented using the software platform described in [45], [46].

7.4.2 Image Pre–Processing

The image pre–processing pipeline is represented in Figure 7.1. The image is processed with a Gaussian filter of size 3 × 3, aiming at attenuating the noise without smearing the image contours. The image is further processed with a median filter with size 5 × 5. This filter is very useful for attenuating impulsive noise while preserving the contours. As the contrast between the left ventricle lumen and the wall could be low due to insuficient X-Rays contrast or non uniform mixture of the contrast and the blood, it is necessary another processing stage that corresponds to an anisotropic diffusion filter [47]. This type of filter has demonstrated reduction of noise while preserving and enhancing the contours. In this case the evolution equation is given by the diffusion equation where the speed term is proportional to the curvature of the contour [48]:

$$I_t = \kappa |\nabla I| \tag{7.47}$$

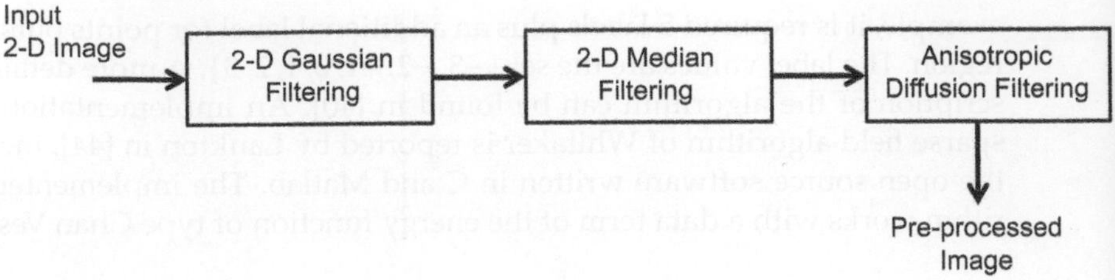

FIGURE 7.1
Image pre-processing.

where κ is the curvature and ∇I is the image gradient. With this filter, the small and noisy contours would tend to disappear due to high diffusion, while strong and smooth contours between objects would be preserved due to low diffusion. The LV contour was traced in each image by a medical doctor. The contours traced by the medical doctor were considered as the reference for validating the segmentation algorithms as ground truth.

7.4.3 Evaluation

Several error measures have been proposed in the literature [49], [50]. Some of these error measures are Dice Similarity (DS), Jaccard Coefficient (JC) and Volume Similarity (VS) in the case of 3-D images. All these error measures take values between 0 and 1. In this research the quality of the segmentation is estimated using the Dice similarity coefficient [51]. This coefficient has been shown to provide good results for evaluation of image segmentation. This coefficient measures the degree of overlap between two binary images. These binary images are the reference image traced by the medical doctor and the segmentation result. The value of this coefficient ranges between 0 when there is not overlap to 1 when there is a perfect overlap between the two binary shapes. Let A and B denote two binary shapes then the Dice coefficient can be estimated as:

$$Dice = \frac{2|A \cap B|}{|A| + |B|} \tag{7.48}$$

where $|A|$, $|B|$ and $|A \cap B|$ represent the number of non zero pixels in each binary set.

7.4.4 Parameter Setting and Tuning

The set of parameters was determined during the training procedure using a set of 20 slices, some of these images are shown in Figure 7.2. Initially the default set of parameters was considered. For each algorithm one of the parameters was varied while the rest remained fixed. For each parameter value,

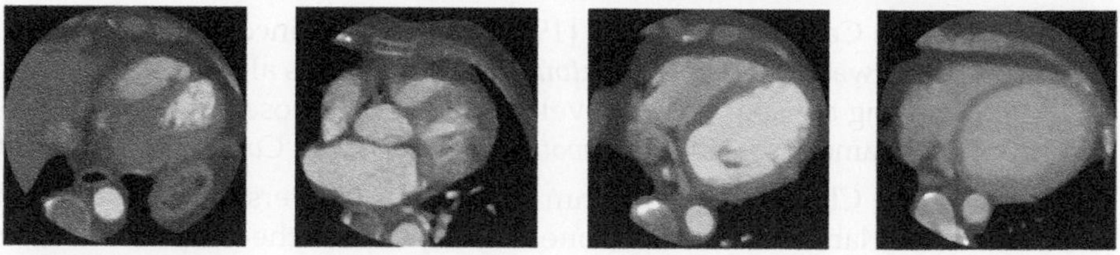

FIGURE 7.2
Some of the images in the training set.

the Dice coefficient was calculated for all the images and the maximum average Dice value attained defined the parameter value. The procedure was repeated for each of the parameters. The algorithms were initialized with a shape traced by the user.

Each of the algorithms compared required a different set of parameters. Such parameters are described in the next section 7.4.5 as well as the values obtained during the tuning stage. All the level set algorithms with the exception the fast marching algorithm, require an additional parameter corresponding to the maximum number of iterations. The maximum number of iterations for each algorithm is shown in Table 7.1.

7.4.5 Algorithms Comparison

Nine segmentation algorithms were compared. The algorithms compared have source code freely available on internet or included in the Matlab software. The set of algorithms compared are the following:

- The Bernard algorithm [23] is the version incorporated in the CREASEG GUI software [26]. In this algorithm the scale parameter is set as $h = 0$, the step size is set as $\alpha_f' = 2.0$ and the number of iterations is 3. The rest of parameters are pre-defined in the set of default parameters.

TABLE 7.1
Maximum Number of Iterations

Algorithm	Maximum Number of Iterations
Bernard Algorithm [23]	4
Caselles [19]	200
Chan Vese [22]	16
Fast Marching [52]	-
Lankton [21]	100
Region Growing [24]	-
Shi [25]	4
Chunming Li [39]	inner=10, outer=4
Sparse Field Model (Lankton version) [44]	120

- The Caselles algorithm [19] is the version incorporated in the Matlab software as the *activecontour(.)* function. This algorithm is implemented using the sparse field level set method proposed by Whitaker [40]. The parameters used are *SmoothFactor* = 1.5 and *ContractionBias* = −0.4.
- The Chan Vese Algorithm [22] is also the version implemented in the Matlab software that is one of the options of the *activecontour(.)* function. The implementation is also based in the sparse level set method [40]. The parameters are similar as the previous case: *SmoothFactor* = 1.5 and *ContractionBias* = −0.4.
- The Fast Marching Method [29,30,52], is also the version incorporated in the Matlab software in the *imsegfmm(.)* function. The function requires a matrix of weights values for each pixel, representing gray level differences between each pixel and the gray level value of pixels included in an input binary mask. The weight matrix is estimated using the *graydiffweight()* function. The algorithm requires a threshold parameter necessary for obtaining the segmentation binary shape from the geodesic distance matrix that is estimated in the *imsegfmm(.)* function. The value for this parameter is *threshold* = 0.0004.
- The Lankton algorithm is a software developed by Lankton for implementing the algorithm reported in [21]. The parameters for this algorithm are the radius of the neighborhood $B(x, y)$ that is set as *rad* = 1[illegible] and the regularization parameter is set as $\lambda = 0.8$.
- A simple and common algorithm for segmentation is the region growing algorithm [24]. Even when this type of algorithm is not within the level set category, it is important their comparison with respect to the level set algorithms because region growing algorithms are widely used for segmentation. The implementation compared is an open source algorithm downloaded from the MathWorks file exchange webpage.
- The Shi algorithm [25] correspond to a level set algorithm oriented to real time operation. In this research the algorithm compared corresponds to the CREASEG GUI software implementation [26] adapted to newer versions of Matlab software. The parameters considered are N that represents the number of iterations for the evolution of the external force term. N_s represents the steps of the smoothing cycle and N_g represents the size of the Gaussian filter used during the smoothing cycle with standard deviation σ. The value of these parameters are N_a = [illegible] $N_s = 3$, $\sigma = 2$ and $N_g = 7$.
- The Chunming Li [39] algorithm compared correspond to the Distance Regularized Level Set Evolution (DRLSE) method. The parameters for this algorithm are μ that represents the weight of the distance regularization term, λ is the weight of the weighted length term, α is the weight of the weighted area term, ϵ is the width of the Dirac delta function and *TimeStep* is the time resolution for the finite difference approach. Th[illegible]

value for these parameters are: $\mu = 0.04$, $\lambda = 6$, $\alpha = -2.9$, $\epsilon = 1.05$ and $TimeStep = 5$.

- An additional Sparse Field Method implementation compared is reported in [44]. The algorithm minimizes the Chan Vese energy. The parameters are λ that is a regularization relative weighting of curve smoothness with values between 0 and 1. Other parameter is the radius of the ball used for localization following the approach described in [21]. The regularization parameter is set as $\lambda = 0.6$ and the radius of localization is set as $rad = 16$.

7.4.6 Initialization

Level set based segmentation requires an initialization binary mask and results are heavily dependent on this shape [53]. If the initialization shape is far from the target contour it could require a large number of iterations and computation time, and eventually, the algorithms could get trapped in a local minimum without attain the actual contour. Initialization is application dependent and several approaches has been reported. A simple approach is semiautomatic segmentation where the user traces manually the initial contour as in [26]. A simple semiautomatic threshold based method is used in [15]. The Otsu threshold method has been used in [54] for segmentation of vertebra CT images. In [53] initial contours are obtained using mean shift clustering without any prior knowledge. A seeded region growing algorithm is used in [55] for the segmentation of hippocampus in Magnetic Resonance Images. The initialization mask is obtained after fitting a convex polygon to the region growing segmentation. Initialization of the level set algorithm is performed in [56], based on fusion of fuzzy C mean clustering and histogram thresholding for segmentation of skin lesions. In general initialization of level sets for left ventricle segmentation is still an open problem that requires research work.

In a previous work reported in [57] an initialization method for level sets segmentation of the left ventricle is described. The algorithm is based on using marker–controlled watershed and region growing segmentation. The algorithm enables initialization for level sets segmentation of the left ventricle in 2-D MSCT images. However, the limitation of this algorithm is the requirement of setting a large number of parameters. For this reason in this research, a simpler initialization algorithm is used. The initialization mask is obtained using a simple seeded region growing algorithm followed by a mathematical morphology operation corresponding to closing with a disk shaped structuring element of radius 3. The mask is then processed using an erosion operation with a disk shaped structuring element of radius 6. The mathematical morphology operations are intended to close small holes in the binary shape, erase small isolated clusters of pixels and keeping the contour slightly inside the actual shape giving room for level set evolution improvements.

7.4.7 Algorithms Comparison on Noisy Images

A test of segmentation was performed on noisy images. A synthetic image showing two concentric disks was generated. Each of the disks had a different gray level value. The image was contaminated with zero mean Gaussian noise for attaining several values of PSNR. All images were segmented without pre–processing filtering using an initialization shape traced by the user as shown in Figure 7.12. A total of ten noise realizations were considered. The Dice similarity coefficient was calculated between the shape of the segmentation obtained and the shape of the target disk.

7.4.8 Left Ventricle External Wall Segmentation

Segmentation of both walls of the left ventricle enables calculation of the left ventricle mass, which is useful for assessment of left ventricular function. In particular, this parameter is used for diagnosis of left ventricle hypertrophy. The segmentation of the left ventricle external wall is challenging [58]. The external wall has low contrast variations between the heart muscle and surrounding structures as well as local contrast variations within the same tissue over time [59]. This fact is complicated with the combination of cardiac and breathing motion. Several attempts to perform the segmentation of myocardium have been proposed. The effort has been centered on MRI images, where several segmentation methods have been reported mainly in 2-D images [60]. In Avendi et al. [61] a method for segmentation of the left ventricle in MRI images is proposed using deep learning algorithms combined with deformable models. The algorithm was trained with the shapes of the left ventricle extracted from a public database but the method required to increase the number of training cases using transformations. The learned shapes were used within the level set Chan Vese algorithm. Tsai et al. [62] proposed a shape-based approach for guiding the evolution of a level set deformable contour. They derive a parametric model for a segmenting curve expressed using an implicit representation. The model is obtained using Principal Component Analysis (PCA) to the training data represented using a signed distance transformation. The formulation used for the level set segmentation algorithm is a modification of the region-based Chan Vese algorithm proposed by Yezzi et al. [63]. This technique is used for 2-D segmentation of the endocardium of the left ventricle shape in MRI images.

A model–based framework for detection of heart structures has been reported by Ecabert *et al.* [9]. The heart is represented as a triangulated mesh model including RV, LV, atria, myocardium, and great vessels. The cardiac model is located near the target heart using the 3-D generalized Hough transform. Finally, in order to detect the cardiac anatomy, parametric deformable adaptations are applied to the model.

In this research, the external wall segmentation is centered around the utilization of a level set algorithm. The segmentation of this anatomical structure is performed in 3-D using the software platform described in [45,46]. The software platform is oriented to research in cardiac segmentation. The platform enables reading DICOM format images, visualization using volumetric rendering and multi-planar reformating techniques. Pre-processing in 3-D using filters implemented in VTK and ITK. Selection of Regions of Interest (ROI) including the left ventricle. Segmentation of the endocardial shape of the left ventricle in 3-D using connected confidence region growing, fast marching algorithms and level set geodesic contour (Caselles) algorithm. Segmentation of the external wall of the left ventricle using a 3-D geodesic contour algorithm. Quantification of volume and mass of the left ventricle as well as tools for interactive manual segmentation.

The pipeline used for the external wall segmentation of the left ventricle is shown in Figure 7.3. The external wall segmentation is performed using a geodesic active contour implemented in ITK using the class *itkGeodesicActiveContourLevelSetImageFilter*. This class implements the level set Caselles active contour algorithm [19]. The algorithm requires two inputs: the seed point or seed region is obtained from the endocardial binary shape after processing with a distance transformation that in this case is performed using the ITK class *itkSignedDanielssonDistanceMapImageFilter*, where the Euclidean distance to the contour shape is calculated [64]. The distance transform assign negative distances for points within the shape and positive distances for

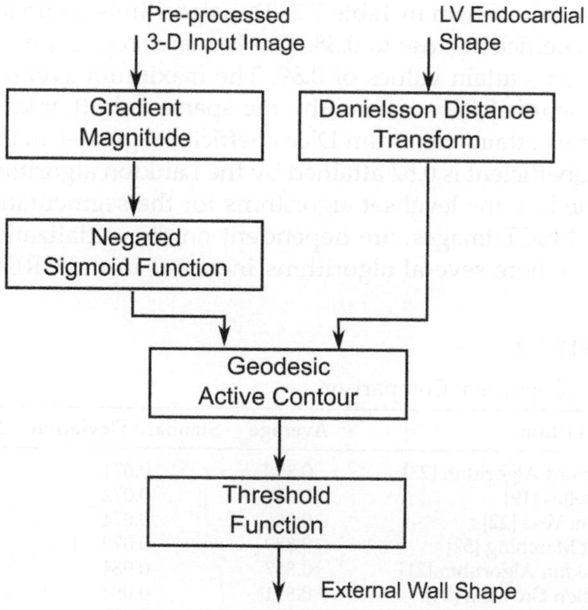

FIGURE 7.3
3-D left ventricle external wall segmentation.

points outside the shape. The second input to the geodesic active contour algorithm is obtained from the pre-processed 3-D input image before ROI extraction. The gradient magnitude is obtained and then processed with a negated sigmoid function for allowing the level set to evolve towards the external left ventricle wall. The final external wall binary shape is obtained by processing the level set function with a threshold function. The left ventricle endocardial shape can be obtained either by using the connected confidence region growing algorithm as detailed in [45] or using a geodesic active contour previously described.

In this research, the segmentation is performed either for the endocardial wall an the externall wall using the level set based method. This enables calculation of the left ventricle wall volume and mass. The accuracy of the segmentation is evaluated using the Dice similarity coefficient with respect to manual segmentation performed by medical staff.

7.5 Results

7.5.1 Performance Comparison on 2-D MSCT Images

The results obtained during the comparison test with respect to the Dice coefficient are shown in Table 7.2. The algorithms attain an average Dice similarity coefficient close to 0.88. The Bernard, region growing and sparse field algorithms attain values of 0.89. The maximum average value for the Dice coefficient is 0.986 obtained by the sparse field (Lankton) algorithm. All algorithms attain maximum Dice coefficients greater than 0.96. The minimum Dice Coefficient is 0.57 attained by the Lankton algorithm. In general, results obtained by the level set algorithms for the segmentation of the left ventricle in MSCT images, are dependent on the initialization. In a previous research where several algorithms included in the CREASEG software were

TABLE 7.2
Dice Coefficient Comparison

Algorithm	Average	Standard Deviation	Minimum	Maximum
Bernard Algorithm [23]	0.890	0.071	0.642	0.975
Caselles [19]	0.880	0.072	0.635	0.978
Chan Vese [22]	0.866	0.074	0.638	0.968
Fast Marching [52]	0.889	0.079	0.604	0.980
Lankton Algorithm [21]	0.887	0.084	0.577	0.985
Region Growing [24]	0.891	0.084	0.584	0.982
Shi Algorithm [25]	0.882	0.073	0.641	0.969
Shunming Li Algorithm [39]	0.887	0.081	0.636	0.983
Sparse Field (lankton) [44]	0.890	0.075	0.634	0.986

compared [57] two type of initialization were used. The first type was a shape traced by the user and the maximum average Dice coefficient attained by the Caselles algorithm was 0.94. Results obtained using the initialization based on marker–controlled watershed and region growing segmentation attained a Dice coefficient of 0.88 for the Caselles algorithm. In that research the image validation set was smaller. One of the limitations of the semi-automatic initialization is the fact that the obtained mask in general excludes the papillary muscles and it could be far from the actual contour. In such cases, the final shape obtained with the level set algorithms could also exclude the papillary muscles and providing segmentation with lower Dice similarity values.

A boxplot for the Dice coefficient is shown on Figure 7.4. All algorithms compared have a median close to 0.90. The data between 25% and 75% quartiles for all methods is located approximately in the range [0.85; 0.95]. There are outliers for all methods representing low Dice coefficients. In general, the low Dice coefficients occur when the image has poor contrast or when the slice has a high density of papillary muscles that prevent the algorithm from attaining the actual contour. Comparison of the obtained results is calculated using the Kruskal-Wallis test [65]. This method is useful for testing whether samples originate from the same distribution. It is a non-parametric method that would be equivalent to the parametric one-way analysis of variance (ANOVA). Results concerning the Dice similarity coefficient show that all algorithm compared have a similar performance with the exception of the Chan Vese algorithm whose performance is different with respect to the rest

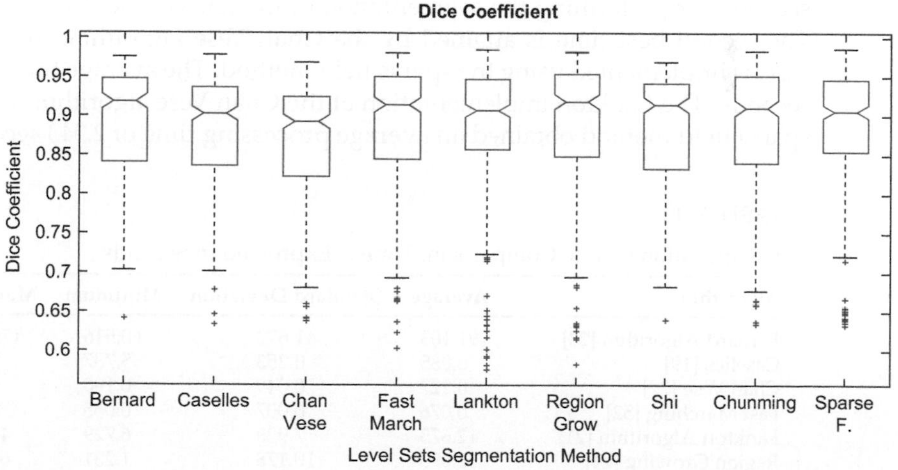

FIGURE 7.4
Boxplot representing the results of the Dice coefficient comparison for the level set algorithms. All algorithms compared have a mean value close to 0.90.

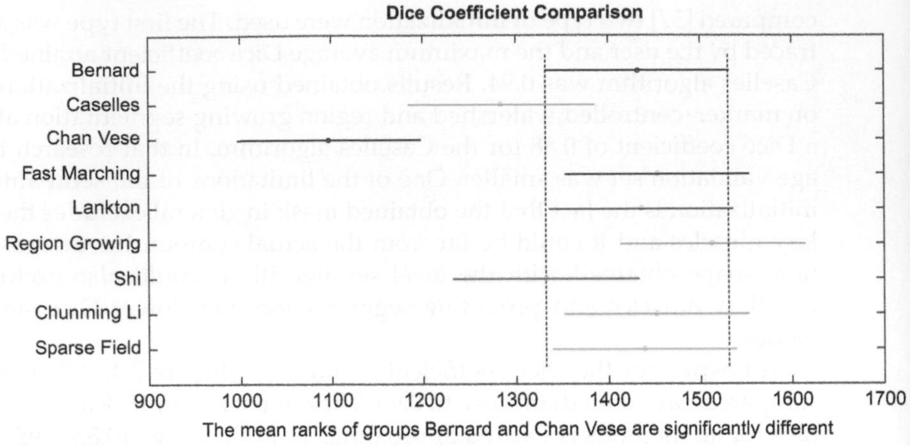

FIGURE 7.5
Dice coefficient comparison for the level set algorithms. Results of the Kruskal-Wallis test that show the ranking obtained by the algorithms. The group including Bernard, Caselles, fast marching, Lankton, region growing, Shi, Chunming Li and sparse field model (Lankton) has a different performance with respect to the Chan Vese algorithm.

of algorithms. Results of the comparison are shown in Figure 7.5. Observe that this difference only implies a small reduction in terms of the Dice similarity coefficient.

The results obtained concerning the execution time are shown in Table 7.3. The corresponding boxplot is shown in Figure 7.6. The fast marching algorithm has the lowest computation time corresponding to an average of 0.076 seconds for performing the segmentation of the left ventricle in one image. The second best time is attained by the Chan Vese algorithm, that in this case, is implemented using the sparse field method. The average time is 0.227 seconds. The Lankton implementation of the Chan Vese algorithm using the sparse field method obtained an average processing time of 2.343 seconds in

TABLE 7.3
Computational Time Comparison. Time is Expressed in Seconds

Algorithm	Average	Standard Deviation	Minimum	Maximum
Bernard Algorithm [23]	91.103	41.672	60.516	170.340
Caselles [19]	6.085	0.253	5.737	7.189
Chan Vese [22]	0.227	0.049	0.190	0.544
Fast Marching [52]	0.076	0.007	0.065	0.153
Lankton Algorithm [21]	12.675	7.923	6.729	44.268
Region Growing [24]	12.693	10.178	1.231	66.071
Shi Algorithm [25]	5.063	3.359	1.472	21.591
Shunming Li Algorithm [39]	5.009	0.296	4.806	5.916
Sparse Field (lankton) [44]	2.343	3.632	0.243	14.828

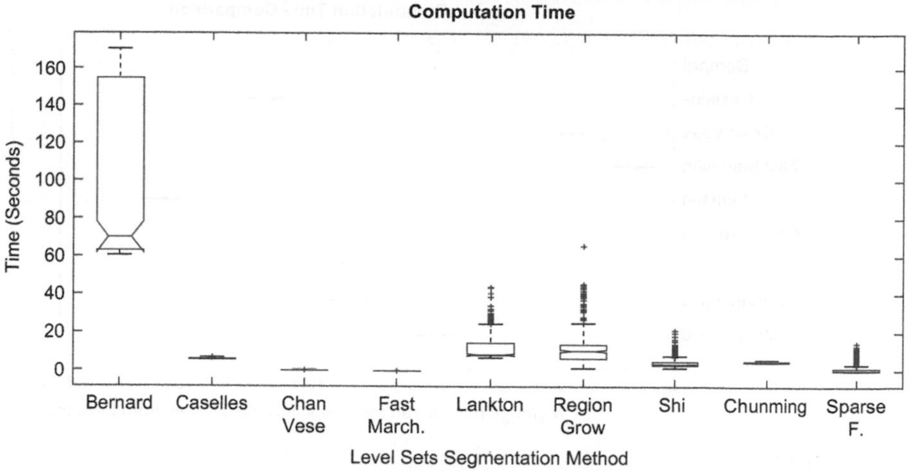

FIGURE 7.6
Boxplot representing the results for the computation time comparison for the level set algorithms. The Bernard algorithm has the highest computational time.

the third place. The Chunming Li algorithm obtained 5.009 seconds, the Shi algorithm had an average time of 5.063 seconds and the Caselles algorithm had a computation time of 6.085 seconds. The Bernard Algorithm attained the highest average computation time of 91.103 seconds. The computation time for the localized Lankton algorithm was 12.675 seconds and 12.693 seconds for the region growing algorithm. The boxplot for this parameter shows that the algorithms Caselles, Chan Vese, fast marching and Chunming Li have lower average computation time with low variance. The comparison of the results concerning the computation time is shown in Figure 7.7. The algorithms Shi and Chunming Li have a similar performance as well as the Lankton and region growing algorithms. The performance obtained for the rest of algorithms is different and its rank is shown in Figure 7.7.

Results of the segmentation of the left ventricle using the Caselles algorithm are shown in Figure 7.8. A subset of slices is extracted from the test set and the segmentation contour is shown overlaid on the corresponding slice. In general the segmentation shape is a good representation of the shape of the left ventricle in each slice. The algorithm is robust and it is able to recover the left ventricle shape even in the slices located at the apex where the contrast is poor and the density of papillary muscles is high. When the slices include a well contrasted left ventricle lumen the differences between results of the compared algorithms are difficult to visualize. However, when the slice represent a low area, poor contrasted or a high density of papillary muscles, the differences between results of the segmentation provided by the compared algorithms could be apparent. In Figures 7.9 and 7.10 the results of the level set algorithms compared are presented for a subset of slices with features that

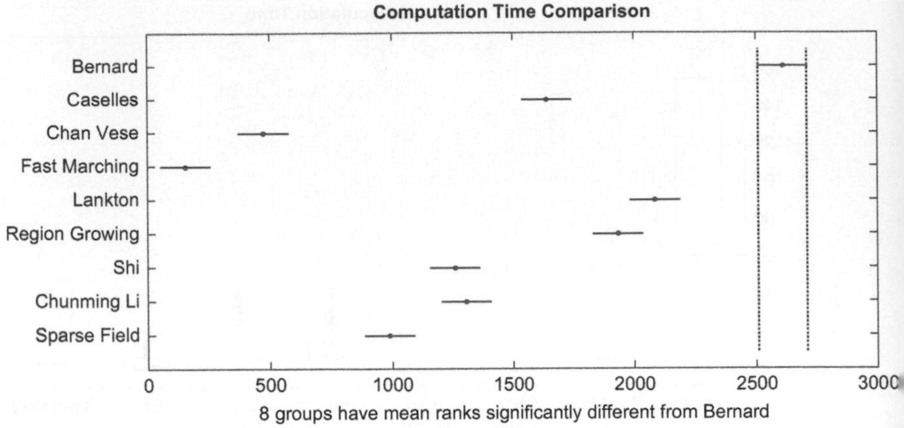

FIGURE 7.7
Computation time comparison for the level set algorithms. The plot shows the results of the Kruskal-Wallis test corresponding to the ranking of each algorithm. The fastest algorithm is fast marching and the slowest is the Bernard algorithm.

make them difficult for segmentation. Each of the rows in Figure 7.9 represents the results of the segmentation for one of the level set methods, from top to bottom the methods are: Bernard, Caselles, Chan Vese, fast marching Lankton and Shi. The methods corresponding to Chunming Li and sparse field (Lankton) are shown in Figure 7.10.

The segmentation methods are initialized using the procedure described in section 7.4.6. Concerning the image in the first column in Figure 7.9 from left to right, most of the algorithms have good results except for the fast marching algorithm and Lankton where the contour does not match the actual contour at the upper right. The image in the second column is difficult and all algorithms with the exception of the Caselles algorithm, fail at obtaining the segmentation. The algorithms get trapped by the papillary muscles. Comparatively, the result provided by the Caselles algorithm is outstanding. The image in the third column is also difficult and in general all algorithms fail as they only recover approximately half of the left ventricle shape. The best results are obtained by the algorithms Bernard, Caselles, Chan Vese and Shi. The rest of algorithms obtain a shape subdivided into smaller portions. Results for the image in the fourth column are sub-optimal except for the Caselles algorithm that is able to recover the entire shape. Results for the Chunming Li and sparse field method (Lankton) are shown in Figure 7.10 the shape obtained for these images is sub-optimal for both algorithms.

The Lankton algorithm that uses a localized approach for the optimization has an important limitation. When the algorithm is initialized with a shape that is to far from the actual contour and the setting for the radius of the localized region is small. The algorithm rather than growing for approaching

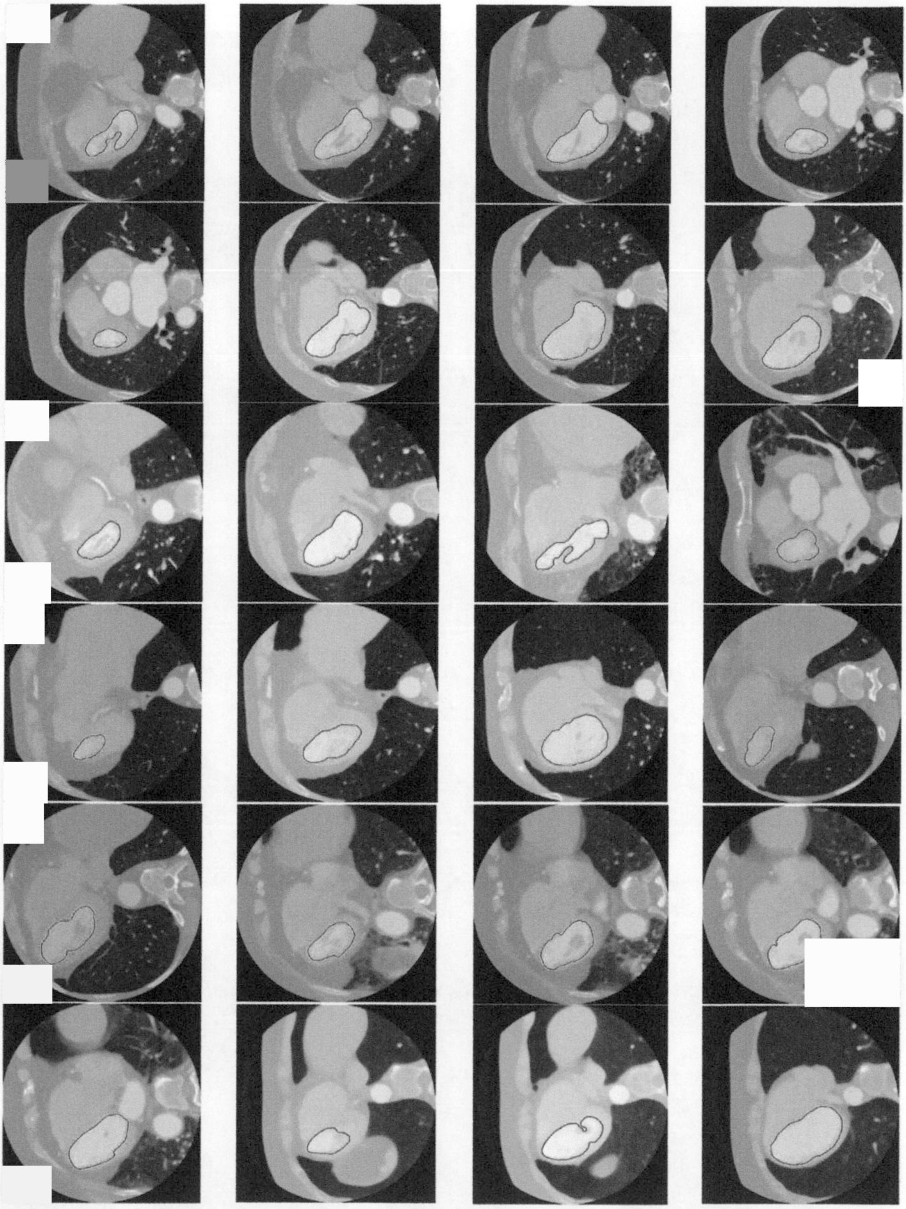

FIGURE 7.8
Results of the segmentation using the Caselles algorithms. The contour of the segmentation of the left ventricle is overlaid on each of the slice. In this figure a subset of the test set is shown. The set of slices shown comes from several 3-D MSCT cardiac images in diastole. The Caselles algorithm in general has an excellent performance as the contour of the segmentation are located over the actual contour of the left ventricle.

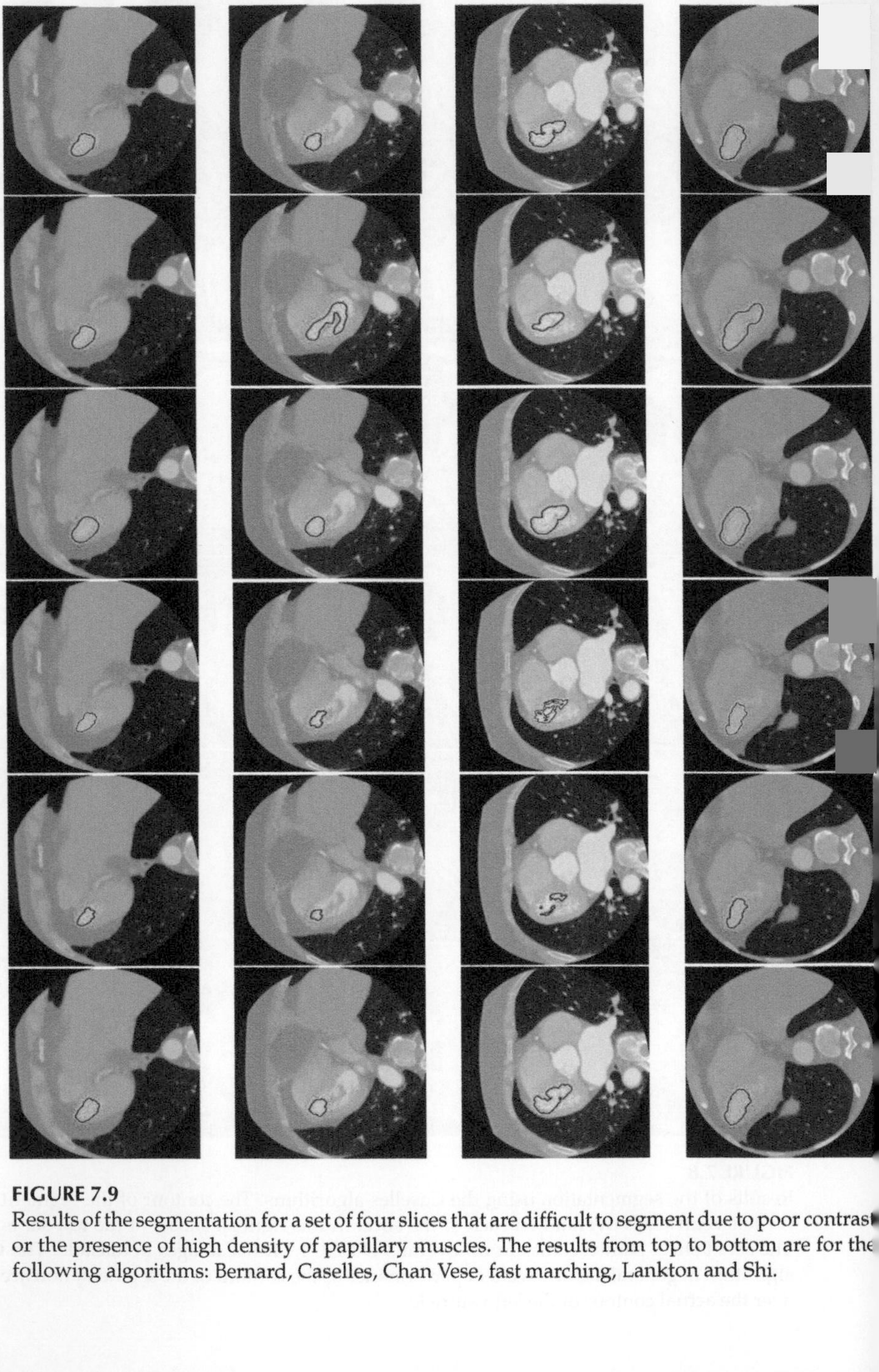

FIGURE 7.9
Results of the segmentation for a set of four slices that are difficult to segment due to poor contrast or the presence of high density of papillary muscles. The results from top to bottom are for the following algorithms: Bernard, Caselles, Chan Vese, fast marching, Lankton and Shi.

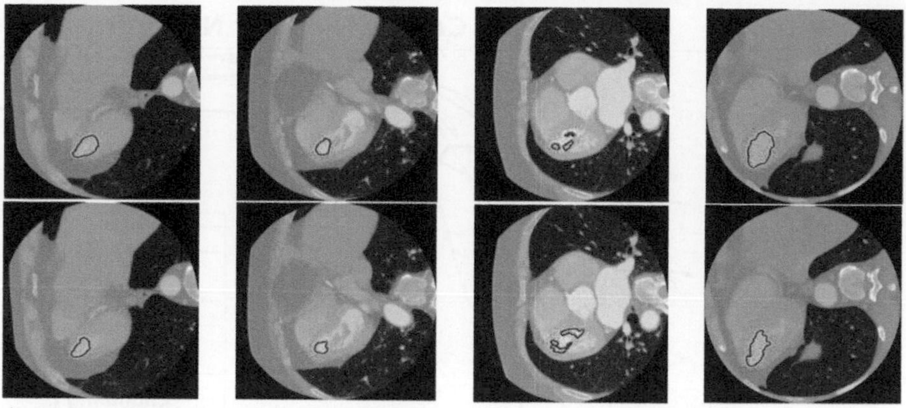

FIGURE 7.10
Results of the segmentation for a set of four slices that are difficult to segment due to poor contrast or the presence of high density of papillary muscles. The results from top to bottom are for the Chunming Li and sparse field model algorithm.

the contour, begin to shrink and eventually collapses without providing any segmentation.

7.5.2 Comparison on Noisy Images

Results of the average Dice coefficient as a function of the PSNR of the image are shown in Figure 7.11. With higher values of PSNR representing low content of noise, the Dice similarity coefficient attained by the algorithms compared is clustered into three groups. The group corresponding to Chunming Li, sparse field (Lankton) and region growing attained the highest value close to 0.99. The second group includes the algorithms Caselles, Chan Vese, Bernard and Shi with Dice values close to 0.98. Then, the fast marching algorithm attains a value close to 0.95. The region growing algorithm is highly sensible to the presence of Gaussian noise and its performance is poor for PSNR values lower than 23 dB. The Caselles algorithm is highly robust as the variation of the Dice value is low when the PSNR decreases. The lower dice coefficient attained for the group including Chan Vese, Bernard, Chunming Li and fast marching is 0.80 when the PSNR decreases to 4.8 dB. The group including Lankton, sparse field (Lankton) and Shi is less robust than the previous group. For the level set algorithms compared, the cut-off PSNR is about 15 dB.

Results of the segmentation for an image with a PSNR=5 dB are shown in Figure 7.12. In Figure 7.12(a) the noisy input image is shown. In Figure 7.12(b) the reference contour is shown. In Figure 7.12(c) the contour used for initialization is shown and the segmentation result using the Caselles algorithm is shown in Figure 7.12(d). The Dice coefficient obtained for this segmentation is 0.96.

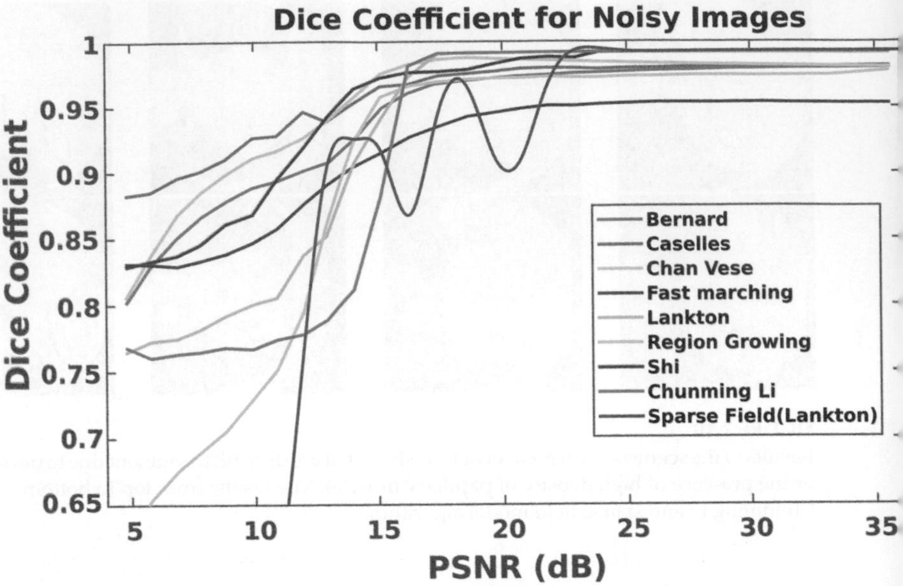

FIGURE 7.11
Average Dice coefficient as a function of the PSNR of the input image. The Caselles algorithm is highly robust as the variation of the Dice coefficient is small even when the change in PSNR is high.

7.5.3 Performance Comparison on a 3-D MSCT Image

An additional comparison test is performed on a 3-D MSCT cardiac image in diastole. The image has a size of 512 × 512 × 393. The pre-processing for this image was performed in 3-D using the software platform described in [45]. The 3-D image is processed with a Gaussian filter considering a standard deviation close to 1. The 3-D image is further processed with a 3-D median filter implemented using the Visualization Toolkit (VTK) [66] with neigborhood

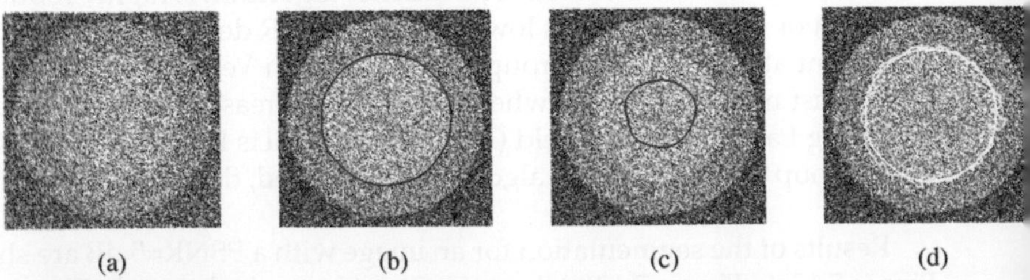

FIGURE 7.12
Results of the Caselles algorithm in a phantom image with a PSNR of 5 dB. (a) Noisy input image, (b) Reference contour overlaid on the input image, (c) Initialization contour and (d) Result of the segmentation compared with the reference contour. The Dice coefficient is 0.96.

of radius 5. This filter is very useful for attenuating impulsive noise while preserving the contours. Another processing stage applied, corresponds to an anisotropic diffusion filter [47]. This filter is implemented in the Insight Toolkit (ITK) [31,42]. This type of filter has demonstrated reduction of noise while preserving and enhancing the contours. In this case the evolution equation is given by the diffusion equation where the speed term is proportional to the curvature of the contour [48]. The last stage of pre-processing is obtaining a ROI including the left ventricle.

The segmentation is performed on a 2-D slice basis, considering the axial view. For each slice the user trace a seed point used for obtaining the initialization mask based on the region growing algorithm. The number of slices segmented for extracting the 3-D left ventricle shape are 128. The segmentation was performed using all the algorithms compared and the Dice similarity coefficient is calculated in 2-D for each of the segmented slices. The Dice similarity coefficient is estimated with respect to a manual segmentation traced by medical staff.

Results of the validation concerning the Dice similarity coefficient are shown in Table 7.4. The highest average Dice similarity coefficient is attained by the Chan Vese algorithm with a value of 0.941 while the lowest value is attained by the sparse field (Lankton) algorithm with a value of 0.866. The localized Lankton algorithm attained an average Dice coefficient of 0.891. The remaining of algorithms attained values of the Dice coefficient higher than 0.90. The Box plot representing the results of the Dice similarity coefficient for the segmentation methods compared is presented in Figure 7.13. All algorithms compared attain a median value of the Dice coefficient larger than 0.90. The best performance in this case is attained by the Chan Vese algorithm with a median value close to 0.95. The comparison performed using the Krustal-Wallis method is shown in Figure 7.14. The Chan Vese algorithm is ranked first, then there is a group with similar performance composed by the algorithms Bernard, Caselles, fast marching, region growing, Shi and Chunming Li. The next rank is for the Lankton algorithm and finally is located the sparse field (Lankton) algorithm.

TABLE 7.4
Dice Coefficient Comparison for the Segmentation of a 3-D MSCT Image

Algorithm	Average	Standard Deviation	Minimum	Maximum
Bernard Algorithm [23]	0.923	0.047	0.808	0.966
Caselles [19]	0.924	0.034	0.833	0.969
Chan Vese [22]	0.941	0.039	0.846	0.977
Fast Marching [52]	0.921	0.050	0.801	0.972
Lankton Algorithm [21]	0.891	0.057	0.738	0.939
Region Growing [24]	0.925	0.049	0.767	0.974
Shi Algorithm [25]	0.924	0.040	0.820	0.964
Shunming Li Algorithm [39]	0.919	0.031	0.843	0.953
Sparse Field (lankton) [44]	0.866	0.069	0.702	0.931

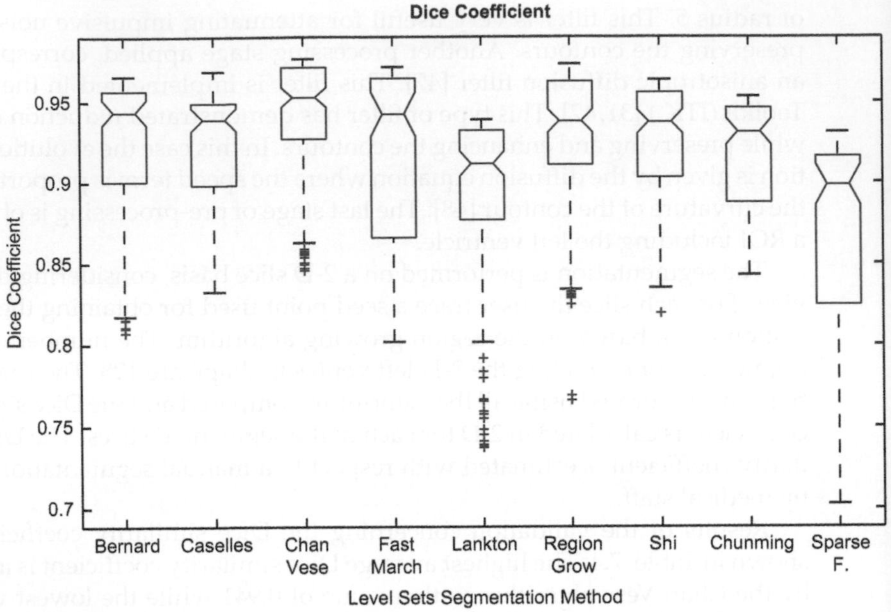

FIGURE 7.13
Boxplot representing the results of the Dice similarity coefficient for the segmentation of the 3-D MSCT image. Almost all algorithms provide a mean Dice coefficient greater than 0.90

The comparison concerning the computation time necessary for segmenting one slice of the 3-D image is shown in Table 7.5. The lowest computation time is attained by the fast marching algorithm with an average time of 0.079 seconds for each slice. In this case, the region growing algorithm has an average time of 0.253 seconds and the sparse field (Lankton) algorithm has an average time of 0.892 seconds. The Chunming Li has an average time of 2.812 seconds, the Chan Vese algorithm has an average time of 3.799 seconds and the Caselles algorithm 5.916 seconds. The slower algorithms are the Bernard algorithm with an average computation time of 53.152 seconds and the Lankton algorithm with 111.491 seconds. The Box plot for results concerning the computation time for the compared algorithm is shown on Figure 7.15. The result for the comparison concerning the computation time is shown in Figure 7.16. The fastest algorithm is the fast marching, then there are three algorithms with computation time quite similar: region growing, Chunming Li and the sparse field (Lankton) algorithm. The next group is formed by the Caselles algorithm and the Chan Vese algorithm and finally the slower algorithms are the Shi, Bernard and Lankton.

Results of the segmentation for the 3-D MSCT diastole image are shown in Figures 7.17 and 7.18. Each row of these figures shows four views of the segmentation representing the 3-D shape of the left ventricle in diastole. In general the shape obtained by each of the algorithms compared has a similar

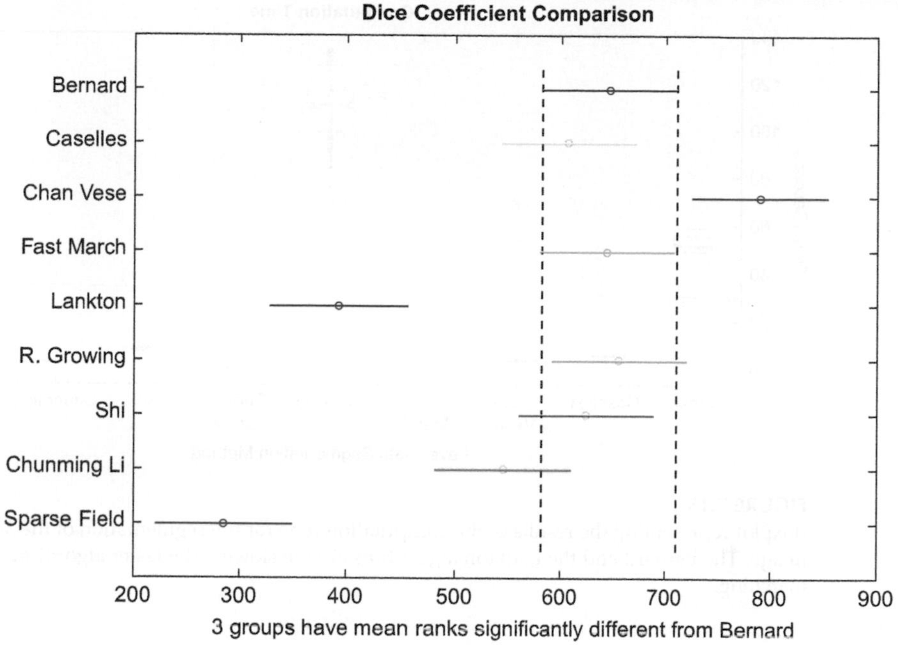

FIGURE 7.14
Krustal-Wallis comparison for the Dice similarity coefficient concerning the segmentation of the 3-D MSCT image. The Chan Vese algorithm obtains the highest rank within this classification.

appearance and the differences are mainly related with the concavities created by the papillary muscles. Results of the segmentation are shown in Figures 7.19 and 7.20 as slices of the left ventricle with the contour of the segmentation overlaid on the slice. The contour of the 3-D segmentation is overlaid on the three standard views of the 3-D image: axial, coronal and sagittal.

TABLE 7.5

Computational Time Comparison on a 3-D MSCT Image. Time is Expressed in Seconds

Algorithm	Average	Standard Deviation	Minimum	Maximum
Bernard Algorithm [23]	53.152	2.511	49.044	58.776
Caselles [19]	5.916	0.223	3.547	6.258
Chan Vese [22]	3.799	0.167	3.647	4.822
Fast Marching [52]	0.079	0.003	0.070	0.088
Lankton Algorithm [21]	111.491	11.523	75.882	134.200
Region Growing [24]	0.253	0.060	0.069	335
Shi Algorithm [25]	8.595	0.844	7.052	10.628
Shunming Li Algorithm [39]	2.812	0.111	2.646	3.058
Sparse Field (lankton) [44]	0.892	0.181	0.619	2.344

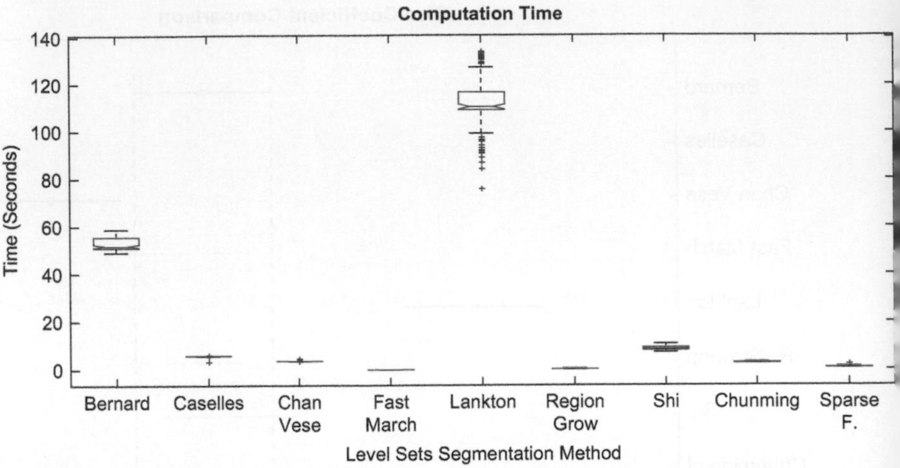

FIGURE 7.15
Boxplot representing the results of the computation time for the segmentation of the 3-D MSCT image. The Bernard and the Lankton algorithms are the slower. The faster algorithm is the fast marching.

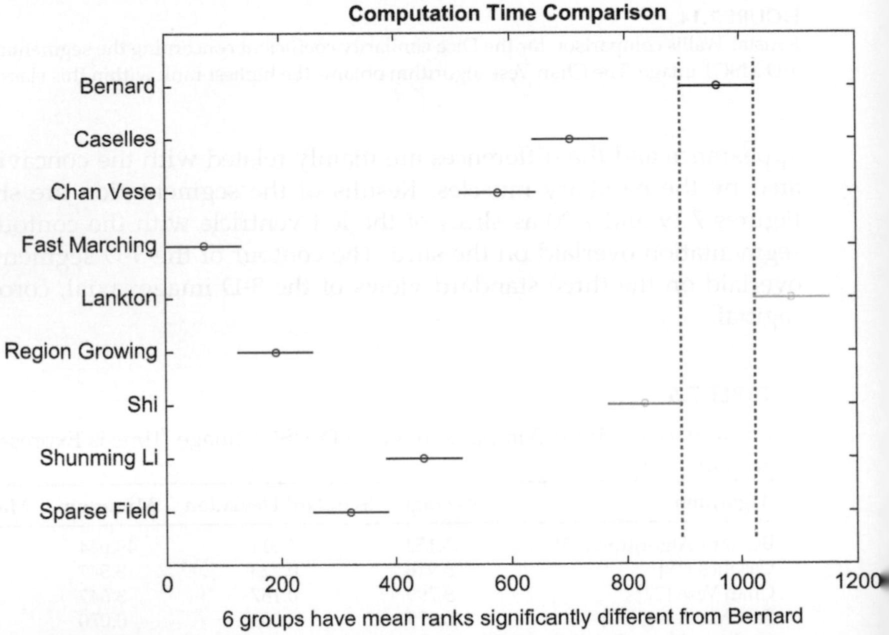

FIGURE 7.16
Krustal-Wallis comparison for the computation time concerning the segmentation of the 3-D MSCT image. The Shi, Bernard and Lankton algorithms are the slower

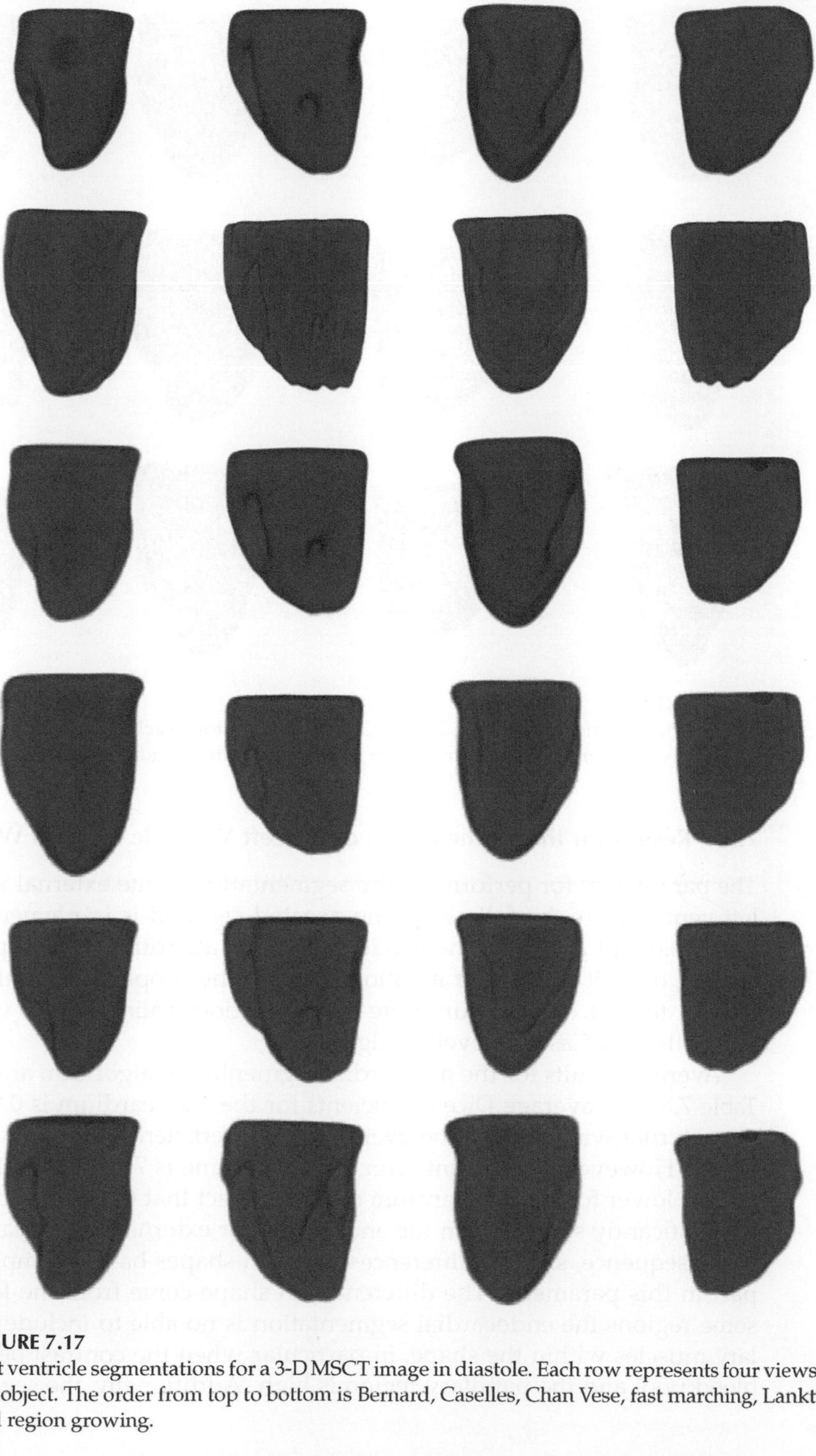

FIGURE 7.17
Left ventricle segmentations for a 3-D MSCT image in diastole. Each row represents four views of the object. The order from top to bottom is Bernard, Caselles, Chan Vese, fast marching, Lankton and region growing.

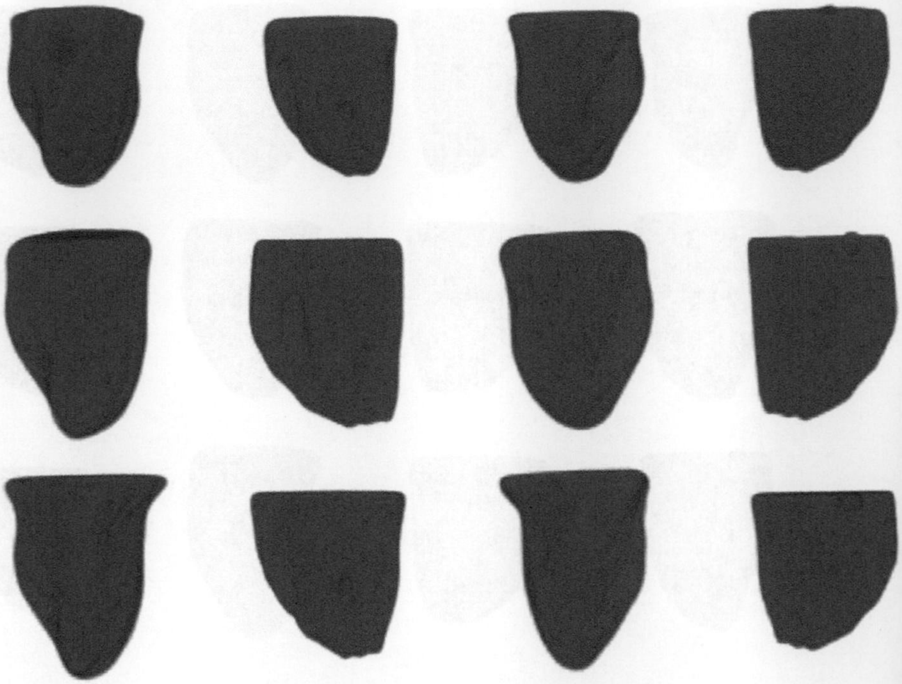

FIGURE 7.18
Left ventricle segmentations for a 3-D MSCT image in diastole. Each row represents four views of the object. The order from top to bottom is Shi, Chunming Li and fast marching (Lankton).

7.5.4 Results for the Segmentation of the Left Ventricle External Wall

The parameters for performing the segmentation of the external wall of the left ventricle are the following: the negated sigmoid is implemented using $\alpha = -0.6$ and $\beta = 0.8$. The geodesic contour algorithm was implemented using a default number of iterations of 140. The propagation scaling factor was set to 10.0, and the curvature and advection scaling factors were set to 1.0 for the 3-D Caselles level set algorithm.

Average results for the myocardial segmentation algorithm are shown in Table 7.6. The average Dice coefficients for the endocardium is 0.91 and for the external wall is 0.92. The average Dice coefficient for the myocardium is 0.80. However, the percent error for the volume is 7.10%. The Dice coefficient is lower for the myocardium due to the fact that the myocardial region is significantly smaller than the endocardial or external wall binary shapes. In consequence, smaller differences between shapes have an important impact in this parameter. The differences in shape come from the fact that in some regions the endocardial segmentation is no able to include the papillary muscles within the shape, in particular when the contrast between the blood pool and the papillary region is high. Additionally, the segmentation

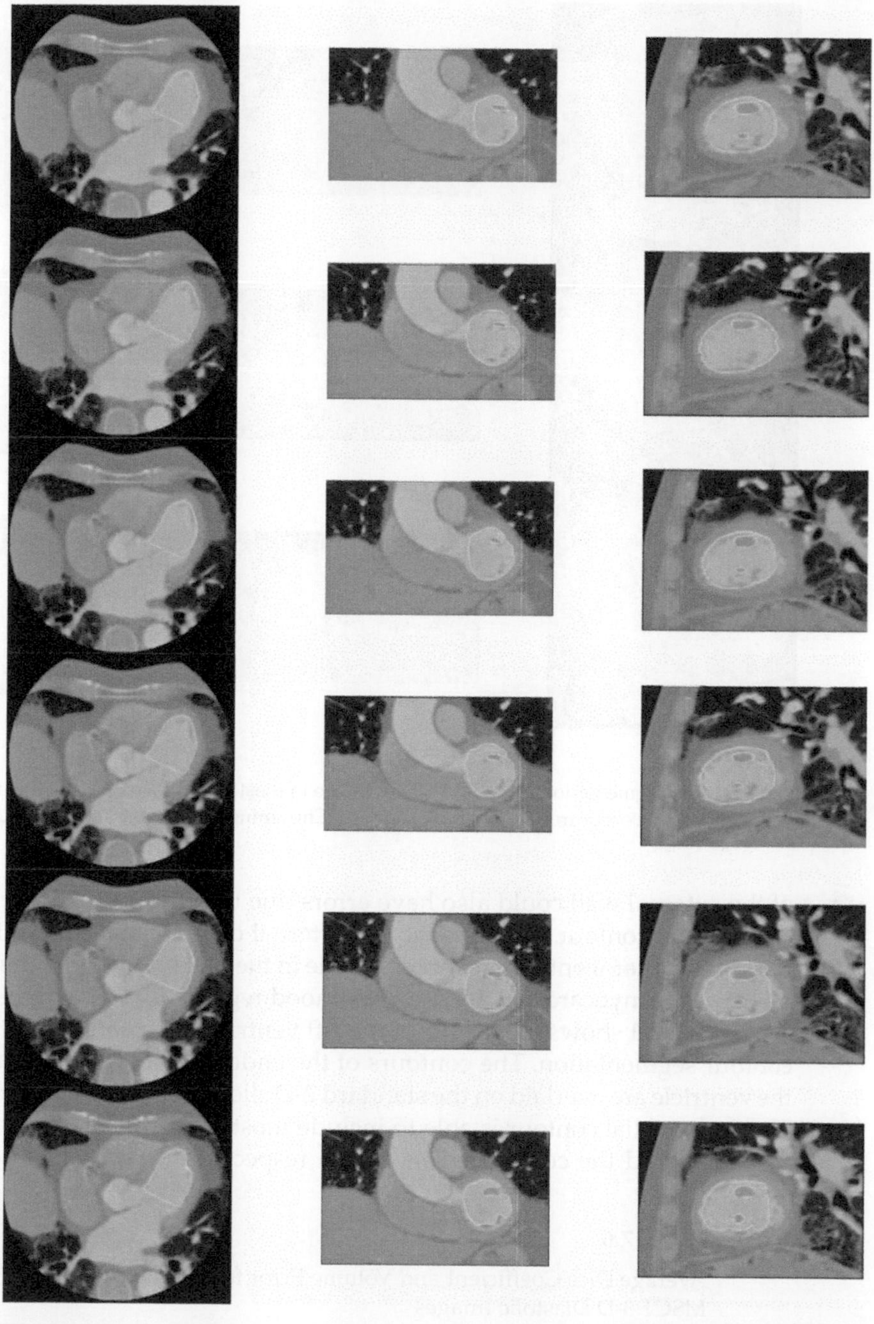

FIGURE 7.19
Left ventricle segmentations for a 3-D MSCT image in diastole. Each row represents four views of the object. The order from top to bottom is Bernard, Caselles, Chan Vese, fast marching, Lankton and region growing.

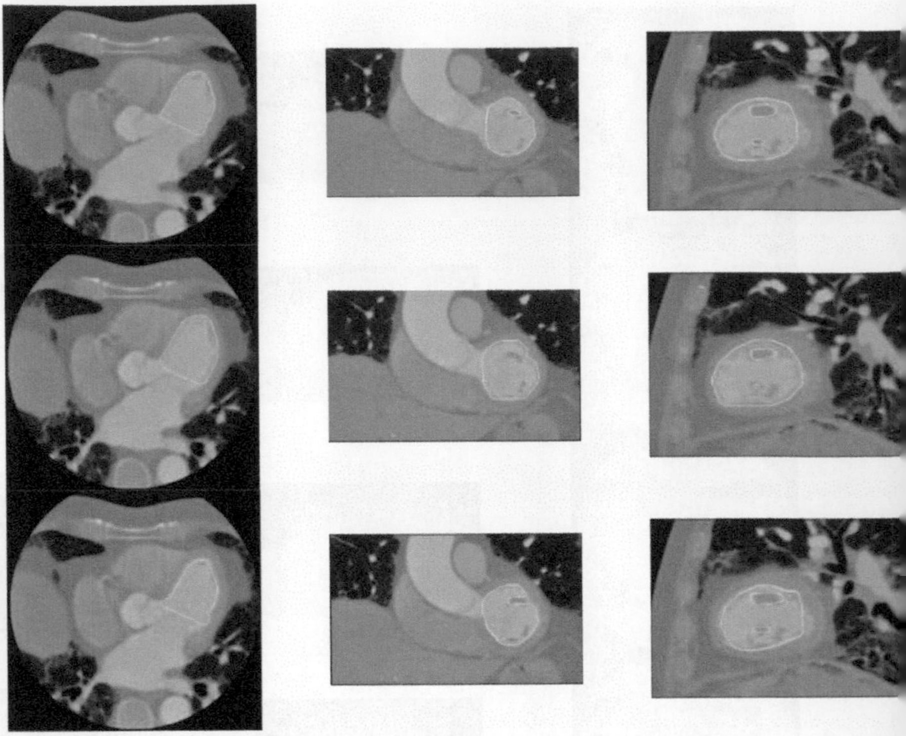

FIGURE 7.20
Left ventricle segmentations for a 3-D MSCT image in diastole. Each row represents four views of the object. The order from top to bottom is Shi, Chunming Li and fast marching (Lankton).

of the external wall could also have errors due to differences in intensity for the external contour. For instance the external contour could have low contrast in the inter–ventricular septum while in the posterior region the contrast between the myocardium and neighborhood regions could be higher.

Figure 7.21 shows the results of the left ventricle endocardial and external contour segmentation. The contours of the endocardial and external wall of the ventricle are overlaid on the standard 2-D slices axial, coronal and sagittal. The endocardial contour is able to include most of papillary muscles within the shape and the correspondence with respect to the actual contour is in

TABLE 7.6

Average Dice Coefficient and Volume Error for the Validation Using MSCT 3-D Diastolic Images

Parameters	LV Endocardium	LV External Wall	LV Myocardium
Dice Coefficient	0.91	0.92	0.80
Volume Error (%)	7.60	1.80	7.10

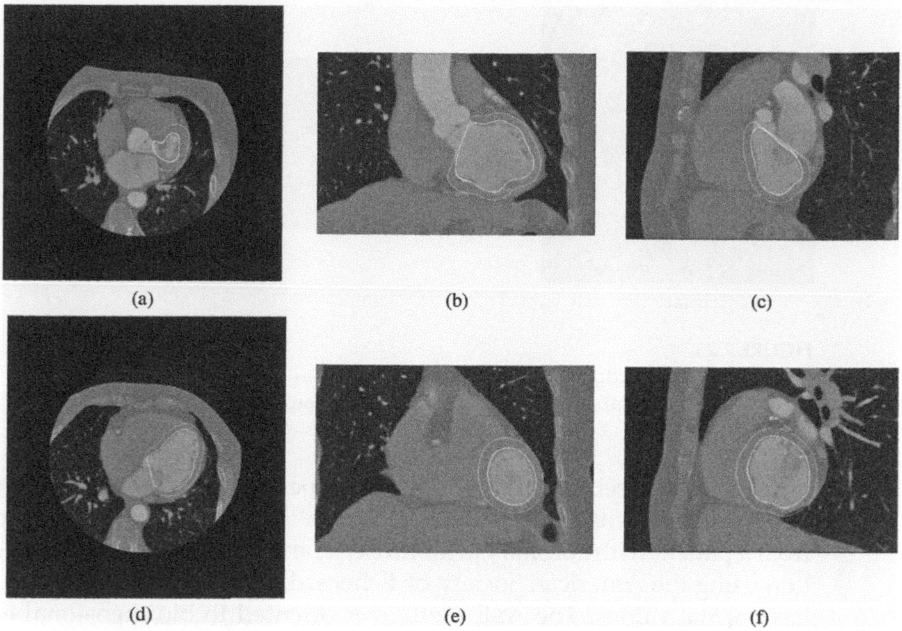

FIGURE 7.21
Left ventricle myocardial segmentation contours overlayed on 2-D slices: (a) Apical region axial slice. (b) Mid-cavity region coronal slice. (c) Basal region sagittal slice. (d) Mid-cavity region axial slice. (e) Apical region coronal slice. (f) Mid-cavity region sagittal slice.

general good. The matching between the segmentation contour and the actual location of the external wall is good even in presence of low contrast images like the one shown in this figure.

In Figure 7.22 the shapes obtained for the left ventricle endocardial wall and external wall are shown overlaid. The myocardium is visualized as the

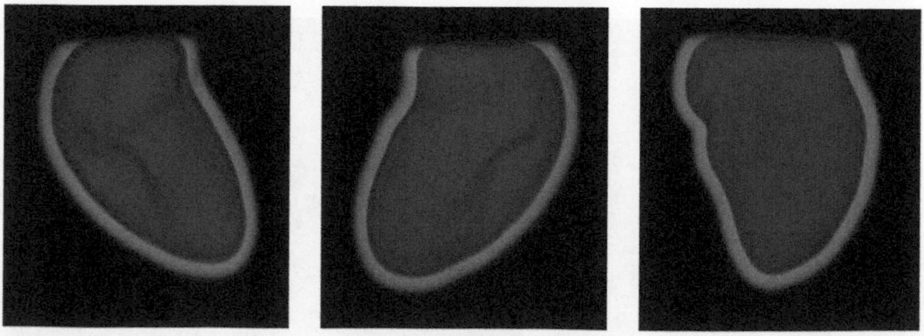

FIGURE 7.22
Three views of the 3-D shape segmentation representing the endocardial and external wall for the left ventricle.

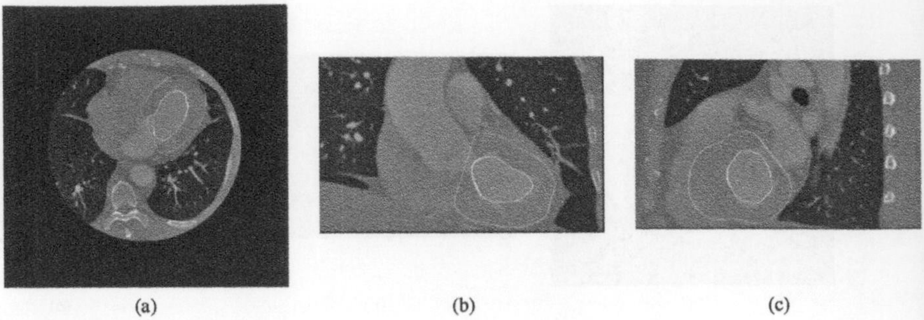

FIGURE 7.23
Left ventricle myocardial segmentation contours overlaid on 2-D slices. The patient has Left Ventricle Hypertrophy: (a) Apical region axial slice. (b) Coronal slice. (c) Sagittal slice.

difference between both shapes. The shapes are shown considering three views of the cardiac structure. In this case the cardiac image was acquired from a patient with coronary artery disease and the left ventricle mass estimation using the American Society of Echocardiography (ASE) method [67,68] has normal values. The ASE method is oriented to bidimensional echocardiography cardiac images. Calculation is based on assuming approximate known geometric shape models such as ellipsoids, cones or truncated polyhedrons. However, the most common method is the method based on cubed formulas that considers only one dimension of the left ventricular cavity and assumes an ellipsoid geometry.

An example for a patient with Left Ventricular Hypertrophy (LVH) is shown in Figures 7.23 and 7.24. The patient has a left ventricle mass of 182 grams and a left ventricle mass index of 141 g/m^2 in the moderately abnormal range with a Relative Wall Thickness (RWT) index of 0.78 corresponding to concentric hypertrophy. The contours obtained with the automatic segmentation are shown in Figure 7.23. In this case the contours are shown overlaid

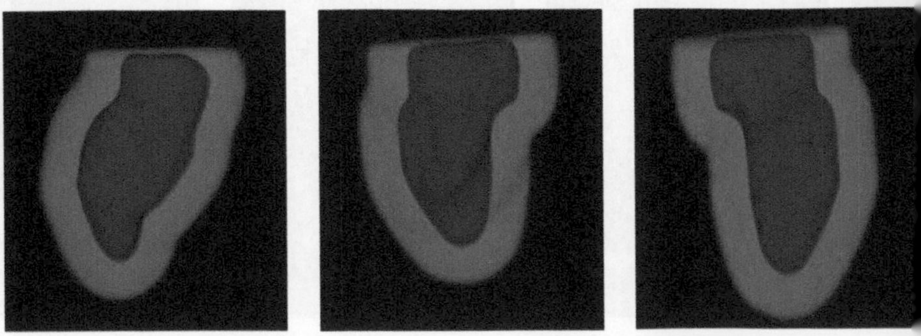

FIGURE 7.24
Three views of the 3-D shape for the left ventricle endocardial and external wall segmentation.

with the input image in three standard views axial, coronal and sagittal. Even when the contrast is poor for determining the actual external wall contour, the level set based algorithm is able to attain a feasible solution that recovers a ventricle shape that matches the anatomical information provided by this 3-D image. The 3-D representation of the myocardial segmentation is shown in Figure 7.24 where the endocardial shape is overlaid with the shape representing the external wall of the left ventricle. Three views of the segmentation results are shown where the width of the left ventricle wall is clearly larger than the cases shown in Figure 7.22.

7.6 Conclusions

Eight level set segmentation algorithms were briefly reviewed. The fast marching algorithm is simple and fast, however the smoothness of the obtained contour cannot be controlled. The Caselles algorithm is implemented by minimizing a contour–based energy function, whereas the Chan Vese algorithm minimizes a region–based energy function. The remaining of algorithms are somehow derived from the Caselles and Chan Vese by introducing other features providing more control about the final segmentation or improvements concerning the computation time.

The level set segmentation algorithms are robust for segmenting noisy images corrupted with Gaussian noise. Within this comparison, the Caselles and Chan Vese algorithms are highly robust even in presence of high noise levels. The comparison also shows that when the PSNR for the image is high and the target shape is uniform, the region growing algorithm can also obtain good results.

The comparison of algorithms on real MSCT images shows that level set algorithms in general attain a Dice coefficient close or higher that 0.90. The differences between algorithms are mainly related to the computation time and the presence of outliers. The Caselles algorithm provides high Dice similarity coefficients and their implementation using sparse field techniques provides low computation times.

The Caselles algorithm was used for performing the 3-D segmentation of the left ventricle external wall. The segmentation of this wall is challenging in MSCT images due to poor contrast and non-uniform gray level in the left ventricle wall. However, the algorithm proposed provided a volume error of 7.10% for the left ventricle wall.

Future research is aimed at performing the segmentation of the remaining cardiac cavities and proposing a simple and robust initialization method for this application.

References

1. A. Frangi, D. Rueckert, and J. Duncan, "Three–dimensional cardiovascular image analysis," *IEEE Transactions on Medical Imaging*, vol. 21, no. 9, pp. 1005–1010, 2002.
2. M. Erdt, S. Steger, and G. Sakas, "Regmentation: A new view of image segmentation and registration," *Journal of Radiation Oncology Informatics*, vol. 4, no. 1, pp. 1–23, 2012.
3. D. L. Pham, C. Xu, and J. L. Prince, "Current methods in medical image segmentation 1," *Annual Review of Biomedical Engineering*, vol. 2, no. 1, pp. 315–337, 2000.
4. O. Ecabert, J. Peters, J. Weese, C. Lorenz, J. von Berg, M. Walker, M. Olszewski, and M. Vembar, "Automatic heart segmentation in ct: current and future applications," *MedicaMundi*, vol. 50, no. 3, pp. 12–17, 2006.
5. J. Fleureau, M. Garreau, A. Hernandez, A. Simon, and D. Boulmier, "Multi–object and N–D segmentation of cardiac MSCT data using SVM classifiers and a connectivity algorithm," *Computers in Cardiology*, vol. 33, no. 1, pp. 817–820, 2006.
6. A. Bravo, M. Vera, M. Garreau, and R. Medina, "Three–dimensional segmentation of ventricular heart chambers from multi–*slice* computerized tomography An hybrid approach," in *DICTAP*, ser. CCIS. Springer, 2011, vol. 166, pp. 287–301
7. G. Mühlenbruch, M. Das, C. Hohl, J. E. Wildberger, D. Rinck, T. G. Flohr, R. Koos C. Knackstedt, R. W. Günther, and A. H. Mahnken, "Global left ventricular function in cardiac ct. evaluation of an automated 3d region-growing segmentation algorithm," *European Radiology*, vol. 16, no. 5, pp. 1117–1123, 2006.
8. M. L. Chuang, P. Gona, G. L. Hautvast, C. J. Salton, S. J. Blease, S. B. Yeon M. Breeuwer, C. J. O'Donnell, and W. J. Manning, "Left ventricular trabeculae and papillary muscles: Correlation with clinical and cardiac characteristics and impact on cardiovascular magnetic resonance measures of left ventricular anatomy and function," *JACC. Cardiovascular Imaging*, vol. 5, no. 11, p. 1115, 2012.
9. O. Ecabert, J. Peters, H. Schramm, C. Lorenz, J. von Berg, M. Walker, M. Vembar M. Olszewski, K. Subramanyan, G. Lavi, and J. Weese, "Automatic model–based segmentation of the heart in CT images," *IEEE Transactions on Medical Imaging* vol. 27, no. 9, pp. 1189–1201, 2008.
10. H. Zhang, A. Wahle, R. Johnson, T. Scholz, and M. Sonka, "4-D cardiac MR image analysis: Left and right ventricular morphology and function," *IEEE Transactions on Medical Imaging*, vol. 29, no. 2, pp. 350–364, 2010.
11. H. Assen, M. Danilouchkine, M. Dirksen, J. Reiber, and B. Lelieveldt, "A 3-D active shape model driven by fuzzy inference: Aplication to cardiac CT and MR," *IEEE Transactions on Information Technology in Biomedicine*, vol. 12, no. 5, pp. 595–605 2008.
12. H. Kirisli, M. Schaap, S. Klein, L. Neefjes, A. Weustink, T. V. Walsum, and W. Niessen, "Fully automatic cardiac segmentation from 3-D CTA data: a multi atlas based approach," *Proceedings of SPIE Medical Imaging*, vol. 7623, no. 1, pp 5–9, 2010.
13. Y. Zheng, A. Barbu, B. Georgescu, M. Scheuering, and D. Comaniciu, "Four chamber heart modeling and automatic segmentation for 3-D cardiac CT volumes using marginal space learning and steerable features," *IEEE Transactions on Medical Imaging*, vol. 27, no. 11, pp. 1668–1681, 2008.

14. M. Lynch, O. Ghita, and P. Whelan, "Segmentation of the left ventricle of the heart in 3-D MRI data using an optimized nonrigid temporal model," *IEEE Transactions on Medical Imaging*, vol. 27, no. 2, pp. 195–203, 2008.
15. P. Yushkevich, J. Piven, H. Cody, S. Ho, J. Gee, and G. Gerig, "User–guided level set segmentation of anatomical structures with ITK–SNAP," *Insight Journal*, vol. 1, pp. 252–264, 2005, special Issue on ISC/NA-MIC/MICCAI Workshop on Open-Source Software.
16. E. Heiberg, L. Wigstrom, M. Carlsson, A. Bolger, and M. Karlsson, "Time resolved three-dimensional automated segmentation of the left ventricle," in *proceedings of IEEE Computers In Cardiology*, vol. 32, Lyon, France, 2005, pp. 559–602.
17. I. Dydenko, F. Jamal, O. Bernard, J. Dhooge, I. Magnin, and D. Friboulet, "A level set framework with a shape and motion prior for segmentation and region tracking in echocardiography," *Medical Image Analysis*, vol. 10, no. 1, pp. 38–59, 2006.
18. W. Bai, W. Shi, D. P. O'Regan, T. Tong, H. Wang, S. Jamil-Copley, N. S. Peters, and D. Rueckert, "A probabilistic patch-based label fusion model for multi-atlas segmentation with registration refinement: application to cardiac mr images," *IEEE Transactions on Medical Imaging*, vol. 32, no. 7, pp. 1302–1315, 2013.
19. V. Caselles, R. Kimmel, and G. Sapiro, "Geodesic active contours," *International Journal of Computer Vision*, vol. 22, no. 1, pp. 61–79, 1997.
20. S. Zhu and A. Yuille, "Region competition: Unifying snakes, region growing, and Bayes–MDL for multiband image segmentation," *IEEE Transactions on Pattern Analysis and Machine Intelligence*, vol. 18, no. 9, pp. 884–900, 1996.
21. S. Lankton and A. Tannenbaum, "Localizing region-based active contours," *IEEE Transactions on Image Processing*, no. 11, pp. 2029–2039, 2008.
22. T. Chan and L. Vese., "Active contours without edges," *IEEE Transactions on Image Processing*, vol. 10, no. 2, pp. 266–277, 2001.
23. O. Bernard, D. Friboulet, P. Thevenaz, and M. Unser, "Variational b-spline level-set: A linear filtering approach for fast deformable model evolution," *Image Processing, IEEE Transactions on*, vol. 18, no. 6, pp. 1179–1191, June 2009.
24. S. C. Zhu and A. Yuille, "Region competition: Unifying snakes, region growing, and bayes–mdl for multiband image segmentation," *IEEE Transactions on Pattern Analysis and Machine Intelligence*, vol. 18, no. 9, pp. 884–900, 1996.
25. Y. Shi and W. Karl, "A real-time algorithm for the approximation of level-set-based curve evolution," *IEEE Transactions on Image Processing*, vol. 17, no. 5, pp. 645–656, May 2008.
26. T. Dietenbeck, M. Alessandrini, D. Friboulet, and O. Bernard, "Creaseg: A free software for the evaluation of image segmentation algorithms based on level-set," in *Image Processing (ICIP), 2010 17th IEEE International Conference on*, Sept 2010, pp. 665–668.
27. S. Osher and J. Sethian, "Fronts propagating with curvature dependent speed: algorithms based on hamilton–jacobi formulations," *Computational Physics*, vol. 1, pp. 17–33, 1988.
28. R. Tsai and S. Osher, "Review article: Level set methods and their applications in image science," *Commun. Math. Sci.*, vol. 1, no. 4, pp. 1–20, 12 2003. [Online]. Available: http://projecteuclid.org/euclid.cms/1119655349
29. J. A. Sethian, "A fast marching level set method for monotonically advancing fronts," *Proceedings of the National Academy of Sciences*, vol. 93, no. 4, pp. 1591–1595, 1996.

30. R. Malladi and J. A. Sethian, "An o (n log n) algorithm for shape modeling," *Proceedings of the National Academy of Sciences*, vol. 93, no. 18, pp. 9389–9392, 1996.
31. L. Ibañez, "The ITK Software Guide," Kitware Inc., Tech. Rep., July 2005.
32. M. Kass, A. Witkin, and D. Terzopoulos, "Snakes: Active contour models," *International Journal of Computer Vision*, vol. 1, no. 4, pp. 321–331, 1988.
33. D. Adalstein and J. Sethian, "A fast level set method for propagating interfaces," *Computational Physics*, vol. 1, pp. 269–277, 1995.
34. J. Yezzi, A. Tsai, and A.Willsky, "A fully global approach to image segmentation via coupled curve evolution equations," *Journal of Visual Communications and Image Representations*, vol. 13, no. 1, pp. 195–216, 2002.
35. A. Bhattacharyya, "On a measure of divergence between two statistical populations defined by their probability distributions," *Bull. Calcutta Mathematical Society*, vol. 35, pp. 99–110, 1943.
36. J. Sethian, *Level set methods and Fast marching methods*. New York, USA: Springer, 1999.
37. G. Aubert, M. Barlaud, O. Faugeras, and S. Jehan-Besson, "Image segmentation using active contours: Calculus of variations or shape gradients?" *SIAM Journal on Applied Mathematics*, vol. 63, no. 6, pp. 2128–2154, 2003.
38. C. Li, C. Xu, J. C. Gore, and Z. Ding, "Minimization of region-scalable fitting energy for image segmentation," *IEEE Transactions on Image Processing*, vol. 17, no. 10, pp. 1940–1949, 2008.
39. C. Li, C.-Y. Kao, C. Gui, and M. D. Fox, "Distance regularized level set evolution and its application to image segmentation," *IEEE Transactions on Image Processing*, vol. 19, no. 12, pp. 3243–3254, 2010.
40. R. Whitaker, "A level-set approach to 3-D reconstruction from range data," *International Journal of Computer Vision*, vol. 29, no. 3, pp. 203–231, 1998.
41. T. Yoo, *Insight into Images Principles and Practice for Segmentation, Registration, and Image Analysis: A companion to the Insight Toolkit*. MA, USA: AK Peters, 2004.
42. T. S. Yoo, M. J. Ackerman, W. E. Lorensen, W. Schroeder, V. Chalana, S. Aylward, D. Metaxas, and R. Whitaker, "Engineering and algorithm design for an image processing api: a technical report on itk-the insight toolkit," *Studies in Health Technology and Informatics*, pp. 586–592, 2002.
43. A. E. Lefohn, J. M. Kniss, C. D. Hansen, and R. T. Whitaker, "A streaming narrowband algorithm: interactive computation and visualization of level sets," *IEEE Transactions on Visualization and Computer Graphics*, vol. 10, no. 4, pp. 422–433, July 2004.
44. S. Lankton, "Sparse field methods-technical report," *Georgia Institute of Technology*, 2009.
45. R. Medina, S. Bautista, and V. Morocho, "Accuracy of connected confidence left ventricle segmentation in 3-d multi-slice computerized tomography images," in *2017 IEEE Second Ecuador Technical Chapters Meeting (ETCM)*, Oct 2017, pp. 1–6.
46. R. Medina, S. Bautista, P. Vanegas, and V. Morocho, "Left ventricle myocardium segmentation in multi-slice computerized tomography," in *IEEE proceedings of ANDESCON–2016*. IEEE, 2016, pp. 1–4.
47. C. Tsiotsios and M. Petrou, "On the choice of the parameters for anisotropic diffusion in image processing," *Pattern Recognition*, vol. 46, no. 5, pp. 1369–1381, 2013.

48. P. Perona and J. Malik, "Scale-space and edge detection using anisotropic diffusion," *IEEE Transactions on Pattern Analysis and Machine Intelligence*, vol. 12, no. 7, pp. 629–639, 1990.
49. R. Cárdenes, R. de Luis-García, and M. Bach-Cuadra, "A multidimensional segmentation evaluation for medical image data," *Computer Methods and Programs in Biomedicine*, vol. 96, no. 2, pp. 108–124, 2009.
50. A. A. Taha and A. Hanbury, "Metrics for evaluating 3d medical image segmentation: analysis, selection, and tool," *BMC Medical Imaging*, vol. 15, no. 1, pp. 1–29, 2015.
51. K. Babalola, B. Patenaude, P. Aljabar, J. Schnabel, D. Kennedy, W. Crum, S. Smith, T. Cootes, M. Jenkinson, and D. Rueckert, "Comparison and evaluation of segmentation techniques for subcortical structures in brain mri," in *Medical Image Computing and Computer-Assisted Intervention – MICCAI 2008*, ser. Lecture Notes in Computer Science, D. Metaxas, L. Axel, G. Fichtinger, and G. Székely, Eds. Springer Berlin Heidelberg, 2008, vol. 5241, pp. 409–416. [Online]. Available: http://dx.doi.org/10.1007/978-3-540-85988-8_49
52. J. A. Sethian, *Level set methods and fast marching methods: evolving interfaces in computational geometry, fluid mechanics, computer vision, and materials science*. Cambridge University Press, 1999, vol. 3.
53. P. R. Bai, Q. Y. Liu, L. Li, S. H. Teng, J. Li, and M. Y. Cao, "A novel region-based level set method initialized with mean shift clustering for automated medical image segmentation," *Computers in Biology and Medicine*, vol. 43, no. 11, pp. 1827–1832, 2013.
54. J. Huang, F. Jian, H. Wu, and H. Li, "An improved level set method for vertebra ct image segmentation," *Biomedical Engineering Online*, vol. 12, no. 1, p. 48, 2013.
55. X. Jiang, Z. Zhou, X. Ding, X. Deng, L. Zou, and B. Li, "Level set based hippocampus segmentation in mr images with improved initialization using region growing," *Computational and Mathematical Methods in Medicine*, vol. 2017, Article ID 5256346, pp. 1–11, 2017.
56. A. Masood, A. A. Al-Jumaily, and Y. Maali, "Level set initialization based on modified fuzzy c means thresholding for automated segmentation of skin lesions," in *International Conference on Neural Information Processing*. Springer, 2013, pp. 341–351.
57. R. Medina, A. La Cruz, A. Ordoñes, D. Pesántez, V. Morocho, and P. Vanegas, "Level set algorithms comparison for multi-slice ct left ventricle segmentation," in *11th International Symposium on Medical Information Processing and Analysis*, vol. 9681. International Society for Optics and Photonics, 2015, p. 96810O.
58. L. Wang, T. Chitiboi, H. Meine, M. Günther, and H. K. Hahn, "Principles and methods for automatic and semi-automatic tissue segmentation in mri data," *Magnetic Resonance Materials in Physics, Biology and Medicine*, vol. 29, no. 2, pp. 95–110, 2016.
59. M. Lynch, O. Ghita, and P. F. Whelan, "Segmentation of the left ventricle of the heart in 3-d+ t mri data using an optimized nonrigid temporal model," *IEEE Transactions on Medical Imaging*, vol. 27, no. 2, pp. 195–203, 2008.
60. C. Petitjean and J.-N. Dacher, "A review of segmentation methods in short axis cardiac mr images," *Medical Image Analysis*, vol. 15, no. 2, pp. 169–184, 2011.
61. M. Avendi, A. Kheradvar, and H. Jafarkhani, "A combined deep-learning and deformable-model approach to fully automatic segmentation of the left ventricle in cardiac mri," *Medical Image Analysis*, vol. 30, pp. 108–119, 2016.

62. A. Tsai, A. Yezzi, W. Wells, C. Tempany, D. Tucker, A. Fan, W. E. Grimson, and A. Willsky, "A shape-based approach to the segmentation of medical imagery using level sets," *IEEE Transactions on Medical Imaging*, vol. 22, no. 2, pp. 137–154, 2003.
63. A. Yezzi, A. Tsai, and A. Willsky, "A statistical approach to snakes for bimodal and trimodal imagery," in *Computer Vision, 1999. The Proceedings of the Seventh IEEE International Conference on*, vol. 2. IEEE, 1999, pp. 898–903.
64. P.-E. Danielsson, "Euclidean distance mapping," *Computer Graphics and Image Processing*, vol. 14, no. 3, pp. 227–248, 1980.
65. W. H. Kruskal and W. A. Wallis, "Use of ranks in one-criterion variance analysis," *Journal of the American Statistical Association*, vol. 47, no. 260, pp. 583–621, 1952.
66. W. J. Schroeder, L. S. Avila, and W. Hoffman, "Visualizing with vtk: a tutorial," *Computer Graphics and Applications, IEEE*, vol. 20, no. 5, pp. 20–27, 2000.
67. S. G. Myerson, H. E. Montgomery, D. J. Pennell *et al.*, "Left ventricular mass reliability of m-mode and 2-dimensional echocardiographic formulas," *Hypertension*, vol. 40, no. 5, pp. 673–678, 2002.
68. M. Foppa, B. B. Duncan, and L. E. Rohde, "Echocardiography-based left ventricular mass estimation. how should we define hypertrophy?" *Cardiovascular Ultrasound*, vol. 3, no. 1, p. 1, 2005.

8

Deformable Models and Image Segmentation

Ahmed ElTanboly, Ali Mahmoud, Ahmed Shalaby, Magdi El-Azab, Mohammed Ghazal, Robert Keynton, Ayman El-Baz, and Jasjit S. Suri

CONTENTS

8.1 Introduction

In computer vision, image segmentation is the process of partitioning an image into multiple segments. In other words, it is the process of labeling every pixel in an image such that pixels with the same label share the same characteristics, such as texture, brightness, or gray level [1]. Segmentation of medical images, in particular, has become of immense importance as a non-invasive tool that provides physicians with a reliable way of diagnosis of the abnormalities found in different organs.

In the field of medical imaging, accurate segmentation of structures is crucial for detecting lesions and abnormalities. It has recently provided great advances to clinicians in assessing abnormalities through computer-aided diagnostic systems. Segmentation, however, is highly challenging due to many factors, such as the low contrast between different tissues types that makes it difficult to segment the desired object even manually, and the motion artifacts associated with the scans which adds noise to images.

In order to formulate the segmentation problem mathematically, consider the finite 2-D arithmetic lattice $\mathbf{R}$, of the size XY supporting pixels, the finite set of intensities $\mathbf{Q}$, and the finite set of region labels $\mathbf{K}$:

$$\mathbf{R} = (r = (x, y): x = 0, 1, \ldots, X-1,\ y = 0,\ 1, \ldots,\ Y-1)$$

$$\mathbf{Q} = (0,\ 1, \ldots, Q-1)$$

$$\mathbf{K} = (0,\ 1, \ldots, K-1)$$

where x, y denote the Cartesian coordinates of the lattice sites. Let g: $\mathbf{R} \rightarrow \mathbf{Q}$ and m: $\mathbf{R} \rightarrow \mathbf{K}$ denote a digital image and a region respectively. If $H(.)$ is a homogeneity predicate for signals from a connected subset of image pixels, the segmentation divides the image g into K connected subimages, g_k: $\mathbf{R}_k \rightarrow \mathbf{Q}$; $k \in \mathbf{K}$; $\mathbf{R}_k \subset \mathbf{R}$ that cover the whole lattice, $\cup_{k \in \mathbf{K}} \mathbf{R}_k = \mathbf{R}$, without overlaps, $\mathbf{R}_k \cap \mathbf{R}_{\mathcal{K}} = \emptyset$ for all pairs $(k, \mathcal{K})$: $k \neq \mathcal{K}$, and keep the homogeneity individually, $H(g_k) = true$ for all $k \in \mathbf{K}$, but not in combination with their immediate neighbors, $H(g_k \cup g_k) = false$ for all the pairs of adjacent regions $\mathbf{R}_k$ and $\mathbf{R}_k$, Figure 8.1.

The segmentation problem has been extensively addressed in the literature, and can be classified into many categories. One possible classification is methods that are either edge-based or region-based. Edge-based

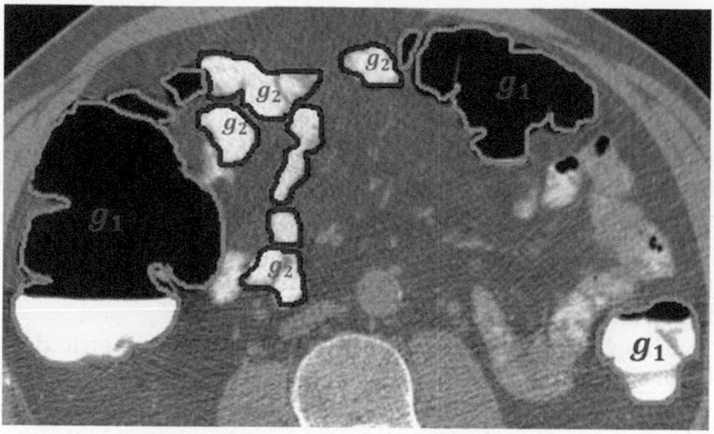

FIGURE 8.1
Sub-images g_1, g_2 under the homogeneity predicate requiring the same grey level for all pixels. g_1 (orange) represents colon segments of a CT slice, whereas g_2 (blue) represent small bowels. The union of any two adjacent regions is inhomogeneous.

segmentation mainly depends on edge detection, which is conducted with many algorithms such as edge relaxation methods [2], border detection methods [3–5], and Hough transform-based methods [6, 7]. In region-based segmentation, pixels that share the same characteristics, e.g. gray level, are clustered together to form homogeneous regions [8–10]. Segmentation can also be classified with respect to the user's intervention. Segmentation could either be manually initialized, semi-automated, or fully-automated. Current advances in the field of image processing seek the full automation of segmentation techniques in order to optimize the process and refrain from manual intervention which is both time consuming and error-prone. Segmentation techniques can also be deformable model-based, where a curve is initialized, and then propagates (deforms) according to an energy function to be minimized. Under this category, numerous techniques have been devised that are either parametric, or geometric, also called level-set based, models. In parametric models, Lagrangian methods are used to deform the initial contour according to some external forces along with some internal properties of the image [11]. Geometric models, on the other hand, are capable of handling the topological changes of the object, as it tackles the minimization problem in higher dimensions without the need for parameterization. Osher and Sethian [12] first proposed the evolving curve, which is represented implicitly using a signed distance function, whose zero level represents the original contour.

Although deformable models have been widely used in the literature with numerous formulae for the segmentation of different body organs, it is impossible to have a generic framework that is suited for any segmentation problem. The algorithm should also be adapted in order to meet each one's characteristics. This chapter focuses on deformable-model based segmentation, due to the many advances it recently has made in the field of medical imaging analysis, the ease of integrating its concepts in any framework, and the high efficiency it provides in convergence to solutions.

The basics of deformable models with its two major categories—parametric and geometric—are detailed. The chapter also provides an overview of the recent advances in image segmentation using deformable models, which have been extensively used in literature for image segmentation. A variety of energy functions and numerical schemes have been proposed to solve their associated partial differential equations. Some of these major energy functions are provided in detail.

This chapter starts with a review of the parametric deformable models in literature. It goes through some of the popular external forces used along with their main drawbacks. It also covers the most widely used numerical schemes for the solution of the energy functions. It then reviews the geometric deformable models that were designed to overcome the limitations of the classical parametric representation. Basics of the level sets method and some of its important concepts are provided in detail and numerical schemes for solving the level sets equation are provided. The general form, namely Hamilton-Jacobi, is discussed. The popular Euler-Lagrange equation is also provided with its derivation as a powerful optimization technique that is used in many applications. The chapter then goes through some of the popular guiding forces in literature, such as the Chan-Vese model that is widely applied in image segmentation techniques, along with some recent improvements of it. Finally, a survey on recent medical imaging segmentation techniques using deformable models is conducted.

8.2 Geometric Deformable Models

In geometric deformable models, the planar curve is implicitly represented by the level set of an appropriate 2-D surface [12–18]. Due to the limitations of classical deformable models [13, 15, 16, 19], the level sets were proposed by Osher and Sethian [12], where topological changes were better handled during curve evolution without the need for parameterization, Figure 8.2.

Before deriving the level sets equation, some concepts need to be highlighted.

Level set is a set of points that represents an isocontour of a function mathematically in $\mathbb{R}^n$ space;

$$L(\varphi) = \{(x_1, x_2, \dots, x_n) | f(x_1, \dots, x_n) = 0\}$$

Principal Curvatures are the maximum and minimum normal curvature k_1, k_2 given at any surface point that measure the amount of surface bending at this point [20].

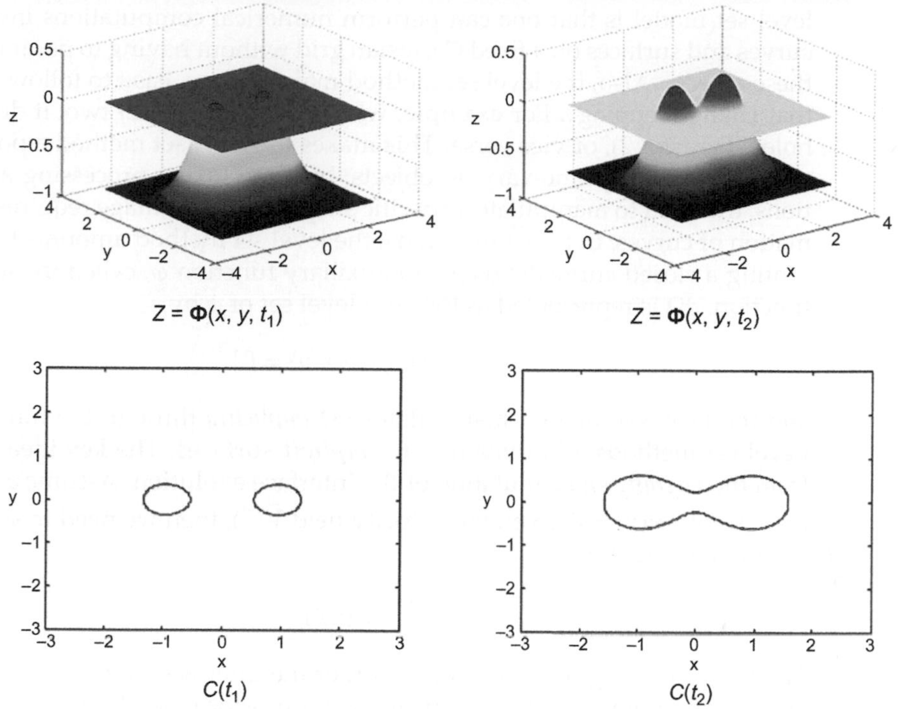

FIGURE 8.2
Illustration of contour deformation with time using the level set method.

The Gaussian curvature is defined as: $K = k_1 k_2$, while the mean curvature is defined as: $H = \frac{1}{2}(k_1 + k_2)$. Both can be used to compute both k_1 and k_2, where

$$k_1 = H + \sqrt{H^2 - k}, \tag{8.1}$$

and

$$k_2 = H - \sqrt{H^2 - k} \tag{8.2}$$

Geodesic Curvature is another form of curve representation. Given a parametric curve **C(S)** embedded into the surface **S**, this curve will have the following acceleration vector:

$$C_{ss} = k_g \hat{T} + k_n \hat{N} \tag{8.3}$$

This means that the acceleration vector is represented in terms of the unit normal vector $\hat{N}$ and the unit tangent vector $\hat{T}$ which lie in the same plane with C_{ss} and the surface normal. Geodesics are planar curves with acceleration only in the normal direction, i.e. $k_g = 0$ [21].

Level set methods (LSM) are a conceptual framework for using level sets as a tool for numerical analysis of surfaces and shapes. The advantage of the level set model is that one can perform numerical computations involving curves and surfaces on a fixed Cartesian grid without having to parameterize these objects. Also, the level set method makes it very easy to follow shapes that change topology. For example, when a shape splits in two, it develops holes (Figure 8.2), or vice versa. This makes the level set method a powerful tool for modeling time-varying objects. In some image processing applications, the need to manipulate a specific shape inside an image requires deformation of curves. In two dimensions, the level set method amounts to representing a closed curve $\partial\Omega$ using an auxiliary function φ, called the level set function. $\partial\Omega$ is represented as the zero level set of φ by

$$\partial\Omega = \{(x, y)|\varphi(x, y) = 0\}, \tag{8.4}$$

and the level set method manipulates $\partial\Omega$ *implicitly* through the function φ. Level set methods add dynamics to ***implicit*** surfaces. The key idea started from the *Lagrangian* formulation of the interface evolution. Assume a point $\vec{x}$ moves with $\varphi(\vec{x}) = 0$ given the velocity field $\vec{V}(\vec{x})$, then we need to solve the differential equation:

$$\frac{d\vec{x}}{dt} = \vec{V}(\vec{x}) \tag{8.5}$$

The use of the Lagrangian formulation of the interface motion given in the last equation along with numerical techniques for smoothing and regularization are collectively referred to as ***front tracking*** methods [22]. In order to avoid problems with instabilities and complicated surgical procedures for topological repair, Osher and Sethian [12] formulate the interface evolution implicitly (from implicit function φ) using the simple convection equation (which defines the evolution of the implicit function φ),

$$\varphi_t + \vec{V} \cdot \nabla\varphi = 0 \tag{8.6}$$

This partial differential equation defines the motion of the interface where $\varphi(\vec{x}) = 0$. The interface here is captured by the implicit function φ as opposed to being tracked by interface elements as was done in the Lagrangian formulation. This last equation is referred to as the *level set equation.*

Consider the following form for curve propagation:

$$C(p, t) = F(k)\hat{N}, \tag{8.7}$$

where $p = (x, y)$. The level set function represents the curve in the form of an implicit surface as follows:

$$\varphi(x, y, t)\colon \mathcal{R}^2 \times [0, T) \to \mathcal{R}, \tag{8.8}$$

that is derived from the initial contour according to the following condition:

$$C(p, 0) = \{(x, y)\colon \varphi(x, y, 0) = 0\}. \tag{8.9}$$

Taking the derivative with respect to time:

$$\varphi(C(p,t),t) = 0 \Longrightarrow \frac{\partial \varphi}{\partial C} \cdot \frac{\partial C}{\partial t} + \frac{\partial \varphi}{\partial t} = 0. \tag{8.10}$$

The level set function has the following relation with the embedded curve:

$$\varphi(C) = 0 \; or \; C = \varphi^{-1}(0). \tag{8.11}$$

The curve $\varphi(x, y, t) = 0$ deforms with time, Figure 8.2. Thus the level set function changes with time as follows:

$$\frac{\partial \varphi}{\partial t}dt + \frac{\partial \varphi}{\partial x}dx + \frac{\partial \varphi}{\partial y}dy = 0. \tag{8.12}$$

$$\frac{\partial \varphi}{\partial t} + \left(\frac{\partial \varphi}{\partial x}, \frac{\partial \varphi}{\partial y}\right) \cdot \left(\frac{dx}{dt}, \frac{dy}{dt}\right) = 0. \tag{8.13}$$

This leads to the fundamental level set equation:

$$\frac{\partial \varphi}{\partial t} + \nabla\varphi.\vec{V} = 0. \tag{8.14}$$

Further analysis may be done to obtain:

$$\frac{\partial \varphi}{\partial t} + |\nabla\varphi|\frac{\nabla\varphi}{|\nabla\varphi|}.\vec{V} = 0. \tag{8.15}$$

$$\frac{\partial \varphi}{\partial t} + |\nabla\varphi|F = 0. \tag{8.16}$$

The velocity vector $\vec{V}$ has a component F in the normal direction, whereas the other tangential component has no effect because the gradient works only in the normal direction.

F is called the speed function, and has several forms. One widely-used form of F is:

$$F = \pm 1 + \varepsilon k, \tag{8.17}$$

where the + sign is for expansion, and the − sign is for contraction. The coefficient K forces the contour to evolve smoothly, and the bending is controlled by ε [23]. The next two sections address the numerical schemes in detail as well as some of the most popular speed functions proposed in literature.

There are plenty of numerical schemes that can be used for solving the level set equation. The numerical solution of the level set equation, however, requires sophisticated techniques. Simple finite difference methods fail quickly. Up-winding methods, such as the Godunov method, fare better; yet the level set method does not guarantee the conservation of the volume or the shape of the level set in an advection field that does conserve the shape and size, for example uniform or rotational velocity field. Instead, the shape of the level set may get severely distorted and it may vanish over several time steps. For this reason, high-order finite difference schemes are generally required, such as high-order essentially non-oscillatory (ENO) schemes.

8.3 Numerical Approaches Solving the Level Set Equation

As was previously mentioned, the level set equation is:

$$\varphi_t + \vec{V} \cdot \nabla\varphi = 0 \tag{8.18}$$

Once φ and $\vec{V}$ are defined at every grid point (or at least sufficiently close to the interface) on our Cartesian grid, we can apply numerical methods to evolve φ forward in time moving the interface across the grid. At some point in time, say time t^n, let $\varphi^n = \varphi(t^n)$ represent the current values of φ. Updating φ in time consists of finding new values of φ at every grid point after some time increment Δt. We denote these new values of φ by $\varphi^{n+1} = \varphi(t^{n+1})$, where $t^{n+1} = t^n + \Delta t$. Then the time discretization of the above level set equation will be

$$\frac{\varphi^{n+1} - \varphi^n}{\Delta t} + \vec{V}^n \cdot \nabla\varphi^n = 0 \tag{8.19}$$

Where $\vec{V}^n =< u^n, v^n, w^n >$ is the given external velocity field at time t^n, and $\nabla\varphi^n$ evaluates the gradient operator using the values of φ at time t^n. One might evaluate the spatial derivatives of φ in a straightforward manner using first order finite difference formulas. Unfortunately, this straightforward approach will fail [24]. One generally needs to exercise great care when numerically discretizing partial differential equations. We begin by writing this equation in expanded form as

$$\frac{\varphi^{n+1} - \varphi^n}{\Delta t} + \left(u^n\varphi_x^n + v^n\varphi_y^n + w^n\varphi_z^n\right) = 0 \tag{8.20}$$

The techniques used to approximate the term $u^n\varphi_x^n$ can then be applied independently to the $v^n\varphi_y^n$ and $w^n\varphi_z^n$ terms in a ***dimension-by-dimension*** manner. For simplicity, consider the one-dimensional (x or y or z-direction) version of the last equation to be

$$\frac{\varphi^{n+1} - \varphi^n}{\Delta t} + u^n\varphi_x^n = 0, \quad \frac{\varphi^{n+1} - \varphi^n}{\Delta t} + v^n\varphi_y^n = 0 \quad or \quad \frac{\varphi^{n+1} - \varphi^n}{\Delta t} + w^n\varphi_z^n = 0$$

where the sign of u^n indicates whether the surface point of interest is moving to the right or to the left. Similarly the sign of v^n *and* w^n indicate forward or backward and up or down, respectively.

For simplicity in writing, $D^-\varphi$ and $D^+\varphi$ are used to denote first order backward and forward differences, respectively as follows: the same abbreviation may be used for y and z dimensions)

$$D^-\varphi = \frac{\partial\varphi}{\partial x} \approx \frac{\varphi_i - \varphi_{i-1}}{\Delta x} \quad and \quad D^+\varphi = \frac{\partial\varphi}{\partial x} \approx \frac{\varphi_{i+1} - \varphi_i}{\Delta x} \tag{8.21}$$

8.3.1 Upwind Differencing

Considering a specific grid point x_i, then we write the one dimensional version to be

$$\frac{\varphi_i^{n+1} - \varphi_i^n}{\Delta t} + u_i^n (\varphi_i)_x^n = 0, \tag{8.22}$$

If $u_i > 0$, the values of φ are moving from left to right, and the method of characteristics tells us to look to the left of x_i to determine what value of φ will land on the point x_i at the end of a time step. Similarly, if $u_i < 0$, the values of φ are moving from right to left, and the method of characteristics implies that we should look to the right to determine an appropriate value of φ_i at time t^{n+1}. Clearly, $D^-\varphi$ from equation (8.45) should be used to approximate φ_x when $u_i > 0$. Because $D^+\varphi$ from equation (8.45) cannot possibly give a good approximation, since it fails to contain the information to the left of x_i that dictates the new value of φ_i Similar reasoning indicates $D^+\varphi$ should be used to approximate φ_x when $u_i < 0$. The numerical explicit solution to the one-dimensional version can be re-written as:

$$\varphi_i^{n+1} = \varphi_i^n - \Delta t\left[\max\left(0, u_i^n\right) D^- \varphi_i^n + \min\left(0, u_i^n\right) D^+ \varphi_i^n\right], \tag{8.23}$$

We summarize the upwind discretization as follows. At each grid point, If $u_i > 0$, approximate φ_x with $D^-\varphi$. If $u_i < 0$, approximate φ_x with $D^+\varphi$. When $u_i = 0$, the $u_i(\varphi_x)_i$ term vanishes, and φ_x does not need to be approximated. This is a first-order accurate discretization of the spatial operator, since $D^-\varphi$ and $D^+\varphi$ are first-order accurate approximations of the derivative; i.e., the errors are of order $O(\Delta x)$. The combination of the forward ***Euler*** time discretization with the upwind difference scheme is a consistent finite difference approximation to the partial differential equation, since the approximation error converges to zero as $\Delta t \to 0$ *and* $\Delta x \to 0$. According to the Lax-Richtmyer equivalence theorem, a finite difference approximation to a linear partial differential equation is convergent (i.e., the correct solution is obtained) as $\Delta t \to 0$ *and* $\Delta x \to 0$, if and only if it is both consistent and stable. Stability guarantees that small errors in the approximation are not amplified as the solution is marched forward in time. Stability can be enforced using the Courant-Friedreichs-Lewy CFL condition, which asserts that the numerical waves should propagate at least as fast as the physical waves. This means that the numerical wave speed of $\Delta x/\Delta t$ must be at least as fast as the physical wave speed $|u|$. This leads us to the CFL *time step restriction* of

$$\Delta t < \frac{\Delta x}{\max\{|u|\}}, \tag{8.24}$$

Where $\max\{|u|\}$ is chosen to be the largest value of $|u|$ over the entire Cartesian grid. In reality, we only need to choose the largest value of $|u|$ on the interface. This condition is usually enforced by choosing a **CFL** number α, [25] as

$$\Delta t\left(\frac{\max\{|u|\}}{\Delta x}\right) = \alpha \tag{8.25}$$

And $0 < \alpha < 1$. A multidimensional **CFL** condition can be written as

$$\Delta t\, max\left\{\frac{|u|}{\Delta x}+\frac{|v|}{\Delta y}+\frac{|w|}{\Delta z}\right\}=\alpha \qquad or \qquad \Delta t\left(\frac{max\{|\vec{V}|\}}{min\{\Delta x,\Delta y,\Delta z\}}\right)=\alpha \tag{8.26}$$

Numerical Solution to the higher order scheme

The numerical solution of the level set equation:

$$\varphi_t+|\nabla\varphi|F=0$$

can be obtained similar to above, and is as follows:

$$\left(\varphi_{ij}^{n+1}\right)=\left(\varphi_{ij}^{n}\right)-\Delta t(\nabla^{+}\ \nabla^{-})\begin{pmatrix}\max(F_{i,j},0)\\ \min(F_{i,j},0)\end{pmatrix}, \tag{8.27}$$

where

$$\nabla^{+}=[\max(A,0)^2+\min(B,0)^2+\max(C,0)^2+\min(D,0)^2]^{0.5}$$
$$\nabla^{-}=[\min(A,0)^2+\max(B,0)^2+\min(C,0)^2+\max(D,0)^2]^{0.5}$$
$$A=D_{ij}^{-x}\varphi+\frac{\Delta x}{2}m\left(D_{ij}^{-x-x}\varphi,D_{ij}^{+x-x}\varphi\right)$$
$$B=D_{ij}^{+x}\varphi-\frac{\Delta x}{2}m\left(D_{ij}^{+x+x}\varphi,D_{ij}^{+x-x}\varphi\right)$$
$$C=D_{ij}^{-y}\varphi+\frac{\Delta y}{2}m\left(D_{ij}^{-y-y}\varphi,D_{ij}^{+y-y}\varphi\right)$$
$$D=D_{ij}^{+y}\varphi-\frac{\Delta y}{2}m\left(D_{ij}^{+y+y}\varphi,D_{ij}^{+y-y}\varphi\right)$$

where the speed function is given by

$$F_{i,j}=v+\varepsilon K_{ij}, \tag{8.28}$$

and the switching function m is given by:

$$m(a,b)=\begin{cases}aH_\alpha(a,b) & if\ \ |a|\le|b|\\ bH_\alpha(a,b) & if\ \ |a|>|b|\end{cases}, \tag{8.29}$$

where $H_\alpha(\varphi)$ is the Heaviside function and is defined as:

$$H_\alpha(\varphi)=\begin{cases}0.5\left(1+\frac{\varphi}{\alpha}+\frac{1}{\pi}\sin\left(\frac{\pi\varphi}{\alpha}\right)\right), & |\varphi|\le\alpha\\ 1, & |\varphi|>\alpha\end{cases} \tag{8.30}$$

Instead of ***upwinding***, the spatial derivatives of image energy could be approximated with the more accurate central differencing. Unfortunately, simple central differencing is unstable with forward Euler time discretization and the usual **CFL** conditions with $\Delta t \sim \Delta x$. Stability can be achieved by using a much more restrictive **CFL** condition with $\Delta t \sim (\Delta x)^2$, although this is too computationally costly. Stability can also be achieved by using a different temporal discretization, e.g., the third-order accurate Runge-Kutta method (discussed later). A third way of achieving stability consists in adding some artificial dissipation to obtain

$$\varphi_t + \vec{V} \cdot \nabla \varphi = \mu \Delta \varphi \tag{8.31}$$

where the viscosity coefficient μ is chosen proportional to Δx, i.e., $\mu \sim \Delta x$, so that the artificial viscosity vanishes as $\Delta x \to 0$, enforcing consistency for this method. While all three of these approaches stabilize central differencing, we instead prefer to use upwind methods, which draw on the highly successful technology developed for the numerical solution of conservation laws.

8.3.2 Hamilton-Jacobi

The first-order accurate upwind scheme described in the last section can be improved upon by using a more accurate approximation for φ_x^- and φ_x^+. The velocity u is still used to decide whether φ_x^- or φ_x^+ is used, but the approximations for φ_x^- or φ_x^+ can be improved significantly. ***Harten*** et al. [26] introduced the idea of ***essentially nonoscillatory*** (**ENO**) polynomial interpolation of data for the numerical solution of conservation laws. Their basic idea was to compute numerical flux functions using the smoothest possible polynomial interpolants. The actual numerical implementation of this idea was improved considerably by Shu and Osher in [27, 28], where the numerical flux functions were constructed directly from a **divided difference table** of the pointwise data. Osher and Sethian realized that Hamilton-Jacobi equations in one spatial dimension are integrals of conservation laws. They used this fact to extend the ENO method for the numerical discretization of conservation laws to Hamilton-Jacobi equations. This Hamilton-Jacobi with the idea of essentially nonoscillatory (**HJENO**) method allows to extend first-order accurate upwind differencing to higher-order spatial accuracy by providing better numerical approximations to φ_x^- or φ_x^+.

We summarize the idea of (**HJ ENO**) method as follows. We use the smoothest possible polynomial interpolation (with Newton polynomial interpolation [29]) to find φ and then differentiate to get φ_x. Define $D_i^0\varphi = \varphi_i$ at each grid node located at x_i. The first divided differences of φ are defined midway between grid nodes as

$$D_{i+1/2}^1\varphi = \frac{D_{i+1}^0\varphi - D_i^0\varphi}{\Delta x} \tag{8.32}$$

Assuming that the mesh spacing is uniformly equals Δx. Note that $D_{i+1/2}^1\varphi = (D^+\varphi)_i$ *and* $D_{i-1/2}^1\varphi = (D^-\varphi)_i$, i.e., ***the first divided differences, are the forward and backward difference approximations to the derivatives***. The second divided differences are defined at the grid nodes as

$$D_i^2\varphi = \frac{D_{i+1/2}^1\varphi - D_{i-1/2}^1\varphi}{2\Delta x} \tag{8.33}$$

while the third divided differences

$$D_{i+1/2}^3\varphi = \frac{D_{i+1}^2\varphi - D_i^2\varphi}{3\Delta x} \tag{8.34}$$

The divided differences are used to reconstruct a polynomial of the form

$$\varphi(x) = Q_0(x) + Q_1(x) + Q_2(x) + Q_3(x) \tag{8.35}$$

that can be differentiated and evaluated at x_i to find $(\varphi_x^+)_i$ and $(\varphi_x^-)_i$. That is,

$$\varphi_x(x_i) = Q_1'(x_i) + Q_2'(x_i) + Q_3'(x_i) \tag{8.36}$$

Note that the constant $Q_0(x)$ vanishes upon differentiation. And to find φ_x^+ we define

$$Q_1(x) = \left(D_{i+1/2}^1\varphi\right)(x - x_i) \quad \textit{so that} \quad Q_1'(x_i) = D_{i+1/2}^1\varphi \tag{8.37}$$

And to define φ_x^-, then we define $Q_1(x) = (D_{i-1/2}^1\varphi)(x - x_{i-1})$ *so* $Q_1'(x_i) = D_{i-1/2}^1\varphi$. Implying that the contribution from the *first-order accurate polynomial interpolation* $Q_1'(x_i)$ is exactly first-order upwinding. Improvements are obtained by including the $Q_2'(x_i)$ and $Q_3'(x_i)$ terms, leading to second- and third-order accuracy, respectively.

Looking at the divided difference table, let $j = i$ *for* φ_x^+ *and* $j = i - 1$ *for* φ_x^-. Then we have two choices for the second-order accurate correction. We could include the next point to the left and use $D_j^2\varphi$, or we could include the next point to the right and use $D_{j+1}^2\varphi$. The key observation is that smooth slowly varying data tend to produce small numbers in divided difference tables, while discontinuous or quickly varying data tend to produce large numbers in divided difference tables. This is obvious in the sense that the differences measure variation in the data. Comparing $|D_j^2\varphi|$ to $|D_{j+1}^2\varphi|$ indicates which of the polynomial interpolants has more variation. We would like to avoid interpolating near large variations such as discontinuities or steep gradients since they cause overshoots in the interpolating function, leading to numerical errors in the approximation of the derivative. Thus, if $|D_j^2\varphi| \leq |D_{j+1}^2\varphi|$, we set $c = D_j^2\varphi$; otherwise, we set $c = D_{j+1}^2\varphi$. Then we define

$$Q_2(x) = c(x - x_j)(x - x_{j+1}) \tag{8.38}$$

So that

$$Q_2'(x_i) = c(2(i - \mathrm{j}) - 1)\Delta x$$

Is the second-order accurate correction to the approximation of φ_x in equation (level set). If we stop here, i.e., omitting the Q_3 term, we have a second-order accurate method for approximating φ_x^+ and φ_x^-. Similar to the second-order accurate correction, the third-order accurate correction is obtained by comparing $|D^3_{k+1/2}\varphi|$ to $|D^2_{k+3/2}\varphi|$. If $|D^3_{k+1/2}\varphi| \le |D^3_{k+3/2}\varphi|$, we set $\hat{c} = D^3_{k+1/2}\varphi$; otherwise, we set $\hat{c} = D^3_{k+3/2}\varphi$. Then we define

$$Q_3(x) = \hat{c}(x - x_k)(x - x_{k+1})(x - x_{k+2}) \tag{8.39}$$

So that

$$Q_3'(x_i) = \hat{c}(3(i - \mathrm{k})^2 - 6(i = k) + 2)(\Delta x)^2$$

Is the third-order accurate correction to the approximation of φ_x.

8.3.3 Hamilton-Jacobi WENO

When calculating $(\varphi_x^-)_i$ *or* $(\varphi_x^+)_i$, the third-order accurate **HJ ENO** scheme uses a subset of $\{\varphi_{i-3}, \varphi_{i-2}, \varphi_{i-1}, \varphi_i, \varphi_{i+1}, \varphi_{i+2}\}$ *or* $\{\varphi_{i-2}, \varphi_{i-1}, \varphi_i, \varphi_{i+1}, \varphi_{i+2}, \varphi_{i+3}\}$ respectively. In fact, there are exactly three possible **HJ ENO** approximations to $(\varphi_x^-)_i$. Defining $\nu_1 = D^-\varphi_{i-2}$, $\nu_2 = D^-\varphi_{i-1}$, $\nu_3 = D^-\varphi_i$, $\nu_4 = D^-\varphi_{i+1}$ *and* $\nu_5 = D^-\varphi_{i+2}$ allows us to write

$$\varphi_x^1 = \frac{\nu_1}{3} - \frac{7\nu_2}{6} + \frac{11\nu_3}{6} \tag{8.40}$$

$$\varphi_x^2 = -\frac{\nu_2}{6} + \frac{5\nu_3}{6} + \frac{\nu_4}{3}$$

and

$$\varphi_x^3 = \frac{\nu_3}{3} + \frac{5\nu_4}{6} - \frac{\nu_5}{6}$$

as the three potential **HJ ENO** approximations to φ_x^-. The goal of **HJ ENO** is to choose the single approximation with the least error by choosing the smoothest possible polynomial interpolation of φ.

In [30], Liu et al. pointed out that the ENO philosophy of picking exactly one of three candidate stencils is overkill in smooth regions where the data are well behaved. They proposed a **weighted ENO (WENO)** method that takes a convex combination of the three ENO approximations. All three approximations are allowed to make a significant contribution in a way that improves the local accuracy from third order to fourth order. Of course, if any of the three approximations interpolates across a discontinuity, it is given minimal weight in the convex combination in order to minimize its contribution and the resulting errors. Later, following the work on **HJ ENO** in [30], Jiang and Peng extended WENO to the Hamilton-Jacobi framework. This Hamilton-Jacobi WENO, or HJ WENO, scheme turns out to be very useful for solving Eq. (8.18), since it reduces the errors by more than an order of magnitude over the third-order accurate HJ ENO scheme for typical applications.

The HJ WENO approximation of $(\varphi_x^-)_i$ is a convex combination of the three approximations in Eq. (8.40) given by

$$\varphi_x = \omega_1 \varphi_x^1 + \omega_2 \varphi_x^2 + \omega_3 \varphi_x^3 \tag{8.41}$$

Where the $0 \leq \omega_k \leq 1$ are the weights with $\omega_1 + \omega_2 + \omega_3 = 1$. The key observation for obtaining high-order accuracy in smooth regions is that weights of $\omega_1 = 0.1, \omega_2 = 0.6$ *and* $\omega_3 = 0.3$ give the optimal fifth-order accurate approximation to φ_x. While this is the optimal approximation, it is valid only in smooth regions. In non-smooth regions this optimal weighting can be very inaccurate, and we are better off with digital ($\omega_k = 0$ *or* $\omega_k = 1$) weights that choose a single approximation to φ_x, i.e., the **HJ ENO** approximation.

In [31], it was pointed out that setting $\omega_1 = 0.1 + O((\Delta x)^2), \omega_2 = 0.6 + O((\Delta x)^2)$ *and* $\omega_3 = 0.3 + O((\Delta x)^2)$ still gives the optimal fifth-order accuracy in smooth regions. In order to see this, we rewrite these as $\omega_1 = 0.1 + C_1(\Delta x)^2$, $\omega_2 = 0.6 + C_2(\Delta x)^2$ *and* $\omega_3 = 0.3 + C_3(\Delta x)^2$ and plug them into Eq. (8.41) to obtain

$$0.1\varphi_x^1 + 0.6\varphi_x^2 + 0.3\varphi_x^3 \tag{8.42}$$

and

$$C_1(\Delta x)^2\varphi_x^1 + C_2(\Delta x)^2\varphi_x^2 + C_3(\Delta x)^2\varphi_x^3 \tag{8.43}$$

as the two terms that are added to give the **HJ WENO** approximation to φ_x. The term given by Eq. (8.42) is the optimal approximation that gives the exact value of φ_x plus an $O((\Delta x)^5)$ error term. Thus, if the term given by Eq. (8.43) is $O((\Delta x)^5)$, then the entire **HJ WENO** approximation is $O((\Delta x)^5)$ in smooth regions. To see that, first note that each of the **HJ ENO** φ_x^k approximations gives the exact value of φ_x, denoted by φ_x^E, plus an $O((\Delta x)^3$ error term (in smooth regions). Thus, the term in Eq. (8.43) is

$$C_1(\Delta x)^2\varphi_x^E + C_2(\Delta x)^2\varphi_x^E + C_3(\Delta x)^2\varphi_x^E \tag{8.44}$$

Plus an $O((\Delta x)^2)O((\Delta x)^3) = O((\Delta x)^5)$ term. Since, each of the C_k *is* $O(1)$, as is φ_x^E, this appears to be an $O((\Delta x)^2)$ term at first glance. However, since $\omega_1 + \omega_2 + \omega_3 = 1$, we have $C_1 + C_2 + C_3 = 0$, implying that the term in Eq. (8.44) is identically zero. Thus, the **HJ WENO** approximation is $O((\Delta x)^5)$ in smooth regions. Note that [48] obtained only fourth-order accuracy, since they chose $\omega_1 = 0.1 + O(\Delta x), \omega_2 = 0.6 + O(\Delta x)$ *and* $\omega_3 = 0.3 + O(\Delta x)$.

In order to define the weights ω_k, we follow [32] and estimate the smoothness of the three stencils in Eq. (8.40) as

$$S_1 = \frac{13}{12}(\nu_1 - 2\nu_2 + \nu_3)^2 + \frac{1}{4}(\nu_1 - 4\nu_2 + 3\nu_3)^2 \tag{8.45}$$

$$S_2 = \frac{13}{12}(\nu_2 - 2\nu_3 + \nu_4)^2 + \frac{1}{4}(\nu_2 - \nu_4)^2$$

$$S_3 = \frac{13}{12}(\nu_3 - 2\nu_3 + \nu_4)^2 + \frac{1}{4}(3\nu_1 - 4\nu_4 + \nu_5)^2,$$

respectively. Using these smoothness estimates, we define

$$\alpha_1 = \frac{0.1}{(S_1+\epsilon)^2} \quad \alpha_2 = \frac{0.6}{(S_2+\epsilon)^2} \quad \alpha_3 = \frac{0.3}{(S_3+\epsilon)^2}, \tag{8.46}$$

with

$$\epsilon = 10^{-6} max\{\nu_1{}^2, \nu_2{}^2, \nu_3{}^2, \nu_4{}^2, \nu_5{}^2\} + 10^{-99}, \tag{8.47}$$

where the 10^{-99} term is set to avoid division by zero in the definition of the α_k. This value for epsilon was first proposed by Fedkiw et al. [33], where the first term is a scaling term that aids in the balance between the optimal fifth-order accurate stencil and the digital HJ ENO weights. In the case that φ is an approximate signed distance function, the ν_k that approximate φ_x are approximately equal to one, so that the first term in Eq. (8.47) can be set to 10^{-6}. This first term can then absorb the second term, yielding $\epsilon = 10^{-6}$ in place of Eq. (8.47) to make this $\nu_k \approx 1$ estimate in higher dimensions as well.

A smooth solution has small variation leading to small S_k. If they are small enough compared to ϵ, then $\alpha_1 \approx 0.1\epsilon^{-2}, \alpha_2 \approx 0.6\epsilon^{-2}$ *and* $\alpha_3 \approx 0.3\epsilon^{-2}$, exhibiting the proper ratios for the optimal fifth-order accuracy. That is, normalizing the α_k to obtain the weights

$$\omega_1 = \frac{\alpha_1}{\alpha_1+\alpha_2+\alpha_3} \qquad \omega_2 = \frac{\alpha_2}{\alpha_1+\alpha_2+\alpha_3} \qquad \omega_3 = \frac{\alpha_3}{\alpha_1+\alpha_2+\alpha_3}, \tag{8.48}$$

gives (approximately) the optimal weights of $\omega_1 = 0.1$, $\omega_2 = 0.6$ *and* $\omega_3 = 0.3$. Nearly optimal weights are also obtained when the S_k are larger than ϵ, as long as all the S_k are approximately the same size, as is the case for sufficiently smooth data. On the other hand, if the data are not smooth as indicated by large S_k, then the corresponding α_k will be small compared to the other α_k's. If two of the S_k are relatively large, then their corresponding α_k's will both be small, and the scheme will rely most heavily on a single stencil similar to the digital behavior of HJ ENO. In the unfortunate instance that all three of the S_k are large, the data are poorly conditioned, and none of the stencils are particularly useful. This case is problematic for the HJ ENO method as well, but fortunately it usually occurs only locally in space and time, allowing the methods to repair themselves after the situation subsides.

The function $(\varphi_x^+)_i$ is constructed with a subset $\{\varphi_{i-2}, \varphi_{i-1}, \varphi_i, \varphi_{i+1}, \varphi_{i+2}, \varphi_{i+3}\}$. Defining $\nu_1 = D^+\varphi_{i+2}$, $\nu_2 = D^+\varphi_{i+1}$, $\nu_3 = D^+\varphi_i$, $\nu_4 = D^+\varphi_{i-1}$ *and* $\nu_5 = D^+\varphi_{i-2}$ allows us to use equations (8.64) as the three HJ ENO approximations to $(\varphi_x^+)_i$. Then the HJ WENO convex combination is given by Eq. (8.41) with the weights given by Eq. (8.48).

8.3.4 TVD Runge-Kutta

Practical experience suggests that level set methods are sensitive to spatial accuracy, implying that the fifth-order accurate **HJ WENO** method is desirable. On the other hand, temporal truncation errors seem to produce significantly less deterioration of the numerical solution, so one can often use the low-order accurate forward Euler method for discretization in time. There are times when a higher-order temporal discretization is necessary in order to obtain accurate numerical solutions. In [27], Shu and Osher proposed **total variation diminishing (TVD) Runge-Kutta (RK)** methods to increase the accuracy to temporal discretization. The approach assumes that the spatial discretization can be separated from the temporal discretization in a manner that allows the temporal discretization of the PDE to be treated independently as an ODE. While there are numerous RK schemes, these TVD RK schemes guarantee that no spurious oscillations are produced as a consequence of the higher-order accurate temporal discretization. The basic first-order accurate TVD RK scheme is just the forward Euler method. We assume that the forward Euler method is TVD in conjunction with the spatial discretization of the PDE. Then higher-order accurate methods are obtained by sequentially taking Euler steps and combining the results with the initial data using a convex combination. The second-order accurate TVD RK scheme is identical to the standard second-order accurate RK scheme. It is also known as the midpoint rule, as the modified Euler method, and as Heun's predictor-corrector method.

First, an Euler step is taken to advance the solution to time $t^n + \Delta t$,

$$\frac{\varphi^{n+1} - \varphi^n}{\Delta t} + \vec{V}^n \cdot \nabla \varphi^n = 0 \tag{8.49}$$

followed by a **second Euler step** to advance the solution to time $t^n + 2\Delta t$,

$$\frac{\varphi^{n+2} - \varphi^{n+1}}{\Delta t} + \vec{V}^{n+1} \cdot \nabla \varphi^{n+1} = 0, \tag{8.50}$$

followed by an averaging step

$$\varphi^{n+1} = \frac{\varphi^n + \varphi^{n+2}}{2}. \tag{8.51}$$

The final averaging step produces the second-order accurate TVD (for HJ ENO and HJ WENO) approximation to φ at time $t^n + \Delta t$. **The third-order accurate** TVD RK scheme proposed in [34] is as follows. First, an Euler step is taken to advance the solution to time $t^n + \Delta t$ Eq. (8.49) and Eq. (8.50) followed by an averaging step

$$\varphi^{n+\frac{1}{2}} = \frac{3\varphi^n + \varphi^{n+2}}{4} \tag{8.52}$$

that produces an approximation to φ at time $t^n + \frac{1}{2}\Delta t$ then another Euler step is taken to advance the solution to time $t^n + \frac{3}{2}\Delta t$

$$\frac{\varphi^{n+\frac{3}{2}} - \varphi^{n+\frac{1}{2}}}{\Delta t} + \vec{V}^{n+\frac{1}{2}} \cdot \nabla\varphi^{n+\frac{1}{2}} = 0, \tag{8.53}$$

followed by a second averaging step

$$\varphi^{n+1} = \frac{\varphi^n + 2\,\varphi^{n+\frac{3}{2}}}{3} \tag{8.54}$$

that produces a **third-order** accurate approximation to φ at time $t^n + \Delta t$. This third-order accurate TVD RK method has a stability region that includes part of the imaginary axis. Thus, a stable (although ill-advised) numerical method results from combining third-order accurate TVD RK with central differencing for the spatial discretization. While fourth-order accurate (and higher) TVD RK schemes exist, this improved temporal accuracy does not seem to make a significant difference in practical calculations. Also, the fourth-order accurate (and higher) TVD RK methods require both upwind and downwind differencing approximations, doubling the computational cost of evaluating the spatial operators. See [27] for fourth- and fifth-order accurate TVD RK schemes. Finally, we note that a rather interesting approach to TVD RK schemes has recently been carried out by Spiteri and Ruuth [35], who proposed increasing the number of internal stages so that this number exceeds the order of the method.

The next section addresses the Hamilton-Jacobi equations, from which the basic level set equation was derived. Numerical solutions to the general form of the Hamilton-Jacobi equations are sought.

8.3.5 Hamilton-Jacobi Equations

The level set representation discussed is a simple instance of the general form of the Hamilton-Jacobi equations [24], with numerous numerical methods proposed in literature for solution. Some of these numerical schemes include Lax-Friedrichs scheme [36], the Roe-Fix scheme [37], and Godunov's scheme [38].

Consider the general form of *Hamilton-Jacobi* equations of the form

$$\varphi_t + H(\nabla\varphi) = 0, \tag{8.55}$$

where H can be a function of both space and time. In three spatial dimensions, we can write

$$\varphi_t + H(\varphi_x, \varphi_y, \varphi_z) = 0$$

as an expanded version of equation (8.79). Convection in an externally generated velocity field equation (8.42) is an example of a Hamilton-Jacobi equation where $H(\nabla\varphi) = \vec{V} \cdot \nabla\varphi$. Hamilton-Jacobi equations depend on (at most) the first derivatives of φ, and these equations are hyperbolic.

From first glance Eq. (8.55) looks different, however in the next paragraph it will be shown that it is a general form to the convection laws.

Consider the one-dimensional scalar conservation law

$$u_t + F(u)_x = 0; \tag{8.56}$$

where u is the conserved quantity and $F(u)$ is the flux function. A well-known conservation law is the continuity equation for conservation of mass

$$\rho_t + (\rho u)_x = 0 \tag{8.57}$$

where ρ is the density of the material. The continuity equation is combined with equations for conservation of momentum and conservation of energy to obtain the compressible Navier-Stokes equations. When viscous effects are ignored, the Navier-Stokes equations reduce to the compressible inviscid Euler equations. The presence of discontinuities in the Euler equations forces one to consider weak solutions where the derivatives of solution variables can fail to exist. Examples include linear contact discontinuities and nonlinear shock waves. The nonlinear nature of shock waves allows them to develop as the solution progresses forward in time even if the data are initially smooth. The Euler equations may not always have unique solutions, and an *entropy condition* is used to pick out the physically correct solution.

Burgers' equation

$$u_t + \left(\frac{u^2}{2}\right)_x = 0 \tag{8.58}$$

Is a scalar conservation law that possesses many of the interesting nonlinear properties contained in the more complex Euler equations. It develops discontinuous shock waves from smooth initial data. Many of the numerical methods developed to solve *Burgers' equation* can be extended to treat both the one-dimensional and the multidimensional Euler equations of gas dynamics.

Consider the one-dimensional *Hamilton-Jacobi* equation

$$\varphi_t + H(\varphi_x) = 0, \tag{8.59}$$

which becomes

$$(\varphi_x)_t + H(\varphi_x)_x = 0 \tag{8.60}$$

after one takes a spatial derivative of the entire equation. Setting $u = \varphi_x$ results in

$$u_t + H(u)_x = 0 \tag{8.61}$$

which is a scalar conservation law; thus, in one spatial dimension we can draw a direct correspondence between Hamilton-Jacobi equations and conservation laws. The solution u to a conservation law is the derivative of a solution φ to a Hamilton-Jacobi equation. Conversely, the solution φ to a Hamilton-Jacobi equation is the integral of a solution u to a conservation law. This allows us to point out a number of useful facts. For example, since the integral of a discontinuity is a kink, or discontinuity in the first derivative, solutions to Hamilton-Jacobi equations can develop kinks in the solution even if the data are initially smooth. In addition, solutions to Hamilton-Jacobi equations cannot generally develop a discontinuity unless the corresponding conservation law develops a delta function. Thus, solutions φ to Eq. (8.55) are typically continuous [24]. Furthermore, since conservation laws can have non-unique solutions, entropy conditions are needed to pick out "physically" relevant solutions to Eq. (8.55) as well. Osher and Sethian [12] used the connection between conservation laws and Hamilton-Jacobi equations to construct higher-order accurate numerical methods. Even though the analogy between conservation laws and Hamilton-Jacobi equations fails in multiple spatial dimensions, many Hamilton-Jacobi equations can be discretized in a dimension by dimension fashion. This culminated in [37], where Osher and Shu proposed a general framework for the numerical solution of Hamilton-Jacobi equations using successful methods from the theory of conservation laws. The next step now is how numerically handling Eqn. (8.16) in higher dimensions which is as numerical discretization.

A forward Euler time discretization of a Hamilton-Jacobi equation can be written as

$$\frac{\varphi^{n+1} - \varphi^n}{\Delta t} + \hat{H}(\varphi_x^-, \varphi_x^+; \varphi_y^-, \varphi_y^+; \varphi_z^-, \varphi_z^+) = 0 \tag{8.62}$$

Where $\hat{H}(\varphi_x^-, \varphi_x^+; \varphi_y^-, \varphi_y^+; \varphi_z^-, \varphi_z^+)$ is a numerical approximation of $H(\varphi_x, \varphi_y, \varphi_z)$ The function $\hat{H}$ is called a numerical *Hamiltonian*, and it is required to be consistent in the sense that $\hat{H} = H$. Spatial derivatives are discretized with either first-order accurate one-sided differencing or the higher-order accurate HJ ENO or HJ WENO schemes. We will discuss the two-dimensional numerical approximation to $H(\varphi_x, \varphi_y)$, with the ability to extend this analysis to three spatial dimensions. An important class of schemes is that of *monotone* schemes. A scheme is *monotone* when φ^{n+1} as defined in Eq. (8.62) is a non-decreasing function of all the φ^n. Crandall and Lions proved that these schemes converge to the correct solution, although they are only first-order accurate. The numerical Hamiltonians associated with monotone schemes are important. The forward Euler time discretization also can be extended to higher-order TVD Runge Kutta in a straightforward manner, as discussed before. The CFL condition for Eq. 8.62 is

$$\Delta t \; max \left\{ \frac{|H_1|}{\Delta x} + \frac{|H_2|}{\Delta y} + \frac{|H_3|}{\Delta z} \right\} < 1 \tag{8.63}$$

where H_1, H_2 and H_3 are the partial derivatives of H with respect to φ_x, φ_y and φ_z. For example, in equation (8.42), where $H(\nabla\varphi) = V \cdot \nabla\varphi$, the partial derivatives of H are $H_1 = u, H_2 = v$, and $H_3 = w$. As another example, consider the level set equation with $H(\nabla\varphi) = V_n|\nabla\varphi|$. Here the partial derivatives are slightly more complicated, with $H_1 = V_n\varphi_x/|\nabla\varphi|, H_2 = V_n\varphi_y/|\nabla\varphi|$, and $H_3 = V_n\varphi_z/|\nabla\varphi|$ assuming that V_n does not depend on φ_x, φ_y or φ_z. otherwise, the partial derivatives can be substantially more complicated.

8.3.5.1 Lax-Friedrichs Schemes

The first approximation to $\hat{H}$ that we consider is the *Lax-Friedrichs* (LF) scheme from [36] given by

$$\hat{H} = H\left(\frac{\varphi_x^- + \varphi_x^+}{2}, \frac{\varphi_y^- + \varphi_y^+}{2}\right) - \alpha^x\left(\frac{\varphi_x^+ - \varphi_x^-}{2}\right) - \alpha^y\left(\frac{\varphi_y^+ - \varphi_y^-}{2}\right), \tag{8.64}$$

where α^x and α^y are dissipation coefficients that control the amount of numerical viscosity,

$$\alpha^x = max|H_1(\varphi_x, \varphi_y)|, \alpha^y = max|H_2(\varphi_x, \varphi_y)| \tag{8.65}$$

These dissipation coefficients are chosen based on the partial derivatives of H. The choice of these dissipation coefficients can be rather subtle. In the traditional implementation of the LF scheme, the maximum is chosen over the entire computational domain. First, the maximum and minimum values of φ_x are identified by considering all the values of φ_x^- and φ_x^+ on the Cartesian mesh. Then one can identify the interval $I^x = [\varphi_x^{min}, \varphi_x^{max}]$. A similar procedure is used to define $I^y = [\varphi_y^{min}, \varphi_x^{max}]$. The coefficients α^x and α^y are set to the maximum possible values of $|H_1(\varphi_x, \varphi_y)|$ and $|H_2(\varphi_x, \varphi_y)|$, respectively with $\varphi_x \in I^x$ and $\varphi_y \in I^y$. Although it is occasionally difficult to evaluate the maximum values of $|H_1|$ and $|H_2|$, it is straightforward to do so in many instances. For example, in Eq. (8.18), both $H_1 = u$ and $H_2 = v$ are independent of φ_x and φ_y, so α^x and α^y can be set to the maximum values of $|u|$ and $|v|$ on the Cartesian mesh. The price we pay for using bounds to choose α larger than it should be is increased numerical dissipation. That is, while the numerical method will be stable and give an accurate solution as the mesh is refined, some details of this solution may be smeared out and lost on a coarse mesh.

Since increasing α increases the amount of artificial dissipation, decreasing the quality of the solution, it is beneficial to choose α as small as possible without inducing oscillations or other nonphysical phenomena into the solution. In approximating $\hat{H}_{i,j}$ at a grid point $\vec{x}_{i,j}$ on a Cartesian mesh, it then makes little sense to do a global search to define the intervals I^x and I^y. In particular, consider the simple convection Eq. (8.18) where $\alpha^x = max|u|$ and $\alpha^y = max|v|$. Suppose that some region had relatively small values of $|u|$ and $|v|$, while another region had relatively large values. Since the LF method chooses α^x as the largest value of $|u|$ and α^y as the largest value of $|v|$, the same values of α will be used in the region where the velocities are small a is used in the region where the velocities are large. In the region where the velocities are large, the large values of α are required to obtain a good solution. But in the region where the velocities are small, these large values of α produce too much numerical dissipation, wiping out small features of the solution. Thus, it is advantageous to use only the grid points sufficiently close to $\vec{x}_{i,j}$ in determining α. A rule of thumb is to include the grid points from $\vec{x}_{i-3,j}$ to $\vec{x}_{i+3,j}$ in the x-direction and from $\vec{x}_{i,j-3}$ to $\vec{x}_{i,j+3}$ in the y-direction in the local search neighborhood for determining α. This includes all the grid nodes that are used to evaluate $\varphi_x^{\pm}$ and $\varphi_y^{\pm}$ at $\vec{x}_{i,j}$ using the HJ WENO scheme. This type of scheme has been referred to as a *Stencil Lax-Friedrichs* (SLF) scheme, since it determines the dissipation coefficient using only the neighboring grid points that are part of the stencil used to determine φ_x and φ_y. An alternative to the dimension-by-dimension neighborhoods is to use the 49 grid points in the rectangle with diagonal corners at $\vec{x}_{i-3,j-3}$ and $\vec{x}_{i+3,j+3}$ to determine α. This idea of searching only locally to determine the dissipation coefficients can be taken a step further. The *Local Lax-Friedrichs* (LLF) scheme proposed for conservation laws by Shu and Osher [28] does not look at any neighboring grid points when calculating the dissipation coefficients in a given direction. In [27], Osher and Shu interpreted this to mean that α^x is determined at each grid point using only the values of φ_x^- and φ_x^+ at that specific grid point to determine the interval I^x. The interval I^y is still determined in the LF or SLF manner (in the SLF case we rename LLF as SLLF). Similarly, α^y uses an interval I^y, defined using only the values of φ_y^- and φ_y^+ at the grid point in question while I^x is still determined in the LF or SLF fashion. Osher and Shu [27] also proposed the *Local Local Lax-Friedrichs* (LLLF) scheme with even less numerical dissipation. At each grid point I^x is determined using the values of φ_x^- and φ_x^+ at that grid point; I^y is determined using the values of φ_y^- and φ_y^+ at that grid point; and then these intervals are used to determine both α^x and α^y. When H is separable, i.e., $H(\varphi_x, \varphi_y) = H_x(\varphi_x) + H_y(\varphi_y)$, LLLF reduces to LLF, since α^x is independent of φ_y and α^y is independent of φ_x. When H not separable, LLF and LLLF are truly distinct schemes. In practice, LLF seems to work better than any of the other options. LF and SLF are usually too dissipative, while LLLF is usually not dissipative enough to overcome the problems introduced by using the centrally averaged approximation to φ_x and φ_y in evaluating H in equation (8.88). Note that LLF is a monotone scheme.

8.3.5.2 The Roe-Fix Scheme

As discussed above, choosing the appropriate amount of artificial dissipation to add to the centrally evaluated H in Eq. (8.64) can be problematic. Therefore, it is often desirable to use upwind-based methods with built-in artificial dissipation. For conservation laws, Shu and Osher [28] proposed using *Roe's* upwind method along with an LLF entropy correction at sonic points where entropy-violating expansion shocks might form. The added dissipation from the LLF entropy correction forces the expansion shocks to develop into continuous rarefaction waves. The method was named *Roe Fix* (RF) and it can be written for Hamilton-Jacobi equations (see [28]) as

$$\hat{H} = H(\varphi_x^*, \varphi_y^*) - \alpha^x \left(\frac{\varphi_x^+ - \varphi_x^-}{2} \right) - \alpha^y \left(\frac{\varphi_y^+ - \varphi_y^-}{2} \right) \tag{8.66}$$

In the RF scheme, I^x and I^y are initially determined using only the nodal values for $\varphi_x^\pm$ and $\varphi_y^\pm$ as in the LLLF scheme. In order to estimate the potential for upwinding, we look at the partial derivatives H_1 and H_2. If $H_1(\varphi_x, \varphi_y)$ has the same sign (either always positive or always negative) for all $\varphi_x \in I^x$ and all $\varphi_y \in I^y$, we know which way information flows and can apply upwinding. Similarly, if $H_2(\varphi_x, \varphi_y)$ has the same sign for all $\varphi_x \in I^x$ and $\varphi_y \in I^y$, we can upwind this term as well. If both H_1 and H_2 do not change sign, we upwind completely, setting both α^x and α^y to zero. If $H_1 > 0$, information is flowing from left to right, then we set $\varphi_x^* = \varphi_x^-$. Otherwise, $H_1 < 0$ and we set $\varphi_x^* = \varphi_x^+$. Similarly, $H_2 > 0$ indicates $\varphi_y^* = \varphi_y^-$, and H2 < 0 indicates $\varphi_y^* = \varphi_y^+$.

If either H_1 or H_2 changes sign, we are in the vicinity of a sonic point where the eigenvalue (in this case H_1 or H_2) is identically zero. This signifies a potential difficulty with non-unique solutions, and artificial dissipation is needed to pick out the physically correct vanishing viscosity solution. We switch from the RF scheme to the LLF scheme to obtain the needed artificial viscosity. If there is a sonic point in only one direction, i.e., x or y, it makes little sense to add damping in both directions. Therefore, we look for sonic points in each direction and add damping only to the directions that have sonic points. This is done using the I^x and I^y defined as in the LLF method.

With the RF scheme, upwinding in the x-direction dictates that either φ_x^- or φ_x^+ be used, but not both. Similarly, upwinding in the y-direction uses either φ_y^- or φ_y^+, but not both. Since evaluating $\varphi_x^\pm$ and $\varphi_y^\pm$ using higher-order accurate HJ ENO or HJ WENO schemes is rather costly, it seems wasteful to do twice as much work in these instances. Unfortunately, one cannot determine whether upwinding can be used (as opposed to LLF) without computing $\varphi_x^\pm$ and $\varphi_y^\pm$. In order to minimize CPU time, one can compute $\varphi_x^\pm$ and $\varphi_y^\pm$ using the first-order accurate forward and backward difference formulas and use these cheaper approximations to decide whether or not upwinding or LLF will be used. After making this decision, the higher-order accurate HJ ENO or HJ WENO method can be used to compute the necessary values of $\varphi_x^\pm$ and $\varphi_y^\pm$ used in the numerical discretization, obtaining the usual high-order accuracy. Sonic points rarely occur in practice, and this strategy reduces the use of the costly HJ WENO method by approximately a factor of two.

8.3.5.3 Godunov's Scheme

In [38], Godunov proposed a numerical method that gives the exact solution to the *Riemann problem* for one-dimensional conservation laws with piecewise constant initial data. The multidimensional Hamilton-Jacobi formulation of this scheme can be written as

$$\hat{H} = ext_x ext_y H(\varphi_x, \varphi_y) \tag{8.67}$$

as was pointed out by Bardi and Osher [39]. This is the canonical monotone scheme. Defining our intervals I^x and I^y in the LLLF manner using only the values of $\varphi_x^{\pm}$ and $\varphi_y^{\pm}$ y at the grid node under consideration, we define ext_x and ext_y as follows. If $\varphi_x^- < \varphi_x^+$, then $ext_x H$ takes on the minimum value of H for all $\varphi_x \in I^x$. If $\varphi_x^- > \varphi_x^+$, then $ext_x H$ takes on the maximum value of H for all $\varphi_x \in I^x$. Otherwise, if $\varphi_x^- = \varphi_x^+$, then $ext_x H$ simply plugs $\varphi_x^-(= \varphi_x^+)$ into H for φ_x. Similarly, If $\varphi_y^- < \varphi_y^+$, then $ext_y H$ takes on the minimum value of H for all $\varphi_y \in I^y$. If $\varphi_y^- > \varphi_y^+$, then $ext_y H$ takes on the maximum value of H for all $\varphi_y \in I^y$. Otherwise, if $\varphi_y^- = \varphi_y^+$, then $ext_y H$ simply plugs $\varphi_y^-(= \varphi_y^+)$ into H for φ_y. In general, $ext_x ext_y H \neq ext_y ext_x H$, so different versions of Godunov's method are obtained depending on the order of operations. Although Godunov's method can sometimes be difficult to implement, there are times when it is straightforward. Consider equation (8.42) for motion in an externally generated velocity field. Here, we can consider the x and y directions independently, since H is separable with $ext_x ext_y H = ext_x(u\varphi_x) + ext_y(v\varphi_y)$ If $\varphi_x^- < \varphi_x^+$, we want the minimum value of $u\varphi_x$. Thus, if $u > 0$, we use φ_x^-, and if $u < 0$, we use φ_x^+. If $u = 0$, we obtain $u\varphi_x = 0$ regardless of the choice of φ_x. On the other hand, If $\varphi_x^- > \varphi_x^+$, we want the maximum value of $u\varphi_x$. Thus, if $u > 0$, we use φ_x^-, and if $u < 0$, we use φ_x^+. Again $u = 0$, gives $u\varphi_x = 0$. Finally, if $\varphi_x^- = \varphi_x^+$, then $u\varphi_x$ is uniquely determined. This can be summarized as follows. If $u > 0$, use φ_x^-; if u < 0, use φ_x^+; and if $u = 0$, set $u\varphi_x = 0$. This is identical to the standard upwind differencing method described in solving basic level set method, Eq. (8.18). That is, for motion in an externally generated velocity field, Godunov's method is identical to simple upwind differencing.

8.4 Optimization Schemes

In this section, the minimization technique followed is the Euler-Lagrange equation [40], and the gradient descent technique [41] that gives the flow that minimizes the energy functions. Light is shed on the basics of Euler-Lagrange equation and the gradient descent technique in the coming section.

8.4.1 Euler-Lagrange Equation

Consider the following problem from calculus of variation: minimize an integral of a twice differentiable Lagrangian $q(x, b, \nabla b)$ over a regular bounded domain Ω with a smooth boundary $\partial\Omega$. q mainly depends on the minimizer b and its gradient ∇b. The minimization problem can thus be formulated as:

$$min_{b:b|\partial\Omega=b_0} E(b), E(b) = \int_{\Omega} q(x, b, \nabla b)dx \tag{8.68}$$

Because a differentiable functional is stationary at its local maxima and minima, the Euler–Lagrange equation is useful for solving optimization problems in which, given some functional, one seeks the function b which minimizes the functional $E(b)$.

In order to derive the Euler equation, consider the variation δb of the minimizer b and the difference $\delta E = E(b + \delta b) - E(b)$. Assuming that this variation is small and twice differentiable, then:

$$\delta b(x + t) = 0, \forall t : |t| > \epsilon, |\nabla(\delta b)| < C_{\epsilon} \forall x, \tag{8.69}$$

where $\epsilon \to 0$.

When q is twice differentiable, the Lagrangian can be linearized as follows:

$$\begin{aligned} q(x, b + \delta b, \nabla(b + \delta b)) &= q(x, b, \nabla b) + \frac{\partial q(x, b, \nabla b)}{\partial b}\delta b \\ &+ \frac{\partial q(x, b, \nabla b)}{\partial \nabla b}\delta \nabla b + O(\|\delta b\|, \|\nabla \delta b\|), \end{aligned} \tag{8.70}$$

where $\frac{\partial q(x,b,\nabla b)}{\partial \nabla b}$ represents the vector of partial derivatives of q with respect to the partial derivatives of b,

$$\frac{\partial q(x, b, \nabla b)}{\partial \nabla b} \left[\frac{\partial q(x, b, \nabla b)}{\partial \left(\frac{\partial b}{\partial x_1}\right)}, \ldots, \frac{\partial q(x, b, \nabla b)}{\partial \left(\frac{\partial b}{\partial x_n}\right)} \right]. \tag{8.71}$$

Substitution of the linearized Lagrangian into the formula for δE results in:

$$\delta E = \int_{\Omega} \left(\frac{\partial q}{\partial b}\delta b + \frac{\partial q}{\partial \nabla b} \cdot \delta \nabla b \right) dx + O(\|\delta b\|, \|\nabla \delta b\|) \tag{8.72}$$

Simplifying Eq. (8.72), performing integration by parts, and interchanging the two linear operators of variation and differentiation results in:

$$\int_{\Omega} \left(\frac{\partial q}{\partial \nabla b} \cdot \nabla(\delta b) \right) dx = -\int_{\Omega} \delta b \left(\nabla . \frac{\partial q}{\partial \nabla b} \right) dx + \int_{\partial\Omega} \delta b \left(\frac{\partial q}{\partial \nabla b} \cdot n \right) ds, \tag{8.73}$$

so that

$$\delta E = \int_{\Omega} \left(\frac{\partial q}{\partial b} - \nabla . \frac{\partial q}{\partial \nabla b} \right) \delta b \, dx + \int_{\partial\Omega} \delta b \left(\frac{\partial q}{\partial \nabla b} \cdot n \right) ds, \tag{8.74}$$

where n is the normal vector. The coefficient by δb in the first integral of Eq. (8.74) is called the variational derivative in Ω, and is called the Euler Lagrange equation:

$$\frac{\partial q}{\partial b} - \nabla . \left(\frac{\partial q}{\partial \nabla b} \right) = 0. \tag{8.75}$$

When b is a function of more than one independent variable; e.g. when q has the form:

$$q = q(x_i, b, b_{x_i}, b_{x_i x_j}), \forall i, j \in [1, L], \tag{8.76}$$

and following the same strategy when having one variable, the following Euler-Lagrange equation can be obtained:

$$\frac{\partial q}{\partial b} - \sum_{i=1}^{L} \frac{d}{dx_i} \frac{\partial q}{\partial b_{x_i}} + \sum_{i=1}^{L} \sum_{j=1}^{L} \frac{d^2}{dx_i dx_j} \frac{\partial q}{\partial b_{x_i x_j}} = 0 \tag{8.77}$$

8.4.1.1 Euler-Lagrange and the Gradient Descent

The gradient descent technique helps solving for the function E and its derivative with respect to a set of variables $S = [S_1 \ldots S_m]^T$:

$$\frac{\partial E}{\partial S} = 0, \tag{8.78}$$

using the following formula:

$$\frac{\partial S}{\partial t} = -\frac{\partial E}{\partial S}, \tag{8.79}$$

where the minus sign denoted that it is a minimization problem, where variables change with time until reaching the steady state at $\frac{\partial E}{\partial S} = 0$.

8.4.1.2 The need for re-initialization

The signed distance function for the level sets equation is:

$$\varphi(X) = \begin{cases} +D(x) & \textit{if point is inside the contour} \\ 0 & \textit{if point is on the boundary} \\ -D(x) & \textit{if point is outsice the contour} \end{cases}, \tag{8.80}$$

where $D(x)$ is the minimum Euclidean distance between the point x and the contour. The distance function needs to be frequently re-initialized after solving the level set PDE. This helps maintain the smoothness of the evolution [42]. Re-initialization of the level set equation can be handled using the following formula:

$$\frac{\partial}{\partial t}\varphi = sgn(\varphi^0)(1 - |\nabla \varphi|) \tag{8.81}$$

The solution of this equation keeps the function close to the signed distance function if it is conducted in parallel with the main equation.

The solution of the re-initialization equation is:

$$\varphi_{i,j}^{n+1} = \varphi_{i,j}^{n} - \Delta t S(\varphi_{i,j}^{0}) G(\varphi)_{i,j}, \tag{8.82}$$

where

$$G(\varphi)_{i,j} = \begin{cases} \sqrt{\max(a_+^2, b_-^2) + \max(c_+^2, d_-^2)} - 1 & \text{if } \varphi_{i,j}^0 > 0 \\ \sqrt{\max(a_-^2, b_+^2) + \max(c_-^2, d_+^2)} - 1 & \text{if } \varphi_{i,j}^0 < 0 \end{cases}$$

$$a = D^{x-}\varphi_{i,j} = \frac{\varphi_{i,j} - \varphi_{i-1,j}}{\Delta x}$$

$$b = D^{x+}\varphi_{i,j} = \frac{\varphi_{i+1,j} - \varphi_{i,j}}{\Delta x}$$

$$c = D^{y-}\varphi_{i,j} = \frac{\varphi_{i,j} - \varphi_{i,j-1}}{\Delta y}$$

$$d = D^{y+}\varphi_{i,j} = \frac{\varphi_{i,j+1} - \varphi_{i,j}}{\Delta y}$$

$$a_+ = \max(a, 0)$$

$$a_- = \min(a, 0)$$

$$S(\varphi) = 2 * \left(H_\alpha(\varphi) - \frac{1}{2}\right),$$

where $H_\alpha(\varphi)$ is the Heaviside function.

A major drawback of the level set method is the extensive computation time. This motivated researchers to speed up its algorithms for convergence. One of these notable ideas is narrow banding. The narrow banding theory was first introduced by Chopp in [42], and was later developed in [43]. The idea of narrow banding is that the interest is mainly in the motion of the zero-level set, and other points are not considered (Figure 8.3). Instead, they are assigned either large positive or large negative values. This limits the computation to fewer points that are around the zero level set, whereas the rest of the domain is considered to be only a sign holder [44]. Narrow banding significantly decreases the computational complexity. The Narrow banding algorithm is summarized in Algorithm 1.

Algorithm 1 Steps of the Narrow Banding Algorithm.

1: Extract the latest position.
2: Define a band within a certain distance.
3: Update the level set function
4: Check the new position with respect to the limits of the band.
5: Update the position of the band regularly and re-initialize the implicit function.

8.5 Guiding Forces

Like parametric deformable models, geometric models can also be either region-based or edge-based. There have been numerous forms for the speed

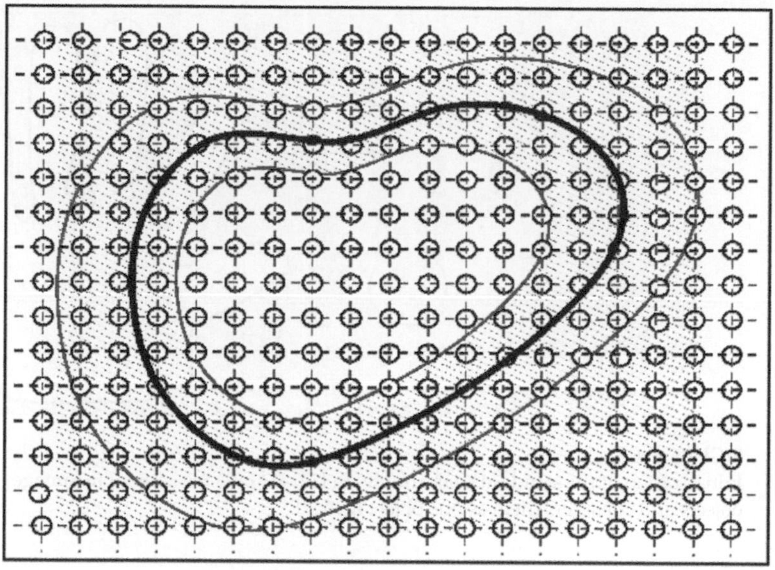

FIGURE 8.3
Illustration of the narrow banding theory. The inward band (red), the front position (black), and the outward band (blue) are the interest in the image. All other points are of no importance.

function F proposed in literature, Eq. (8.17), which can be roughly categorized into either region-based or edge-based functions. Some of the most popular forms for F in both categories are outlined below.

8.5.1 Edge-based Forces

8.5.1.1 Geodesic Active Contour (GAC) Model

This can be alternatively referred to as variational edge-based segmentation and is considered to be a geometric alternative for the snake model. This model is known to be geometrically intrinsic because the energy function is invariant with respect to the curve parameterization [13, 45]. The model is defined by the following minimization problem:

$$min_C \left\{ E_{GAC}(C) = \int_0^{L(C)} g(|\nabla I_0(C(s))|)ds \right\}, \tag{8.83}$$

where ds is the Euclidean element of length and $L(C)$ is the length of the curve C defined by $L(C) = \int_0^{L(C)} ds$. The function g is an edge indicator function that does not exist at object boundaries and is given by:

$$g(|\nabla I_0|) = \frac{1}{1 + \beta|\nabla I_0|^2}, \tag{8.84}$$

where I_0 is the original image and β is an arbitrary positive constant.

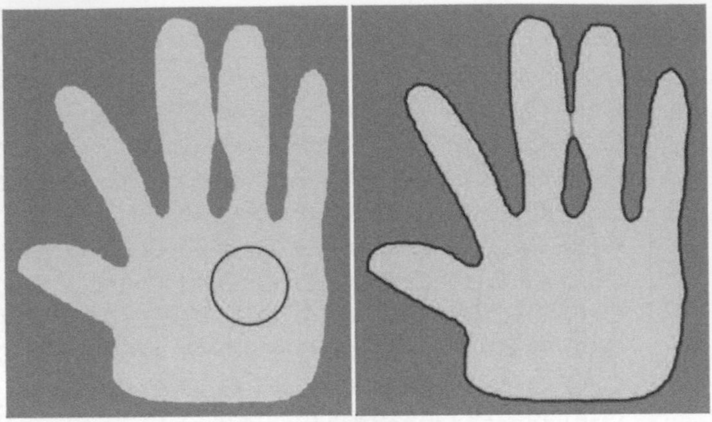

FIGURE 8.4
Initialization of the standard snake model in [32, 48] fails to segment the image (left) into its two objects and considers them as one object instead.

Although this model provides good results, it is highly sensitive to the initial condition [46, 47]. This is due to the non-convex nature of the energy functional to be minimized, E_{GAC}, which leads to the existence of local minima, Figure 8.4. This drawback is not specific to this model because variational models in image processing often suffer from local minima.

8.5.1.2 Gradient Vector Flow Fast GAC

Paragios et al. [47] proposed a fast evolution model where boundaries are extracted using a front propagation flow that combines GAC [13] and GVF [48] models and is implemented using a level set approach. It is thus capable of dealing with topological changes, along with shape deformations. In [47] the GVF energy function was slightly modified as follows:

$$E(V) = \iint \mu\left(u_x{}^2 + v_x{}^2 + u_y{}^2 + u_y{}^2\right) + f|\nabla f|^2|(V - \nabla f)|^2 dx\,dy. \quad (8.85)$$

The only difference in Eq. (8.85) is that image boundaries as well as the gradients are involved, thus enabling the strong edges to overcome the flow generated by weak edges.

The flow in [47] was then determined by obtaining the inner product of the modified GVF $\hat{v}$ and the unit normal $\mathcal{N}$ as follows:

$$C_t = (\hat{v}.\,\mathcal{N})\mathcal{N}. \quad (8.86)$$

Inspired by the work of Osher et al. in [12], the front in Eq. (8.86) evolves according to the following level set implicit representation:

$$C_t(p,t) = F(p)\mathcal{N}(p), \quad (8.87)$$

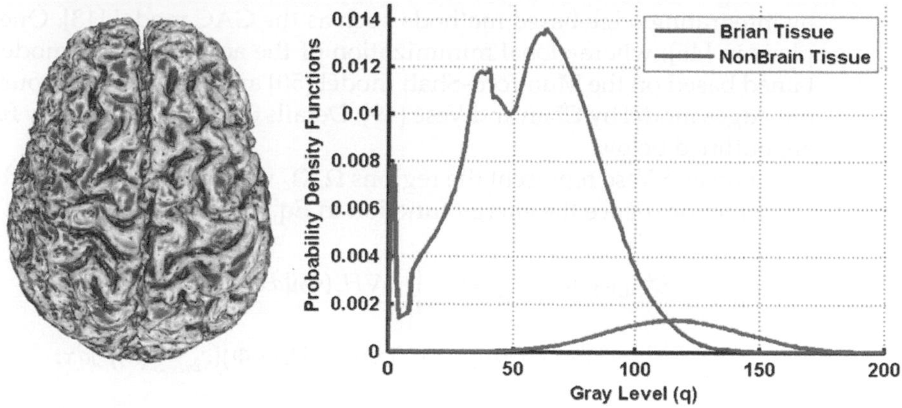

FIGURE 8.5
A human brain (left), with intensity distribution of the two terms c_{in} (brain tissue) and c_{out} (non-brain tissue) in Eq. (8.89).

given that the implicit level set function deforms according to:

$$\varphi_t(p,t) = F(p)|\nabla\varphi(p,t)|. \tag{8.88}$$

8.5.2 Region-based Forces

8.5.2.1 Chan-Vese Model (Active Contour without Edges) for Image Segmentation

An example of a segmentation model is the well-known Chan-Vese model, also known as the Active Contour without Edges (ACWE) [49] that is based on the Mumford-Shah model [50]. The energy function for ACWE comes in the following form:

$$min_{\Omega_c,c_1,c_2}\{E_{ACWE}(\Omega_c,c_1,c_2,\lambda) = per(\Omega_c)\lambda\int_{\Omega_c}(c_1 - f(x))^2dx + \lambda\int_{\Omega\backslash\Omega_c}(c_2 - f(x))^2dx\}, \tag{8.89}$$

This model finds two regions in the image domain Ω. These two regions are designated as object and background, where mean intensities are as disjoint as possible. The first term is the length of the boundary of Σ, where $\Sigma \subset \Omega$. c_{in} and c_{out} are the mean intensities in $\Omega\backslash\Sigma$ and Σ respectively, Figure 8.5.

The minimization in Eq. (8.89) does not enable the solution to assume continuous values, lending itself to a non-convex formulation.

For the limitation above, there have been various recent attempts in literature to obtain global solutions from such non-convex energy functions by integrating edge-based methods such as the GAC model [13]. One example is in [46], where global minimization of the active contour model is obtained based on the Mumford-Shah model [50] and the active contours without edges model by Chan and Vese [49]. Details of this global energy function are outlined below.

Chan and Vese represent the regions Ω, Ω_c with the Heaviside of the level sets function; hence the energy function in Eq. (8.89) can be rewritten as:

$$E^2{}_{ACWE}(\Phi, c_1, c_2, \lambda) = \int_\Omega |\nabla H_\epsilon(\Phi)| dx + \lambda \int_\Omega (H_\epsilon(\Phi)(c_1 - f(x))^2 + H_\epsilon(-\Phi)(c_2 - f(x))^2) dx, \tag{8.90}$$

where $H_\epsilon(\Phi)$ is the regularization of the Heaviside function. The steady state solution of the gradient flow becomes:

$$\partial_t \varphi = div\left(\frac{\nabla\varphi}{|\nabla\varphi|}\right) - \lambda r_1(x, c_1, c_2), \tag{8.91}$$

where $r_1(x, c_1, c_2) = ((c_1 - f(x))^2 - (c_2 - f(x))^2)$. Eq. (8.91) is the gradient descent flow of the following energy:

$$E^3{}_{ACWE}(\varphi, c_1, c_2, \lambda) = \int_\Omega |\nabla\varphi| dx + \lambda \int_\Omega r_1(x, c_1, c_2)\varphi\, dx. \tag{8.92}$$

Based on this, Bresson et al. [46] proposed to minimize the following energy function to obtain the global minimum solution for any parameter > 0:

$$E_1(u, c_1, c_2, \lambda) = TV_g(u) + \lambda \int r_1(x, c_1, c_2) u\, dx, \tag{8.93}$$

where the difference between Eq. (8.92) and Eq. (8.93) is based on the weighted total variation (TV) of a function u [51], with a weight function g, that contains information concerning the boundaries of an image I_0 [13] and is given by Eq. (8.84).

Eq. (8.93) provides the link between ACWE and GAC when g is an edge indicator function and u is a characteristic function, 1_{Ω_c}. The following relation thus stands:

$$TV_g(u = 1_{\Omega_c}) = \int_\Omega g(x)|\nabla 1_{\Omega_c}| dx = \int_C g(s) ds = E_{GAC}(C). \tag{8.94}$$

Eq. (8.93) could thus be re-written as:

$$E_2(u = 1_{\Omega_c}, c_1, c_2, \lambda) = TV_g(1_{\Omega_c}) + \lambda \int r_1(x, c_1, c_2) 1_{\Omega_c} dx, \tag{8.95}$$

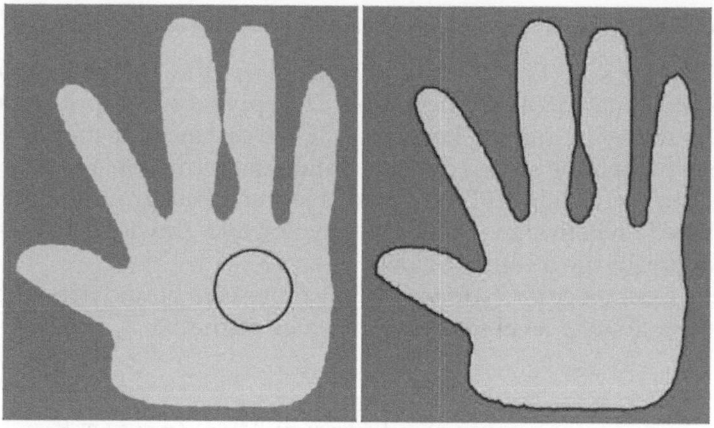

FIGURE 8.6
The proposed deformable-model based segmentation model [46] which provides a global solution to the standard snake model segments the image on the left into 2 objects.

where E_2 is homogeneous of degree 1 in u. This means that for any minimizer u of E_2 got with any minimization framework, the set of points in the function u such that u is a positive constant, defines a set whose boundary is a global minimum of the snake model. The constrained minimization problem for the segmentation problem is then:

$$min_{0\leq u\leq 1} = \left\{ E_2(u, c_1, c_2, \lambda) = TV_g(u) + \lambda \int r_1(x, c_1, c_2) u \, dx. \right\} \tag{8.96}$$

which has the same set of minimizers as the following convex, unconstrained minimization problem:

$$min_u \left\{ TV_g(u) + \lambda \int r_1(x, c_1, c_2) u + \alpha v(u) dx. \right\} \tag{8.97}$$

where $v(\xi) = \max\{0, 2|\xi - \frac{1}{2}| - 1\}$ is an exact penalty function provided that α is large enough compared to λ. The function in Eq. (8.97) is not strictly convex, thus does not possess local minima that are not global. Now the convex formulation for Eq. (8.97) guarantees the segmentation framework to have a global minimizer [46] (Figure 8.6).

The global solution obtained for the convex formulation of the GAC model in [46] using region-based functions such as the ACWE model [49] and the Mumford-Shah model [50] does not guarantee good segmentation however. Such models are not mainly concerned with feature detection unlike the segmentation models based on shape priors as in [51, 52].

8.5.2.2 Level Set Segmentation using Statistical Shape Priors

The work by El Baz et al. [52] proposed the use of level sets with shape constraints for 3D segmentation. The approach uses prior shape information from a set of training images. A signed distance function is assigned to each shape, and the signed distance values are formed in a histogram. Probability density functions (PDFs) of the object and background are then determined based on both signed distance function and gray level values. Details of this approach are outlined below:

Given a curve/surface M that represents boundaries of a certain shape, the following level set function can be defined:

$$\varphi(x,y,z) = \begin{cases} 0 & (x,y,z) \in M \\ d((x,y,z),M) & (x,y,z) \in R_M \\ -d((x,y,z),M) & otherwise \end{cases}, \tag{8.98}$$

where R_M is the region defined by the shape and $d((x,y,z),M)$ is the minimum Euclidean distance between the image location (x,y,z) and the curve/surface M.

Using Eq. (8.98), a database of curves and signed distance functions can be constructed, representing shape variations. From this information, a histogram of the occurrences of signed distance values which characterizes the shape and its local variations can be extracted.

The evolving surface is a propagating front embedded as the zero level of a scalar function $\varphi(x,y,z,t)$. The continuous change of $\varphi(x,y,z,t)$ can be described by the partial differential equation:

$$\frac{\partial\varphi(x,y,z,t)}{\partial t} + F(x,y,z)|\nabla\varphi(x,y,z,t)| = 0, \tag{8.99}$$

where $F(x,y,z)$ is a velocity function and $\nabla = [\frac{\partial}{\partial x}, \frac{\partial}{\partial y}, \frac{\partial}{\partial z}]^T$.

The function $\Phi(x,y,z,t)$ deforms iteratively according to $F(x,y,z)$, and the position of the 2D/3D front is given at each iteration by solving the equation $\Phi(x,y,z,t)$.

Finally, the speed function $F(x,y,z)$ is formulated as:

$$F(x,y,z) = \upsilon - \epsilon \mathbf{k}(x,y,z), \tag{8.100}$$

where $\upsilon = 1$ or -1 for the contracting or expanding front respectively, ϵ is a smoothing coefficient which is always small with respect to 1, and $k(x,y,z)$ is the local curvature of the front. The latter parameter acts as a regularization term. A segmentation example is shown in Figure 8.7.

This section addressed the geometric deformable models that emerged in the late eighties to overcome the limitations of the parametric deformation which does not have the ability to handle topological changes of the evolving contour such as merging and splitting. The basic level set, its numerica

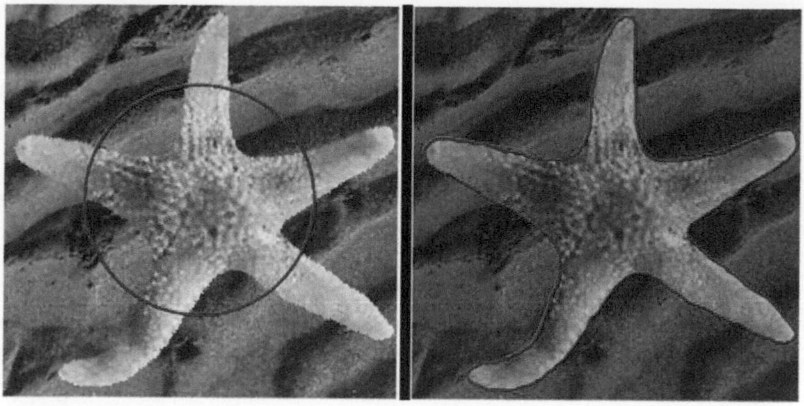

FIGURE 8.7
The proposed geometric deformable segmentation model in [52] showing the initial segmentation in left and the final segmentation in right. Image is courtesy of [53]. Summary on geometric deformable models.

schemes, and some of its popular guiding forces in literature were provided in detail.

The extensive computations required for the convergence of the level set equation could be partially remedied by applying the narrow banding theorem. However, there is no guarantee to find a global solution with level set evolution, and there is a high tendency to get stuck in local minima.

8.6 Applications in Medical Imaging

This section surveys the recent work in medical image deformable-model based segmentation. A countless number of research studies have exploited the deformable models, whether geometric or parametric, in segmenting different body structures such as the brain, heart, kidney, colon, lung, and prostate. As mentioned earlier, it is very hard to generalize a segmentation framework for all medical imaging segmentation problems. There would be different stopping criteria and guiding forces on the evolving contour in order to converge to the desired solution at each case [54]. For example, He et al. [55] conducted a comparative study reviewing eight parametric and geometric deformable models and applying them to different structures such as the knee, brain, blood cells, kidney, and brain's corpus callosum and sulci. The key was to select the appropriate approach for each application. The study highlighted the advantages and disadvantages of each one of the eight deformable models. In [56], a shape-based approach for the segmentation of medical images was proposed. A parametric model for an implicit representation of the segmenting curve was derived by applying principal component analysis to a collection of signed distance representations of the training data. The parameters of this representation were then used to minimize the segmentation objective function.

8.6.1 Heart

Segmentation of cardiac images was heavily conducted in literature using deformable models. For example, Pluempitiwiriyawej et al. [57] proposed a stochastic active contour model for the segmentation of cardiac MR images to overcome the limitations of boundary of topology and extensive computations. Montagnat et al. [58] proposed a 4D deformable model for heart segmentation, where simplex meshes were constructed and the mean curvature at each vertex was estimated. In [59–61], the heart was segmented using a level set-based deformable model where evolution is controlled by a stochastic speed function.

A framework that combines the benefits of both the deformable models and graph cuts was constructed in [62] to segment the epicardium and the myocardium of the left ventricle of the heart from magnetic resonance images. A good initialization scheme for the deformable model was exploited, which resulted in smooth segmentation results with lower interaction costs than using only graph cut segmentation. The deformable model was defined as a region defined by two nested contours in order to segment the epicardium and endocardium by optimizing a single energy functional. In [63], an automated framework for analyzing the wall thickness and thickening function on cine cardiac magnetic resonance images was proposed that included the segmentation as a first step. The inner and outer wall borders were segmented using a geometric deformable model guided by a special stochastic speed relationship. Gopal et al. [64] segmented the left ventricle (LV) from cardiac MR images using an approach that combined statistical and deterministic deformable models. A 3D Active Appearance Model (AAM) was also incorporated. Cardiac first-pass MR images were analyzed in [65–68], where the left ventricle (LV) was segmented using a level-set based function. A shape-based framework for the segmentation of the left ventricle (LV) wall on cardiac first-pass magnetic resonance imaging (FP-MRI) using level sets was proposed. The level set evolution was constrained using three features: a weighted probabilistic shape prior, the first-order pixel-wise image intensities, and a second-order Markov-Gibbs random field (MGRF) spatial interaction model. The left ventricle was also segmented using level-set based functions in [66, 69–72] for the assessment of myocardium function.

8.6.2 Brain

As to brain segmentation, numerous researchers made use of deformable models. Ho et al., for example, segmented the brain tumors using level-set evolution with region competition [73]. A signed local statistical force that replaced the constant propagation term was proposed to avoid boundary leakage problems. The probabilities for background and tumor regions were computed from a pre- and post-contrast image and mixture-modeling of the histogram. Goldenberg et al. [74] used a shape-based level set approach that exploited the coupled surfaces model to segment the brain cortex. A neonatal image segmentation method was proposed [94], where local intensity information, atlas spatial prior, and cortical thickness constraint were combined in a single level-set framework. A longitudinally guided level-sets method for neonatal image segmentation was done by the same group [95], combining local intensity information, atlas spatial prior, cortical thickness constraint, and longitudinal information into a variational framework. A novel patch-driven level set method for the segmentation of neonatal brain MR images using sparse representation techniques was later proposed by the same group [96]. After building an atlas, the probability maps were integrated into a coupled level set framework. In [97–99], the brain was extracted using a hybrid approach that integrates geometrical and statistical models. The brain is parceled to a set of nested iso-surfaces using the fast marching level-set method in order to accurately discriminate between brain and non-brain tissues.

8.6.3 Colon

Colon segmentation using deformable models was also addressed in the literature. A hybrid segmentation procedure, which can handle both air- and fluid-filled parts of the colon, was adopted [100]. The proposed hybrid algorithm uses modified region growing, fuzzy connectedness, and level set segmentation as key components. A level set approach was also developed [101] for automatic segmentation of the colon's haustral folds based on their boundaries.

8.6.4 Kidney

Kidney segmentation has also been conducted using deformable models [102–111]. The kidney borders were extracted using a geometric deformable model guided by a special stochastic speed relationship. This accounts for a shape prior and appearance features in terms of voxel-wise image intensities and their pair-wise spatial interactions integrated into a two-level joint Markov-Gibbs random field (MGRF) model of the kidney and its background. Kidney segmentation was also conducted using an evolving deformable model that is based on two density functions [112–121]; the first function describes the distribution of the gray level inside and outside the kidney region, and the second function describes the prior shape of the kidney. The gray level density is calculated for a given kidney image using a modified expectation maximization (EM) algorithm.

In order to get the kidney's shape prior, an average kidney shape is constructed from a dataset of previously segmented kidneys, and an average signed distance map density is then obtained.

8.6.5 Liver

As to liver segmentation, Cvancarova et al. [122] modified the original GVF algorithm for segmenting ultrasound images of liver tumors by coupling the smoothness of the edge map to the contour's initial size. The tuning parameters of the GVF model were also adjusted, and the numerical discretization was improved as well. An automated liver segmentation method was proposed [123], where the level set-based contour evolution from T2 weighted magnetic resonance data sets was approximated. The method avoided solving partial differential equations and was applied to all slices with a constant number of iterations. The method also did not require any manual initialization. A level set model was also proposed [124] to integrate image gradient, region competition, and prior information for CT liver tumor segmentation. The probabilistic distribution of liver tumors was used to enhance the object indication function, formulate the directional balloon force, and regulate region competition.

8.6.6 Lung

Lung segmentation was also heavily considered in literature using deformable models. A segmentation framework was developed [125] to capture the high curvature features of the lung cavities from the magnetic resonance images. It computed an external force field based on the solution of partial differential equations with boundary condition defined by the initial positions of the evolving contours. An algorithm for isolating lung nodules from spiral CT scans was proposed [126]. The proposed algorithm exploited four different types of deformable templates describing typical geometry and gray level distribution of lung nodules. These four types are (*i*) a solid spherical model of large-size calcified and non-calcified nodules appearing in several successive slices; (*ii*) a hollow spherical model of large lung cavity nodules; (*iii*) a circular model of small nodules appearing in only a single slice; and (*iv*) a semicircular model of lung wall nodules. Each template had a specific gray level pattern which was analytically estimated in order to fit the available empirical data. Finally, the detection combined the normalized cross-correlation template matching by genetic optimization and Bayesian post-classification. A level-set based method for automatic medical image segmentation was adopted [127]. The intensity distribution of the organic structures was investigated, and a calibrating mechanism was conducted in order to automatically weight image intensity and gradient information in the level set speed function. Lung segmentation was also conducted [128], where two adaptive probability models of visual appearance of small 2D and large 3D pulmonary nodules were used to control the evolution of deformable boundaries. An algorithm for unsupervised segmentation of the lung tissues from Low Dose Computed Tomography (LDCT) was adopted [129–130]. It used a joint Markov-Gibbs random field model (MGRF) of independent image signal and interdependent region labels. Lung segmentation was performed [131] using a 3D generalized Gauss-Markov Random Field (GGMRF) model of voxel intensities with pairwise interaction to model the 3D appearance of the lung tissues. Segmentation of lung was also conducted using deformable models [132–139]. In order to isolate pulmonary nodules from background in chest images, adaptive probability models of the visual appearance of small 2D and large 3D pulmonary nodules have been jointly incorporated to control the evolution of the de-formable model. The appearance prior was modeled with a translation and rotation invariant Markov-Gibbs random field (MGRF) of voxel intensities with pairwise interaction. The model was then analytically identified from a set of training nodule images with normalized intensity ranges.

8.6.7 Prostate

Prostate segmentation techniques using deformable models have also been addressed. A deformable model for automatic segmentation of prostate from three-dimensional ultrasound images was proposed [140]. A set of Gabor-support vector machines (G-SVMs) was positioned on different patches of the model surface and trained to capture texture priors of ultrasound images in order to classify tissues as prostate or non-prostate. These G-SVMs were used to label voxels around the surface of deformable model as prostate or non-prostate tissues using a statistical texture matching. This resulted in driving the surface of the deformable model to the boundary between the prostate and non-prostate tissues. An automatic method for the coupled 3D localization and segmentation of lower abdomen structures was proposed [141]. The approach allowed for easily adapting to high shape variation and to intensity inhomogeneities. Also, a statistical shape prior was enforced on the prostate. A statistical shape model was used as prior information for the segmentation of prostate [142], and gray level distribution was modeled by fitting histogram modes with a Gaussian mixture. Markov fields were used to introduce contextual information for the voxels' neighborhoods. Final labeling optimization was conducted based on Bayesian a-posteriori classification. An approach for segmenting the prostate region from Dynamic Contrast Enhancement Magnetic Resonance Images (DCE-MRI) based on using deformable models was adopted [143–149]. They combined three descriptors: (*i*) first-order visual appearance descriptors of the DCE-MRI; (*ii*) a spatially invariant second-order homogeneity descriptor, and (*iii*) a prostate shape descriptor. In [150, 151], prostate segmentation was conducted using a level-set deformable model and non-negative matrix factorization (NMF) techniques. In the proposed framework, the level-set was guided by a novel speed function that was derived using NMF, which extracts meaningful features from a large dimensional feature space.

To summarize, pattern recognition in image processing was the origin of the exploration of the space of images. Simplistic digital techniques used at the beginning of the sixties for gray image processing operations have been now replaced with complex mathematical frameworks that aim to exploit and understand images in two and three dimensions. The medical sector is also a major area for the use of images. The evolution of the acquisition devices led to new ways of capturing information not visible to the human eye. Medical imaging is probably the most established market for processing visual information. Visualization of complex structures and automated processing of computer aided diagnosis is used more and more by physicians in the diagnostic process. Image segmentation is perhaps the well-studied topic in image processing and computer vision. Evolving an initial curve towards the boundaries of the structure of interest is a method that can be used to deal with this problem.

Deformable models have been widely used in the literature for a vast majority of medical imaging problems. The introduction of the snake model presented by Kass et al. aimed at evolving an initial curve towards the lowest potential of a cost function. Level set techniques have proved to be the most suitable method to track moving interfaces. Being implicit, intrinsic, and parametric free, level sets can deal with topological changes while for tracking moving interfaces. Recent work in the literature aims at combining level set method with other techniques to better manipulate it. Li et al., for example [152], proposed a fuzzy level set algorithm that is able to evolve from the initial segmentation by spatial fuzzy clustering. The controlling parameters of the level set evolution are also estimated from the results of fuzzy clustering. Also, the fuzzy level set algorithm is enhanced with locally regularized evolution. Topological graph prior information was considered [153], in order to evolve the contour within a multi-level set formulation. The use of graph priors allowed for segmenting adjacent objects with similar intensity levels that were impossible to segment with the ordinary level set formulation.

8.7 Conclusion and Future Trends

This chapter discussed the deformable models with their explicit and implicit representations in detail. It started with the parametric deformable models, which were introduced in the late 1980s and showed many advances in the field of image processing. Due to their poor performance in some aspects, geometric deformable models were later introduced that could successfully handle most of these problems.

Future work includes many promising aspects. The combination of the benefits of both parametric and geometric deformable models in a hybrid framework can be useful with certain problems which require the speed of the parametric models as well as the capabilities of the implicit representation of the geometric ones. Also, one useful trend could be obtaining the convex formulation of complex level-set based functions. Another useful trend could be integrating the spatial, intensity, and shape models. This would address the drawbacks of getting stuck in local minima and obtaining global solutions to the problem. In the 2000s the shift towards parallel programming and cloud computing of level set methods has also been rapidly growing in order to speed up the convergence and optimize solutions, especially when dealing with large volumes in medical imaging problems. Also, recent work in the literature is aiming at improving and easily manipulating level sets, which could eventually lead to more robust segmentation, such as the integration with fuzzy clustering and topological prior information.

This work could also be applied to various other applications in medical imaging, such as the kidney, the heart, the prostate, the lung, and the retina. One application is renal transplant functional assessment. Chronic kidney disease (CKD) affects about 26 million people in the United States, with 17,000 transplants being performed each year. In renal transplant patients, acute rejection is the leading cause of renal dysfunction. Given the limited number of donors, routine clinical post- transplantation evaluation is of immense importance to help clinicians initiate timely interventions with appropriate treatment and thus prevent graft loss. In recent years, an increased area of research has been dedicated to developing noninvasive CAD systems for renal transplant function assessment, utilizing different image modalities (e.g., ultrasound, computed tomography (CT), MRI, etc.). Accurate assessment of renal transplant function is critically important for graft survival. Although transplantation can improve a patient's wellbeing, there is a potential post-transplantation risk of kidney dysfunction that, if not treated in a timely manner, can lead to the loss of the entire graft, and even patient death. Thus, accurate assessment of renal transplant function is crucial for the identification of proper treatment. In particular, dynamic and diffusion MRI-based systems have been clinically used to assess transplanted kidneys with the advantage of providing information on each kidney separately. For more details about renal transplant functional assessment, please read [75–100]. The heart also has important relevance to this work. The clinical assessment of myocardial perfusion plays a major role in the diagnosis, management, and prognosis of ischemic heart disease patients. Thus, there have been ongoing efforts to develop automated systems for accurate analysis of myocardial perfusion using first-pass images [101–117]. Another application for this work could be the detection of retinal abnormalities. Majority of ophthalmologists depend on visual interpretation for the identification of diseases types. However, inaccurate diagnosis will affect the treatment procedure which may in turn lead to fatal results. Hence, there is a crucial need for computer automated diagnosis systems that yield highly accurate results. Optical coherence tomography (OCT) has become a powerful modality for the non-invasive diagnosis of various retinal abnormalities such as glaucoma, diabetic macular edema, and macular degeneration. The problem with diabetic retinopathy (DR) is that the patient is not aware of the disease until changes in the retina have progressed to a level that treatment tends to be less effective. Therefore, automated early detection could limit the severity of the disease and assist ophthalmologists in investigating and treating it more efficiently [118,119]. Abnormalities of the lung could also be another promising area of research and a related application to this work. Radiation-induced lung injury is the main side effect of radiation therapy for lung cancer patients. Although higher radiation doses increase the radiation therapy effectiveness for tumor control, this can lead to lung injury since a greater quantity of normal lung tissues is included in the treated area. Almost one-third of patients who undergo radiation therapy develop lung injury following radiation treatment. The severity of radiation-induced lung injury ranges from ground-glass opacities and consolidation at the early phase to fibrosis and traction bronchiectasis in the late phase. Early detection of lung injury will thus help to improve management of the treatment [120–160]. This work can also be applied to other brain abnormalities, such as dyslexia and autism. Dyslexia is one of the most complicated developmental brain disorders that affect children's learning abilities. Dyslexia leads to the failure to develop age-appropriate reading skills in spite of normal intelligence level and adequate reading instructions. Neuropathological studies have revealed an abnormal anatomy of some structures, such as the Corpus Callosum in dyslexic brains. There has been a lot of work in the literature that aims at developing CAD systems for diagnosing such disorders, along with other disorders of the brain [161–183].

References

1. N. Sharma and L. M. Aggarwal,"Automated medical image segmentation techniques," *Journal of Medical Physics/Association of Medical Physicists of India*, vol. 35, no. 1, p. 3, 2010.
2. E. R. Hancock and J. Kittler, "Edge-labeling using dictionary-based relaxation," *IEEE Transactions on Pattern Analysis & Machine Intelligence*, no. 2, pp. 165–181, 1990.
3. Y.-T. Liow, "A contour tracing algorithm that preserves common boundaries between regions," *CVGIP: Image Understanding*, vol. 53, no. 3, pp. 313–321, 1991.
4. T. Law, H. Itoh, and H. Seki, "Image filtering, edge detection, and edge tracing using fuzzy reasoning," *IEEE Transactions on Pattern Analysis & Machine Intelligence*, no. 5, pp. 481–491, 1996.
5. H. Ney, "A comparative study of two search strategies for connected word recognition: Dynamic programming and heuristic search," *IEEE Transactions on Pattern Analysis & Machine Intelligence*, no. 5, pp. 586–595, 1992.
6. E. Oja and L. Xu, "Randomized Hough transform (RHT): basic mechanisms, algorithms, and computational complexities," *CVGIP: Image Understanding*, vol. 57, no. 2, pp. 131–154, 1993.

7. H. Kalviainen, P. Hirvonen, L. Xu, and E. Oja, "Probabilistic and non-probabilistic Hough transforms: overview and comparisons," *Image and Vision Computing*, vol. 13, no. 4, pp. 239–252, 1995.
8. H. T. Nguyen, M. Worring, and R. Van Den Boomgaard, "Watersnakes: Energy-driven watershed segmentation," *IEEE Transactions on Pattern Analysis and Machine Intelligence*, vol. 25, no. 3, pp. 330–342, 2003.
9. L. Najman and M. Schmitt, "Geodesic saliency of watershed contours and hierarchical segmentation," *IEEE Transactions on Pattern Analysis and Machine Intelligence*, vol. 18, no. 12, pp. 1163–1173, 1996.
10. A. M. López, F. Lumbreras, J. Serrat, and J. J. Villanueva, "Evaluation of methods for ridge and valley detection," *IEEE Transactions on Pattern Analysis and Machine Intelligence*, vol. 21, no. 4, pp. 327–335, 1999.
11. M. Kass, A. Witkin, and D. Terzopoulos, "Snakes: Active contour models," *International Journal of Computer Vision*, vol. 1, no. 4, pp. 321–331, 1988.
12. S. Osher and J. A. Sethian, "Fronts propagating with curvature-dependent speed: algorithms based on Hamilton-Jacobi formulations," *Journal of Computational Physics*, vol. 79, no. 1, pp. 12–49, 1988.
13. V. Caselles, R. Kimmel, and G. Sapiro, "Geodesic active contours," *International Journal of Computer Vision*, vol. 22, no. 1, pp. 61–79, 1997.
14. C. Xu, A. Yezzi, and J. L. Prince, "On the relationship between parametric and geometric active contours," in *Signals, Systems and Computers, 2000. Conference Record of the Thirty-Fourth Asilomar Conference on*, 2000, vol. 1, pp. 483–489: IEEE.
15. R. Malladi, J. A. Sethian, and B. C. Vemuri, "Shape modeling with front propagation: A level set approach," *IEEE transactions on pattern analysis and machine intelligence*, vol. 17, no. 2, pp. 158–175, 1995.
16. A. Chakraborty, L. H. Staib, and J. S. Duncan, "Deformable boundary finding in medical images by integrating gradient and region information," *IEEE Transactions on Medical Imaging*, vol. 15, no. 6, pp. 859–870, 1996.
17. J. A. Sethian, *Level set methods and fast marching methods: evolving interfaces in computational geometry, fluid mechanics, computer vision, and materials science*. Cambridge University Press, 1999.
18. G. Sapiro, *Geometric partial differential equations and image analysis*. Cambridge university press, 2006.
19. L. H. Staib and J. S. Duncan, "Boundary finding with parametrically deformable models," *IEEE Transactions on Pattern Analysis & Machine Intelligence*, no. 11, pp. 1061–1075, 1992.
20. J. J. Koenderink and A. J. Van Doorn, "Surface shape and curvature scales," *Image and Vision Computing*, vol. 10, no. 8, pp. 557–564, 1992.
21. R. Kimmel, "Intrinsic scale space for images on surfaces: The geodesic curvature flow," in *International Conference on Scale-Space Theories in Computer Vision*, 1997, pp. 212–223: Springer.
22. G. Tryggvason *et al.*, "A front-tracking method for the computations of multiphase flow," *Journal of Computational Physics*, vol. 169, no. 2, pp. 708–759, 2001.
23. S. Osher and N. Paragios, *Geometric level set methods in imaging, vision, and graphics*. Springer Science & Business Media, 2003.
24. S. Osher and R. Fedkiw, *Level set methods and dynamic implicit surfaces*. Springer Science & Business Media, 2006.
25. J. C. Strikwerda, *Finite difference schemes and partial differential equations*. Siam, 2004.

26. A. Harten, B. Engquist, S. Osher, and S. R. Chakravarthy, "Uniformly high order accurate essentially non-oscillatory schemes, III," in *Upwind and high-resolution schemes*: Springer, 1987, pp. 218–290.
27. C.-W. Shu and S. Osher, "Efficient implementation of essentially non-oscillatory shock-capturing schemes," *Journal of Computational Physics*, vol. 77, no. 2, pp. 439–471, 1988.
28. C.-W. Shu and S. Osher, "Efficient implementation of essentially non-oscillatory shock-capturing schemes, II," in *Upwind and High-Resolution Schemes*: Springer, 1989, pp. 328–374.
29. L. M. Milne-Thomson, *The calculus of finite differences*. American Mathematical Soc., 2000.
30. X.-D. Liu, S. Osher, and T. Chan, "Weighted essentially non-oscillatory schemes," *Journal of Computational Physics*, vol. 115, no. 1, pp. 200–212, 1994.
31. G.-S. Jiang and C.-W. Shu, "Efficient implementation of weighted ENO schemes," *Journal of Computational Physics*, vol. 126, no. 1, pp. 202–228, 1996.
32. G.-S. Jiang and D. Peng, "Weighted ENO schemes for Hamilton–Jacobi equations," *SIAM Journal on Scientific Computing*, vol. 21, no. 6, pp. 2126–2143, 2000.
33. R. P. Fedkiw, B. Merriman, and S. Osher, "Simplified discretization of systems of hyperbolic conservation laws containing advection equations," *Journal of Computational Physics*, vol. 157, no. 1, pp. 302–326, 2000.
34. C. Hu and C.-W. Shu, "Weighted essentially non-oscillatory schemes on triangular meshes," *Journal of Computational Physics*, vol. 150, no. 1, pp. 97–127, 1999.
35. R. J. Spiteri and S. J. Ruuth, "A new class of optimal high-order strong-stability-preserving time discretization methods," *SIAM Journal on Numerical Analysis*, vol. 40, no. 2, pp. 469–491, 2002.
36. M. G. Crandall and P.-L. Lions, "Two Approximations of Solutions of Hamilton-Jacobi Equations," WISCONSIN UNIV-MADISON MATHEMATICS RESEARCH CENTER1982.
37. S. Osher and C.-W. Shu, "High-order essentially nonoscillatory schemes for Hamilton–Jacobi equations," *SIAM Journal on Numerical Analysis*, vol. 28, no. 4, pp. 907–922, 1991.
38. S. Godunov, "A finite difference method for the computation of discontinuous solutions of the equations of fluid dynamics," *Sbornik: Mathematics*, vol. 47, no. 8–9, pp. 357–393, 1959.
39. M. Bardi and S. Osher, "The nonconvex multidimensional Riemann problem for Hamilton–Jacobi equations," *SIAM Journal on Mathematical Analysis*, vol. 22, no. 2, pp. 344–351, 1991.
40. O. P. Agrawal, "Formulation of Euler–Lagrange equations for fractional variational problems," *Journal of Mathematical Analysis and Applications*, vol. 272, no. 1, pp. 368–379, 2002.
41. M. Sussman, P. Smereka, and S. Osher, "A level set approach for computing solutions to incompressible two-phase flow," *Journal of Computational Physics*, vol. 114, no. 1, pp. 146–159, 1994.
42. D. L. Chopp, "Computing minimal surfaces via level set curvature flow," 1991.
43. D. Adalsteinsson and J. A. Sethian, "A fast level set method for propagating interfaces," *Journal of Computational Physics*, vol. 118, no. 2, pp. 269–277, 1995.
44. R. Goldenberg, R. Kimmel, E. Rivlin, and M. Rudzsky, "Fast geodesic active contours," *IEEE Transactions on Image Processing*, vol. 10, no. 10, pp. 1467–1475, 2001.

45. S. Kichenassamy, A. Kumar, P. Olver, A. Tannenbaum, and A. Yezzi, "Conformal curvature flows: from phase transitions to active vision," *Archive for Rational Mechanics and Analysis*, vol. 134, no. 3, pp. 275–301, 1996.
46. X. Bresson, S. Esedoḡlu, P. Vandergheynst, J.-P. Thiran, and S. Osher, "Fast global minimization of the active contour/snake model," *Journal of Mathematical Imaging and Vision*, vol. 28, no. 2, pp. 151–167, 2007.
47. N. Paragyios, O. Mellina-Gottardo, and V. Ramesh, "Gradient vector flow fast geodesic active contour," ed: Google Patents, 2003.
48. C. Xu and J. L. Prince, "Generalized gradient vector flow external forces for active contours1," *Signal Processing*, vol. 71, no. 2, pp. 131–139, 1998.
49. T. F. Chan and L. A. Vese, "Active contours without edges," *IEEE Transactions on Image Processing*, vol. 10, no. 2, pp. 266–277, 2001.
50. D. Mumford and J. Shah, "Optimal approximations by piecewise smooth functions and associated variational problems," *Communications on pure and Applied Mathematics*, vol. 42, no. 5, pp. 577–685, 1989.
51. A. Chambolle, "An algorithm for total variation minimization and applications," *Journal of Mathematical Imaging and Vision*, vol. 20, no. 1–2, pp. 89–97, 2004.
52. A. S. El-Baz, A. A. Farag, H. A. El Munim, and S. E. Yuksel, "Level set segmentation using statistical shape priors," in *Computer Vision and Pattern Recognition Workshop, 2006. CVPRW'06. Conference on*, 2006, pp. 78–78: IEEE.
53. A. El-Baz and G. Gimel'farb, "Image segmentation with a parametric deformable model using shape and appearance priors," in *Computer Vision and Pattern Recognition, 2008. CVPR 2008. IEEE Conference on*, 2008, pp. 1–8: IEEE.
54. D. Jayadevappa, S. Srinivas Kumar, and D. Murty, "Medical image segmentation algorithms using deformable models: a review," *IETE Technical Review*, vol. 28, no. 3, pp. 248–255, 2011.
55. L. He *et al.*, "A comparative study of deformable contour methods on medical image segmentation," *Image and Vision Computing*, vol. 26, no. 2, pp. 141–163, 2008.
56. A. Tsai *et al.*, "A shape-based approach to the segmentation of medical imagery using level sets," *IEEE Transactions on Medical Imaging*, vol. 22, no. 2, pp. 137–154, 2003.
57. C. Pluempitiwiriyawej, J. M. Moura, Y.-J. L. Wu, and C. Ho, "STACS: New active contour scheme for cardiac MR image segmentation," *IEEE transactions on Medical Imaging*, vol. 24, no. 5, pp. 593–603, 2005.
58. J. Montagnat and H. Delingette, "4D deformable models with temporal constraints: application to 4D cardiac image segmentation," *Medical Image Analysis*, vol. 9, no. 1, pp. 87–100, 2005.
59. F. Khalifa, G. Beache, A. El-Baz, and G. Gimel'farb, "Deformable model guided by stochastic speed with application in cine images segmentation," in *Image Processing (ICIP), 2010 17th IEEE International Conference on*, 2010, pp. 1725–1728: IEEE.
60. F. Khalifa, G. M. Beache, G. Gimel'farb, and A. El-Baz, "A novel approach for accurate estimation of left ventricle global indexes from short-axis cine MRI," in *Image Processing (ICIP), 2011 18th IEEE International Conference on*, 2011, pp. 2645–2648: IEEE.
61. F. Khalifa, G. M. Beache, M. Nitzken, G. Gimel'Farb, G. Giridharan, and A. El-Baz, "Automatic analysis of left ventricle wall thickness using short-axis cine

CMR images," in *Biomedical Imaging: From Nano to Macro, 2011 IEEE International Symposium on*, 2011, pp. 1306–1309: IEEE.
62. M. G. Uzunbaş, S. Zhang, K. M. Pohl, D. Metaxas, and L. Axel, "Segmentation of myocardium using deformable regions and graph cuts," in *Biomedical Imaging (ISBI), 2012 9th IEEE International Symposium on*, 2012, pp. 254–257: IEEE.
63. F. Khalifa, G. M. Beache, G. Gimelrfarb, G. A. Giridharan, and A. El-Baz, "Accurate automatic analysis of cardiac cine images," *IEEE Transactions on Biomedical Engineering*, vol. 59, no. 2, pp. 445–455, 2012.
64. S. Gopal, Y. Otaki, R. Arsanjani, D. Berman, D. Terzopoulos, and P. Slomka, "Combining active appearance and deformable superquadric models for LV segmentation in cardiac MRI," in *Medical Imaging 2013: Image Processing*, 2013, vol. 8669, p. 86690G: International Society for Optics and Photonics.
65. F. Khalifa, G. M. Beache, G. Gimel'farb, and A. El-Baz, "A novel CAD system for analyzing cardiac first-pass MR images," in *Pattern Recognition (ICPR), 2012 21st International Conference on*, 2012, pp. 77–80: IEEE.
66. F. Khalifa *et al.*, "A new shape-based framework for the left ventricle wall segmentation from cardiac first-pass perfusion MRI," in *Biomedical Imaging (ISBI), 2013 IEEE 10th International Symposium on*, 2013, pp. 41–44: IEEE.
67. F. Khalifa, G. M. Beache, A. Firjani, K. C. Welch, G. Gimel'farb, and A. El-Baz, "A new nonrigid registration approach for motion correction of cardiac first-pass perfusion MRI," in *Image Processing (ICIP), 2012 19th IEEE International Conference on*, 2012, pp. 1665–1668: IEEE.
68. G. M. Beache, F. Khalifa, A. El-Baz, and G. Gimel'farb, "Fully automated framework for the analysis of myocardial first-pass perfusion MR images," *Medical Physics*, vol. 41, no. 10, 2014.
69. H. Sliman *et al.*, "A novel 4D PDE-based approach for accurate assessment of myocardium function using cine cardiac magnetic resonance images," in *Image Processing (ICIP), 2014 IEEE International Conference on*, 2014, pp. 3537–3541: IEEE.
70. H. Sliman *et al.*, "A new segmentation-based tracking framework for extracting the left ventricle cavity from cine cardiac MRI," in *Proceedings of IEEE International Conference on Image Processing, (ICIP'13)*, 2013, pp. 685–689.
71. H. Sliman *et al.*, "Accurate segmentation framework for the left ventricle wall from cardiac cine MRI," in *AIP Conference Proceedings*, 2013, vol. 1559, no. 1, pp. 287–296: AIP.
72. H. Sliman *et al.*, "Myocardial borders segmentation from cine MR images using bidirectional coupled parametric deformable models," *Medical Physics*, vol. 40, no. 9, 2013.
73. S. Ho, E. Bullitt, and G. Gerig, "Level-set evolution with region competition: automatic 3-D segmentation of brain tumors," in *Pattern Recognition, 2002. Proceedings. 16th International Conference on*, 2002, vol. 1, pp. 532–535: IEEE.
74. R. Goldenberg, R. Kimmel, E. Rivlin, and M. Rudzsky, "Cortex segmentation: A fast variational geometric approach," *IEEE Transactions on Medical Imaging*, vol. 21, no. 12, pp. 1544–1551, 2002.
75. Ali, A.M., Farag, A.A., El-Baz, A.: Graph cuts framework for kidney segmentation with prior shape constraints. In: *Proceedings of International Conference on Medical Image Computing and Computer-Assisted Intervention, (MICCAI'07)*. Volume 1., Brisbane, Australia, October 29–November 2 (2007) 384–392.
76. Chowdhury, A.S., Roy, R., Bose, S., Elnakib, F.K.A., El-Baz, A.: Non-rigid biomedical image registration using graph cuts with a novel data term. In

Proceedings of IEEE International Symposium on Biomedical Imaging: From Nano to Macro, (ISBI'12), Barcelona, Spain, May 2–5 (2012) 446–449.
77. El-Baz, A., Farag, A.A., Yuksel, S.E., El-Ghar, M.E.A., Eldiasty, T.A., Ghoneim, M.A.: Application of deformable models for the detection of acute renal rejection. In Farag, A.A., Suri, J.S., eds.: *Deformable Models*. Volume 1. (2007) 293–333.
78. El-Baz, A., Farag, A., Fahmi, R., Yuksel, S., El-Ghar, M.A., Eldiasty, T.: Image analysis of renal DCE MRI for the detection of acute renal rejection. In: *Proceedings of IAPR International Conference on Pattern Recognition (ICPR'06)*, Hong Kong, August 20–24 (2006) 822–825.
79. El-Baz, A., Farag, A., Fahmi, R., Yuksel, S., Miller, W., El-Ghar, M.A., El-Diasty, T., Ghoneim, M.: A new CAD system for the evaluation of kidney diseases using DCE-MRI. In: *Proceedings of International Conference on Medical Image Computing and Computer-Assisted Intervention, (MICCAI'08)*, Copenhagen, Denmark, October 1–6 (2006) 446–453.
80. El-Baz, A., Gimel'farb, G., El-Ghar, M.A.: A novel image analysis approach for accurate identification of acute renal rejection. In: *Proceedings of IEEE International Conference on Image Processing, (ICIP'08)*, San Diego, California, USA, October 12–15 (2008) 1812–1815.
81. El-Baz, A., Gimel'farb, G., El-Ghar, M.A.: Image analysis approach for identification of renal transplant rejection. In: *Proceedings of IAPR International Conference on Pattern Recognition, (ICPR'08)*, Tampa, Florida, USA, December 8–11 (2008) 1–4.
82. El-Baz, A., Gimel'farb, G., El-Ghar, M.A.: New motion correction models for automatic identification of renal transplant rejection. In: *Proceedings of International Conference on Medical Image Computing and Computer-Assisted Intervention, (MICCAI'07)*, Brisbane, Australia, October 29–November 2 (2007) 235–243.
83. Farag, A., El-Baz, A., Yuksel, S., El-Ghar, M.A., Eldiasty, T.: A framework for the detection of acute rejection with Dynamic Contrast Enhanced Magnetic Resonance Imaging. In: *Proceedings of IEEE International Symposium on Biomedical Imaging: From Nano to Macro, (ISBI'06)*, Arlington, Virginia, USA, April 6–9 (2006) 418–421.
84. Khalifa, F., Beache, G.M., El-Ghar, M.A., El-Diasty, T., Gimel'farb, G., Kong, M., El-Baz, A.: Dynamic contrast-enhanced MRI-based early detection of acute renal transplant rejection. *IEEE Transactions on Medical Imaging* 32(10) (2013) 1910–1927 Prostate Cancer Diagnosis using SNCAE 23.
85. Khalifa, F., El-Baz, A., Gimel'farb, G., El-Ghar, M.A.: Non-invasive image-based approach for early detection of acute renal rejection. In: *Proceedings of International Conference Medical Image Computing and Computer-Assisted Intervention, (MICCAI'10)*, Beijing, China, September 20–24 (2010) 10–18.
86. Khalifa, F., El-Baz, A., Gimel'farb, G., Ouseph, R., El-Ghar, M.A.: Shapeappearance guided level-set deformable model for image segmentation. In: *Proceedings of IAPR International Conference on Pattern Recognition, (ICPR'10)*, Istanbul, Turkey, August 23–26 (2010) 4581–4584.
87. Khalifa, F., El-Ghar, M.A., Abdollahi, B., Frieboes, H., El-Diasty, T., El-Baz, A.: A comprehensive non-invasive framework for automated evaluation of acute renal transplant rejection using DCE-MRI. *NMR in Biomedicine* 26(11) (2013) 1460–1470.
88. Khalifa, F., El-Ghar, M.A., Abdollahi, B., Frieboes, H.B., El-Diasty, T., El-Baz, A.: Dynamic contrast-enhanced MRI-based early detection of acute renal transplant rejection. In: *2014 Annual Scientific Meeting and Educational Course Brochure of the*

Society of Abdominal Radiology, (SAR'14), Boca Raton, Florida, March 23–28 (2014) CID: 1855912.

89. Khalifa, F., Elnakib, A., Beache, G.M., Gimel'farb, G., El-Ghar, M.A., Sokhadze, G., Manning, S., McClure, P., El-Baz, A.: 3D kidney segmentation from CT images using a level set approach guided by a novel stochastic speed function. In: *Proceedings of International Conference Medical Image Computing and Computer-Assisted Intervention, (MICCAI'11)*, Toronto, Canada, September 18–22 (2011) 587–594.
90. Khalifa, F., Gimel'farb, G., El-Ghar, M.A., Sokhadze, G., Manning, S., McClure, P., Ouseph, R., El-Baz, A.: A new deformable model-based segmentation approach for accurate extraction of the kidney from abdominal CT images. In: *Proceedings of IEEE International Conference on Image Processing, (ICIP'11)*, Brussels, Belgium, September 11–14 (2011) 3393–3396.
91. Mostapha, M., Khalifa, F., Alansary, A., Soliman, A., Suri, J., El-Baz, A.: Computer-aided diagnosis systems for acute renal transplant rejection: Challenges and methodologies. In El-Baz, A., saba J. Suri, L., eds.: *Abdomen and thoracic imaging*. Springer (2014) 1–35.
92. Shehata, M., Khalifa, F., Hollis, E., Soliman, A., Hosseini-Asl, E., El-Ghar, M.A., El-Baz, M., Dwyer, A.C., El-Baz, A., Keynton, R.: A new non-invasive approach for early classification of renal rejection types using diffusion-weighted mri. In: *IEEE International Conference on Image Processing (ICIP)*, 2016, IEEE (2016) 136–140.
93. Khalifa, F., Soliman, A., Takieldeen, A., Shehata, M., Mostapha, M., Shaffie, A., Ouseph, R., Elmaghraby, A., El-Baz, A.: Kidney segmentation from CT images using a 3D NMF-guided active contour model. In: *IEEE 13th International Symposium on Biomedical Imaging (ISBI)*, 2016, IEEE (2016) 432–435.
94. Shehata, M., Khalifa, F., Soliman, A., Takieldeen, A., El-Ghar, M.A., Shaffie, A., Dwyer, A.C., Ouseph, R., El-Baz, A., Keynton, R.: 3d diffusion mri-based cad system for early diagnosis of acute renal rejection. In: *Biomedical Imaging (ISBI), 2016 IEEE 13th International Symposium on, IEEE* (2016) 1177–1180.
95. Shehata, M., Khalifa, F., Soliman, A., Alrefai, R., El-Ghar, M.A., Dwyer, A.C., Ouseph, R., El-Baz, A.: A level set-based framework for 3d kidney segmentation from diffusion mr images. In: *IEEE International Conference on Image Processing (ICIP)*, 2015, IEEE (2015) 4441–4445. 24 Authors Suppressed Due to Excessive Length.
96. Shehata, M., Khalifa, F., Soliman, A., El-Ghar, M.A., Dwyer, A.C., Gimelfarb, G., Keynton, R., El-Baz, A.: A promising non-invasive cad system for kidney function assessment. In: *International Conference on Medical Image Computing and Computer-Assisted Intervention*. Springer (2016) 613–621.
97. Khalifa, F., Soliman, A., Elmaghraby, A., Gimelfarb, G., El-Baz, A.: 3d kidney segmentation from abdominal images using spatial-appearance models. *Computational and mathematical methods in medicine* 2017 (2017).
98. Hollis, E., Shehata, M., Khalifa, F., El-Ghar, M.A., El-Diasty, T., El-Baz, A.: Towards non-invasive diagnostic techniques for early detection of acute renal transplant rejection: A review. *The Egyptian Journal of Radiology and Nuclear Medicine* 48(1) (2016) 257–269.
99. Shehata, M., Khalifa, F., Soliman, A., El-Ghar, M.A., Dwyer, A.C., El-Baz, A.: Assessment of renal transplant using image and clinical-based biomarkers. In: *Proceedings of 13th Annual Scientific Meeting of American Society for Diagnostics and*

Interventional Nephrology (ASDIN'17), New Orleans, LA, USA, February 10–12, 2017. (2017).

100. Shehata, M., Khalifa, F., Soliman, A., El-Ghar, M.A., Dwyer, A.C., El-Baz, A.: Early assessment of acute renal rejection. In: *Proceedings of 12th Annual Scientific Meeting of American Society for Diagnostics and Interventional Nephrology (ASDIN'16)*, Pheonix, AZ, USA, February 19–21, 2016. (2017).
101. Khalifa, F., Beache, G., El-Baz, A., Gimel'farb, G.: Deformable model guided by stochastic speed with application in cine images segmentation. In: *Proceedings of IEEE International Conference on Image Processing, (ICIP'10)*, Hong Kong, September 26–29 (2010) 1725–1728.
102. Khalifa, F., Beache, G.M., Elnakib, A., Sliman, H., Gimel'farb, G., Welch, K.C., El-Baz, A.: A new shape-based framework for the left ventricle wall segmentation from cardiac first-pass perfusion MRI. In: *Proceedings of IEEE International Symposium on Biomedical Imaging: From Nano to Macro, (ISBI'13)*, San Francisco, CA, April 7–11 (2013) 41–44.
103. Khalifa, F., Beache, G.M., Elnakib, A., Sliman, H., Gimel'farb, G., Welch, K.C., El-Baz, A.: A new nonrigid registration framework for improved visualization of transmural perfusion gradients on cardiac first–pass perfusion MRI. In: *Proceedings of IEEE International Symposium on Biomedical Imaging: From Nano to Macro, (ISBI'12)*, Barcelona, Spain, May 2–5 (2012) 828–831.
104. Khalifa, F., Beache, G.M., Firjani, A., Welch, K.C., Gimel'farb, G., El-Baz, A.: A new nonrigid registration approach for motion correction of cardiac first-pass perfusion MRI. In: *Proceedings of IEEE International Conference on Image Processing, (ICIP'12)*, Lake Buena Vista, Florida, September 30–October 3 (2012) 1665–1668.
105. Khalifa, F., Beache, G.M., Gimel'farb, G., El-Baz, A.: A novel CAD system for analyzing cardiac first-pass MR images. In: *Proceedings of IAPR International Conference on Pattern Recognition (ICPR'12)*, Tsukuba Science City, Japan, November 11–15 (2012) 77–80.
106. Khalifa, F., Beache, G.M., Gimel'farb, G., El-Baz, A.: A novel approach for accurate estimation of left ventricle global indexes from short-axis cine MRI. In: *Proceedings of IEEE International Conference on Image Processing, (ICIP'11)*, Brussels, Belgium, September 11–14 (2011) 2645–2649.
107. Khalifa, F., Beache, G.M., Gimel'farb, G., Giridharan, G.A., El-Baz, A.: A new image-based framework for analyzing cine images. In El-Baz, A., Acharya, U.R., Mirmedhdi, M., Suri, J.S., eds.: *Handbook of multi modality state-of prostate cancer diagnosis using SNCAE 25 the-art medical image segmentation and registration methodologies*. Volume 2. Springer, New York (2011) 69–98.
108. Khalifa, F., Beache, G.M., Gimel'farb, G., Giridharan, G.A., El-Baz, A.: Accurate automatic analysis of cardiac cine images. *IEEE Transactions on Biomedical Engineering* 59(2) (2012) 445–455.
109. Khalifa, F., Beache, G.M., Nitzken, M., Gimel'farb, G., Giridharan, G.A., El-Baz, A.: Automatic analysis of left ventricle wall thickness using short-axis cine CMR images. In: *Proceedings of IEEE International Symposium on Biomedical Imaging: From Nano to Macro, (ISBI'11)*, Chicago, Illinois, March 30–April 2 (2011) 1306–1309.
110. Nitzken, M., Beache, G., Elnakib, A., Khalifa, F., Gimel'farb, G., El-Baz, A.: Accurate modeling of tagged cmr 3D image appearance characteristics to improve cardiac cycle strain estimation. In: *Image Processing (ICIP), 2012 19th IEEE*

International Conference on, Orlando, Florida, USA, IEEE (September 2012) 521–524.

111. Nitzken, M., Beache, G., Elnakib, A., Khalifa, F., Gimel'farb, G., El-Baz, A.: Improving full-cardiac cycle strain estimation from tagged cmr by accurate modeling of 3D image appearance characteristics. In: *Biomedical Imaging (ISBI), 2012 9th IEEE International Symposium on, Barcelona, Spain, IEEE* (May 2012) 462–465 (Selected for oral presentation).
112. Nitzken, M.J., El-Baz, A.S., Beache, G.M.: Markov-gibbs random field model for improved full-cardiac cycle strain estimation from tagged cmr. *Journal of Cardiovascular Magnetic Resonance* 14(1) (2012) 1–2.
113. Sliman, H., Elnakib, A., Beache, G., Elmaghraby, A., El-Baz, A.: Assessment of myocardial function from cine cardiac MRI using a novel 4D tracking approach. *J Comput Sci Syst Biol* 7 (2014) 169–173.
114. Sliman, H., Elnakib, A., Beache, G.M., Soliman, A., Khalifa, F., Gimel'farb, G., Elmaghraby, A., El-Baz, A.: A novel 4D PDE-based approach for accurate assessment of myocardium function using cine cardiac magnetic resonance images. In: *Proceedings of IEEE International Conference on Image Processing (ICIP'14)*, Paris, France, October 27–30 (2014) 3537–3541.
115. Sliman, H., Khalifa, F., Elnakib, A., Beache, G.M., Elmaghraby, A., El-Baz, A.: A new segmentation-based tracking framework for extracting the left ventricle cavity from cine cardiac MRI. In: *Proceedings of IEEE International Conference on Image Processing, (ICIP'13)*, Melbourne, Australia, September 15–18 (2013) 685–689.
116. Sliman, H., Khalifa, F., Elnakib, A., Soliman, A., Beache, G.M., Elmaghraby, A., Gimel'farb, G., El-Baz, A.: Myocardial borders segmentation from cine MR images using bi-directional coupled parametric deformable models. *Medical Physics* (9) (2013) 1–13.
117. Sliman, H., Khalifa, F., Elnakib, A., Soliman, A., Beache, G.M., Gimel'farb, G., Emam, A., Elmaghraby, A., El-Baz, A.: Accurate segmentation framework for the left ventricle wall from cardiac cine MRI. In: *Proceedings of International Symposium on Computational Models for Life Science, (CMLS'13)*. Volume 1559., Sydney, Australia, November 27–29 (2013) 287–296.
118. N. Eladawi, M. Elmogy, M.G.O.H.A.A.A.R.S.S.A.E.B.: Classification of retina diseases based on oct images. *Frontiers in Bioscience Landmark Journal* (2017).
119. A. ElTanboly, M. Ismail, A.S.A.S.S.S.G.G.M.E.A.E.B.: A computer aided diagnostic system for detecting diabetic retinopathy in optical coherence tomography images. *Medical Physics* (2016) 26 Authors Suppressed Due to Excessive Length.
120. Abdollahi, B., Civelek, A.C., Li, X.F., Suri, J., El-Baz, A.: PET/CT nodule segmentation and diagnosis: A survey. In Saba, L., Suri, J.S., eds.: *Multi detector CT imaging*. Taylor, Francis (2014) 639–651.
121. Abdollahi, B., El-Baz, A., Amini, A.A.: A multi-scale non-linear vessel enhancement technique. In: *Engineering in medicine and biology society*, EMBC, 2011 Annual International Conference of the IEEE, IEEE (2011) 3925–3929.
122. Abdollahi, B., Soliman, A., Civelek, A., Li, X.F., Gimel'farb, G., El-Baz, A.: A novel gaussian scale space-based joint MGRF framework for precise lung segmentation. In: *Proceedings of IEEE International Conference on Image Processing, (ICIP'12)* IEEE (2012). 2029–2032.

123. Abdollahi, B., Soliman, A., Civelek, A., Li, X.F., Gimelfarb, G., El-Baz, A.: A novel 3D joint MGRF framework for precise lung segmentation. In: *Machine learning in medical imaging*. Springer (2012) 86–93.
124. Ali, A.M., El-Baz, A.S., Farag, A.A.: A novel framework for accurate lung segmentation using graph cuts. In: *Proceedings of IEEE International Symposium on Biomedical Imaging: From Nano to Macro, (ISBI'07)*, IEEE (2007) 908–911.
125. El-Baz, A., Beache, G.M., Gimel'farb, G., Suzuki, K., Okada, K.: Lung imaging data analysis. *International Journal of Biomedical Imaging* 2013 (2013).
126. El-Baz, A., Beache, G.M., Gimel'farb, G., Suzuki, K., Okada, K., Elnakib, A., Soliman, A., Abdollahi, B.: Computer-aided diagnosis systems for lung cancer: Challenges and methodologies. *International Journal of Biomedical Imaging* 2013 (2013).
127. El-Baz, A., Elnakib, A., Abou El-Ghar, M., Gimel'farb, G., Falk, R., Farag, A.: Automatic detection of 2D and 3D lung nodules in chest spiral CT scans. *International Journal of Biomedical Imaging* 2013 (2013).
128. El-Baz, A., Farag, A.A., Falk, R., La Rocca, R.: A unified approach for detection, visualization, and identification of lung abnormalities in chest spiral CT scans. In: *International Congress Series*. Volume 1256., Elsevier (2003) 998–1004.
129. El-Baz, A., Farag, A.A., Falk, R., La Rocca, R.: Detection, visualization and identification of lung abnormalities in chest spiral CT scan: Phase-I. In: *Proceedings of International conference on Biomedical Engineering*, Cairo, Egypt. Volume 12. (2002).
130. El-Baz, A., Farag, A., Gimel'farb, G., Falk, R., El-Ghar, M.A., Eldiasty, T.: A framework for automatic segmentation of lung nodules from low dose chest CT scans. In: *Proceedings of International Conference on Pattern Recognition, (ICPR'06)*. Volume 3., IEEE (2006) 611–614.
131. El-Baz, A., Farag, A., Gimelfarb, G., Falk, R., El-Ghar, M.A.: A novel level set-based computer-aided detection system for automatic detection of lung nodules in low dose chest computed tomography scans. *Lung Imaging and Computer Aided Diagnosis* 10 (2011) 221–238.
132. El-Baz, A., Gimel'farb, G., Abou El-Ghar, M., Falk, R.: Appearance-based diagnostic system for early assessment of malignant lung nodules. In: *Proceedings of IEEE International Conference on Image Processing, (ICIP'12)*, IEEE (2012) 533–536.
133. El-Baz, A., Gimel'farb, G., Falk, R.: A novel 3D framework for automatic lung segmentation from low dose CT images. In El-Baz, A., Suri, J.S., eds.: *Lung imaging and computer aided diagnosis*. Taylor, Francis (2011) 1–16.
134. El-Baz, A., Gimel'farb, G., Falk, R., El-Ghar, M.: Appearance analysis for diagnosing malignant lung nodules. In: *Proceedings of IEEE International Symposium on Biomedical Imaging: From Nano to Macro (ISBI'10)*, IEEE (2010) 193–196 Prostate Cancer Diagnosis using SNCAE 27.
135. El-Baz, A., Gimel'farb, G., Falk, R., El-Ghar, M.A.: A novel level set-based CAD system for automatic detection of lung nodules in low dose chest CT scans. In El-Baz, A., Suri, J.S., eds.: Lung Imaging and Computer Aided Diagnosis. Volume 1. Taylor, Francis (2011) 221–238.
136. El-Baz, A., Gimel'farb, G., Falk, R., El-Ghar, M.A.: A new approach for automatic analysis of 3D low dose CT images for accurate monitoring the detected lung nodules. In: *Proceedings of International Conference on Pattern Recognition, (ICPR'08)*, IEEE (2008) 1–4.

137. El-Baz, A., Gimel'farb, G., Falk, R., El-Ghar, M.A.: A novel approach for automatic follow-up of detected lung nodules. In: *Proceedings of IEEE International Conference on Image Processing, (ICIP'07)*. Volume 5., IEEE (2007) V–501.
138. El-Baz, A., Gimel'farb, G., Falk, R., El-Ghar, M.A.: A new CAD system for early diagnosis of detected lung nodules. In: *Image Processing, 2007. ICIP 2007. IEEE International Conference on*. Volume 2., IEEE (2007) II–461.
139. El-Baz, A., Gimel'farb, G., Falk, R., El-Ghar, M.A., Refaie, H.: Promising results for early diagnosis of lung cancer. In: *Proceedings of IEEE International Symposium on Biomedical Imaging: From Nano to Macro, (ISBI'08)*, IEEE (2008) 1151–1154.
140. El-Baz, A., Gimel'farb, G.L., Falk, R., Abou El-Ghar, M., Holland, T., Shaffer, T.: A new stochastic framework for accurate lung segmentation. In: *Proceedings of Medical Image Computing and Computer-Assisted Intervention, (MICCAI'08)*. (2008) 322–330.
141. El-Baz, A., Gimel'farb, G.L., Falk, R., Heredis, D., Abou El-Ghar, M.: A novel approach for accurate estimation of the growth rate of the detected lung nodules. In: *Proceedings of International Workshop on Pulmonary Image Analysis*. (2008) 33–42.
142. El-Baz, A., Gimel'farb, G.L., Falk, R., Holland, T., Shaffer, T.: A framework for unsupervised segmentation of lung tissues from low dose computed tomography images. In: *Proceedings of British Machine Vision, (BMVC'08)*. (2008) 1–10.
143. El-Baz, A., Gimelfarb, G., Falk, R., El-Ghar, M.A.: 3D MGRF-based appearance modeling for robust segmentation of pulmonary nodules in 3D LDCT chest images. In: *Lung imaging and computer aided diagnosis*. chapter (2011) 51–63.
144. El-Baz, A., Gimelfarb, G., Falk, R., El-Ghar, M.A.: Automatic analysis of 3D low dose CT images for early diagnosis of lung cancer. *Pattern Recognition* 42(6) (2009) 1041–1051.
145. El-Baz, A., Gimelfarb, G., Falk, R., El-Ghar, M.A., Rainey, S., Heredia, D., Shaffer, T.: Toward early diagnosis of lung cancer. In: *Proceedings of Medical Image Computing and Computer-Assisted Intervention, (MICCAI'09)*, Springer (2009) 682–689.
146. El-Baz, A., Gimelfarb, G., Falk, R., El-Ghar, M.A., Suri, J.: Appearance analysis for the early assessment of detected lung nodules. In: *Lung imaging and computer aided diagnosis*. chapter (2011) 395–404.
147. El-Baz, A., Khalifa, F., Elnakib, A., Nitkzen, M., Soliman, A., McClure, P., Gimel'farb, G., El-Ghar, M.A.: A novel approach for global lung registration using 3D Markov Gibbs appearance model. In: *Proceedings of International Conference Medical Image Computing and Computer-Assisted Intervention, (MICCAI' 12)*, Nice, France, October 1–5 (2012) 114–121.
148. El-Baz, A., Nitzken, M., Elnakib, A., Khalifa, F., Gimel'farb, G., Falk, R., El-Ghar, M.A.: 3D shape analysis for early diagnosis of malignant lung nodules. In: *Proceedings of International Conference Medical Image Computing and Computer-Assisted Intervention, (MICCAI'11)*, Toronto, Canada, September 18–22 (2011) 175–182.
149. El-Baz, A., Nitzken, M., Gimelfarb, G., Van Bogaert, E., Falk, R., El-Ghar, M.A., Suri, J.: Three-dimensional shape analysis using spherical harmonics for early assessment of detected lung nodules. In: *Lung imaging and computer aided diagnosis* chapter (2011) 421–438.
150. El-Baz, A., Nitzken, M., Khalifa, F., Elnakib, A., Gimel'farb, G., Falk, R. El-Ghar, M.A.: 3D shape analysis for early diagnosis of malignant lung nodules. In: Proceedings of International Conference on Information Processing ir

Medical Imaging, (IPMI'11), Monastery Irsee, Germany (Bavaria), July 3–8 (2011) 772–783.

151. El-Baz, A., Nitzken, M., Vanbogaert, E., Gimel'Farb, G., Falk, R., Abo El-Ghar, M.: A novel shape-based diagnostic approach for early diagnosis of lung nodules. In: *Biomedical Imaging: From Nano to Macro, 2011 IEEE International Symposium on,* IEEE (2011) 137–140.
152. El-Baz, A., Sethu, P., Gimel'farb, G., Khalifa, F., Elnakib, A., Falk, R., El-Ghar, M.A.: Elastic phantoms generated by microfluidics technology: Validation of an imaged-based approach for accurate measurement of the growth rate of lung nodules. *Biotechnology Journal* 6(2) (2011) 195–203.
153. El-Baz, A., Sethu, P., Gimel'farb, G., Khalifa, F., Elnakib, A., Falk, R., El-Ghar, M.A.: A new validation approach for the growth rate measurement using elastic phantoms generated by state-of-the-art microfluidics technology. In: *Proceedings of IEEE International Conference on Image Processing, (ICIP'10),* Hong Kong, September 26–29 (2010) 4381–4383.
154. El-Baz, A., Sethu, P., Gimel'farb, G., Khalifa, F., Elnakib, A., Falk, R., Suri, M.A.E.G.J.: Validation of a new imaged-based approach for the accurate estimating of the growth rate of detected lung nodules using real CT images and elastic phantoms generated by state-of-the-art microfluidics technology. In El-Baz, A., Suri, J.S., eds.: *Handbook of lung imaging and computer aided diagnosis.* Volume 1. Taylor & Francis, New York (2011) 405–420.
155. El-Baz, A., Soliman, A., McClure, P., Gimel'farb, G., El-Ghar, M.A., Falk, R.: Early assessment of malignant lung nodules based on the spatial analysis of detected lung nodules. In: *Proceedings of IEEE International Symposium on Biomedical Imaging: From Nano to Macro, (ISBI'12),* IEEE (2012) 1463–1466.
156. El-Baz, A., Yuksel, S.E., Elshazly, S., Farag, A.A.: Non-rigid registration techniques for automatic follow-up of lung nodules. In: *Proceedings of Computer Assisted Radiology and Surgery, (CARS'05).* Volume 1281., Elsevier (2005) 1115–1120.
157. El-Baz, A.S., Suri, J.S.: *Lung imaging and computer aided diagnosis.* CRC Press (2011).
158. Soliman, A., Khalifa, F., Shaffie, A., Liu, N., Dunlap, N., Wang, B., Elmaghraby, A., Gimelfarb, G., El-Baz, A.: Image-based cad system for accurate identification of lung injury. In: *Proceedings of IEEE International Conference on Image Processing, (ICIP'16),* IEEE (2016) 121–125.
159. Soliman, A., Khalifa, F., Dunlap, N., Wang, B., El-Ghar, M., El-Baz, A.: An isosurfaces based local deformation handling framework of lung tissues. In: *Biomedical Imaging (ISBI), 2016 IEEE 13th International Symposium on,* IEEE (2016) 1253–1259.
160. Soliman, A., Khalifa, F., Shaffie, A., Dunlap, N., Wang, B., Elmaghraby, A., El-Baz, A.: Detection of lung injury using 4d-ct chest images. In: *Biomedical Imaging (ISBI), 2016 IEEE 13th International Symposium on,* IEEE (2016) 1274–1277 Prostate Cancer Diagnosis using SNCAE 29.
161. Dombroski, B., Nitzken, M., Elnakib, A., Khalifa, F., El-Baz, A., Casanova, M.F.: Cortical surface complexity in a population-based normative sample. *Translational Neuroscience* 5(1) (2014) 17–24.
162. El-Baz, A., Casanova, M., Gimel'farb, G., Mott, M., Switala, A.: An MRI-based diagnostic framework for early diagnosis of dyslexia. *International Journal of Computer Assisted Radiology and Surgery* 3(3–4) (2008) 181–189.
163. El-Baz, A., Casanova, M., Gimel'farb, G., Mott, M., Switala, A., Vanbogaert, E., McCracken, R.: A new CAD system for early diagnosis of dyslexic brains.

In: *Proc. International Conference on Image Processing (ICIP'2008)*, IEEE (2008) 1820–1823.

164. El-Baz, A., Casanova, M.F., Gimel'farb, G., Mott, M., Switwala, A.E.: A new image analysis approach for automatic classification of autistic brains. In: *Proc. IEEE International Symposium on Biomedical Imaging: From Nano to Macro (ISBI'2007)*, IEEE (2007) 352–355.
165. El-Baz, A., Elnakib, A., Khalifa, F., El-Ghar, M.A., McClure, P., Soliman, A., Gimel'farb, G.: Precise segmentation of 3-D magnetic resonance angiography. *IEEE Transactions on Biomedical Engineering* 59(7) (2012) 2019–2029.
166. El-Baz, A., Farag, A.A., Gimel'farb, G.L., El-Ghar, M.A., Eldiasty, T.: Probabilistic modeling of blood vessels for segmenting mra images. In: *ICPR* (3). (2006) 917–920.
167. El-Baz, A., Farag, A.A., Gimelfarb, G., El-Ghar, M.A., Eldiasty, T.: A new adaptive probabilistic model of blood vessels for segmenting mra images. In: *Medical image computing and computer assisted intervention–MICCAI 2006*. Volume 4191., Springer (2006) 799–806.
168. El-Baz, A., Farag, A.A., Gimelfarb, G., Hushek, S.G.: Automatic cerebrovascular segmentation by accurate probabilistic modeling of tof-mra images. In: *Medical image computing and computer-assisted intervention–MICCAI 2005*. Springer (2005) 34–42.
169. El-Baz, A., Farag, A., Elnakib, A., Casanova, M.F., Gimel'farb, G., Switala, A.E., Jordan, D., Rainey, S.: Accurate automated detection of autism related corpus callosum abnormalities. *Journal of Medical Systems* 35(5) (2011) 929–939.
170. El-Baz, A., Farag, A., Gimelfarb, G.: Cerebrovascular segmentation by accurate probabilistic modeling of tof-mra images. In: *Image Analysis*. Volume 3540., Springer (2005) 1128–1137.
171. El-Baz, A., Gimelfarb, G., Falk, R., El-Ghar, M.A., Kumar, V., Heredia, D.: A novel 3D joint Markov-gibbs model for extracting blood vessels from PC–mra images. In: *Medical image computing and computer-assisted intervention– MICCAI 2009*. Volume 5762., Springer (2009) 943–950.
172. Elnakib, A., El-Baz, A., Casanova, M.F., Gimel'farb, G., Switala, A.E.: Image based detection of corpus callosum variability for more accurate discrimination between dyslexic and normal brains. In: *Proc. IEEE International Symposium on Biomedical Imaging: From Nano to Macro (ISBI'2010)*, IEEE (2010) 109–112.
173. Elnakib, A., Casanova, M.F., Gimel'farb, G., Switala, A.E., El-Baz, A.: Autism diagnostics by centerline-based shape analysis of the corpus callosum. In: *Proc. IEEE International Symposium on Biomedical Imaging: From Nano to Macro (ISBI'2011)*, IEEE (2011) 1843–1846.
174. Elnakib, A., Nitzken, M., Casanova, M., Park, H., Gimel'farb, G., El-Baz, A.: Quantification of age-related brain cortex change using 3D shape analysis. In: *Pattern Recognition (ICPR)*, 2012 21st International Conference on, IEEE (2012) 41–44. 30 Authors Suppressed Due to Excessive Length.
175. Mostapha, M., Soliman, A., Khalifa, F., Elnakib, A., Alansary, A., Nitzken, M., Casanova, M.F., El-Baz, A.: A statistical framework for the classification of infant dt images. In: *Image Processing (ICIP)*, 2014 IEEE International Conference on, IEEE (2014) 2222–2226.
176. Nitzken, M., Casanova, M., Gimel'farb, G., Elnakib, A., Khalifa, F., Switala, A., El-Baz, A.: 3D shape analysis of the brain cortex with application to dyslexia. In: *Image Processing (ICIP)*, 2011 18th IEEE International Conference on, Brussels

Belgium, IEEE (September 2011) 2657–2660 (Selected for oral presentation. Oral acceptance rate is 10 percent and the overall acceptance rate is 35 percent).

177. El-Gamal, F.E.Z.A., Elmogy, M., Ghazal, M., Atwan, A., Barnes, G., Casanova, M., Keynton, R., El-Baz, A.: A novel cad system for local and global early diagnosis of alzheimers disease based on pib-pet scans. In: *Image Processing (ICIP), 2017 IEEE International Conference on, Beijing, China,* IEEE (2017).
178. Ismail, M., Soliman, A., Ghazal, M., Switala, A.E., Gimel'farb, G., Barnes, G.N., Khalil, A. and El-Baz, A., 2017. A fast stochastic framework for automatic MR brain images segmentation. PloS one, 12(11), p.e0187391.
179. Ismail, M.M., Keynton, R.S., Mostapha, M.M., ElTanboly, A.H., Casanova, M.F., Gimel'farb, G.L., El-Baz, A.: Studying autism spectrum disorder with structural and diffusion magnetic resonance imaging: a survey. *Frontiers in Human Neuroscience* 10 (2016).
180. Alansary, A., Ismail, M., Soliman, A., Khalifa, F., Nitzken, M., Elnakib, A., Mostapha, M., Black, A., Stinebruner, K., Casanova, M.F., et al.: Infant brain extraction in t1-weighted mr images using bet and refinement using lcdg and mgrf models. *IEEE Journal of Biomedical and Health Informatics* 20(3) (2016) 925–935.
181. Ismail, M., Barnes, G., Nitzken, M., Switala, A., Shalaby, A., Hosseini-Asl, E., Casanova, M., Keynton, R., Khalil, A. and El-Baz, A., 2017, September. A new deep-learning approach for early detection of shape variations in autism using structural mri. In 2017 IEEE International Conference on Image Processing (ICIP) (pp. 1057–1061). IEEE.
182. Ismail, M., Soliman, A., ElTanboly, A., Switala, A., Mahmoud, M., Khalifa, F., Gimel'farb, G., Casanova, M.F., Keynton, R., El-Baz, A.: Detection of white matter abnormalities in mr brain images for diagnosis of autism in children. (2016) 6–9.
183. Ismail, M., Mostapha, M., Soliman, A., Nitzken, M., Khalifa, F., Elnakib, A., Gimel'farb, G., Casanova, M., El-Baz, A.: Segmentation of infant brain mr images based on adaptive shape prior and higher-order mgrf. (2015) 4327–4331.

9

Cardiac Image Segmentation Using Generalized Polynomial Chaos Expansion and Level Set Function

Yuncheng Du and Dongping Du

CONTENTS

9.1 Introduction

Heart diseases are the leading cause of death and claim more than 18 million lives worldwide per year [1]. Diagnosis and treatment of heart diseases can rely on numerous cardiac imaging modalities such as echocardiography [2], computerized tomography [3], coronary angiography [4], and cardiac magnetic resonance (CMR) images [5]. It is well recognized that CMR, as a noninvasive assessment of cardiac functions, can provide accurate information about morphology, muscle perfusion, tissue viability, and blood flow. Thus, CMR has recently become a useful technique in clinical cardiology practice [6] and can be used for precise diagnosis of cardiovascular diseases and evaluation of heart functions in order to reduce mortality and improve personalized cardiac care.

CMR can produce a series of images generating a volume of data that can be screened by clinicians for patient diagnosis and treatment planning. For example, contractile functions can be quantified with ventricle volumes, ejection fraction, and masses by separating the left ventricle (LV) and right ventricle (RV) from CMR images. Also, the segmentation of CMR images can provide detailed information about the normality of cardiac function, as well as the possible type and severity of heart disease. These applications require the segmentation of cardiac chambers, such as LV and RV from CMR images, which is not trivial task. As previously reported, manual segmentation is a time-consuming task, which may require on average approximately 20 minutes by a clinician [1]. Thus, there is a growing demand for automated image segmentation. Commercialized software packages such as Argus [7] were developed for automatic CMR image segmentation. Although the processing time has been greatly reduced, the accuracy of segmentation still requires further improvements [8].

The main idea of CMR image segmentation is to identify the boundaries of cardiac chambers and separate them from the background. Due to various restrictions involved in image acquisitions [9], CMR images are often of high complexity and ambiguity, rich in measurement noise, and low in contrast [10]. These can make the segmentation and analysis of CMR images a challenging task. In addition, CMR images often involve a great amount of uncertainties due to the characteristics of CMR images and the heterogeneities and variabilities among patients. Measurement noise and uncertainty in CMR images can significantly affect the accuracy and reliability of automatic image segmentation.

CMR images are the results of physical measurement and stored as multi-dimensional matrix, for which elements can be defined with pixel values [11, 12]. For example, Figure 9.1 (a) shows a typical CMR image in which the blood pools in the LV and RV appear bright and their surrounding structures appear dark. Figure 9.1 (b) shows the pixel values of a small inset in the

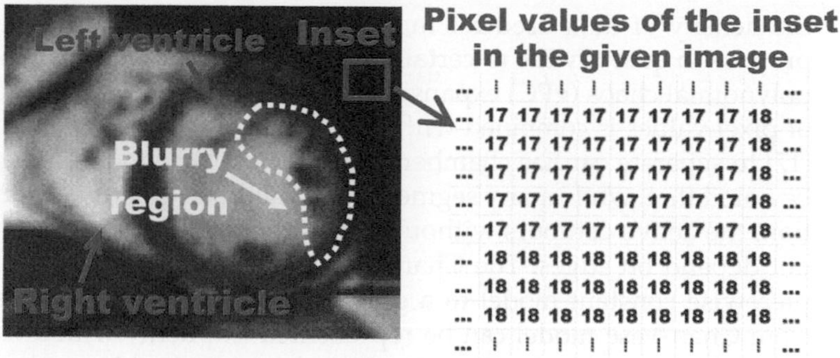

FIGURE 9.1
(a) CMR image of the heart, (b) Pixel values of an inset in CMR image. The CMR image used in Figure 9.1 is from patient 1 in [41].

surrounding of the CMR image. As seen, the pixel values in the surrounding are different due to the characteristic of image and uncertainty resulting from measurement limitations. For most of the image segmentation techniques, the pixel values are assumed to be deterministic quantities, i.e., pixels have fixed deterministic gray values. Such an approximation generally ignores the fact that pixel values can be contaminated by uncertainty such as noise. It would be a good scientific practice to provide a probability description of pixel values. However, this is typically omitted in the literature as reported in [13].

To improve the robustness of image segmentation, techniques were previously developed to quantify uncertainty and measurement noise in images, which leads to the definition of stochastic image segmentation [11, 13]. As compared to image segmentation with fixed pixel values, probability density functions (PDF) are used to describe the distribution of pixel values and to quantify the effect of uncertainty on image segmentation. Note that any small variations in pixel values may result in different segmentation results. For example, as shown in Figure 9.1 (a), the boundary of the left ventricle is blurry. Different image segmentation techniques to find the boundaries will lead to different heart models. Without properly considering these uncertainties (e.g., blurry boundary and noise), image analysis may provide inaccurate estimations of the cardiac parameters, and ultimately lead to false diagnosis, prognosis, and inappropriate treatment strategy. Following the idea of stochastic image segmentation, the PDF of pixel values will be used to distinguish cardiac chambers from the background of the CMR images.

The key step of the stochastic image segmentation is the efficient quantification of uncertainty in pixel values and the rapid evaluation of its effect on image segmentation algorithm. Previous works describe the pixel values as probability distributions [13, 15, 16], but most of them require the calibration of a segmentation model. The performance of such methods greatly rely on the density of data used for model training. To improve the accuracy, we propose to quantify the uncertainty in each CMR image using a generalized polynomial chaos (gPC) expansion [17]. Following this idea, the gPC model of pixel values is combined with the active contours without edges method [17] to separate cardiac chambers from the background of images. It should be noted that, while many segmentation methods greatly rely on edge detection, the active contours without edges method (or Chan-Vese model) does not depend on edges. The Chan-Vese model can optimally fit a two-phase piecewise constant model to a given CMR image. The boundary obtained from Chan-Vese model can be represented implicitly with a level set function, which enables the Chan-Vese model to deal with topological changes more easily than other available methods [18].

This chapter is organized as follows. Section 9.2 briefly summarizes the CMR image segmentation and the challenges. Using the level set functions, three commonly used segmentation methods are presented in Section 9.3. The formulation and the numerical implementation of the stochastic image segmentation are given in Section 9.4. Analysis and discussion of results are present in Section 9.5, followed by conclusions in Section 9.6.

9.2 Cardiac Magnetic Resonance (CMR) Image Processing

9.2.1 Description of CMR Image Segmentation

The segmentation of heart chambers and myocardium greatly relies on heart anatomy and CMR image acquisition specificity. A standard CMR image on the short axis plane is shown in Figure 9.2. Generally, images of the heart in CMR covers the whole heart with approximately 8 $\sim$ 10 short axis images as shown in Figure 9.2, and the distance between two adjacent images ranges from 10 to 20 mm. The left ventricle (LV) can pump the oxygenated blood to the aorta and consequently to the systemic circuit, which has a shape of ellipsoid and is surrounded by myocardium, as seen in Figure 9.2. The normal thickness of the myocardium varies approximately from 6 to 16 mm, due to the heterogeneities and variabilities among patients. As compared to the LV, the right ventricle (RV) often has a complex crescent shape. It can face lower pressure to eject blood to the lungs and is 3 to 6 times thinner than the LV, which reaches the limit of the CMR resolution. Since the function of the RV is less vital than the LV and the CMR resolution is low, most of the research effort has focused on the segmentation of the LV, although it has been proven that accurate quantification of the RV mass can be obtained with CMR images [19]. It should be noted that the ventricles only cover a small area in CMR images, and image analysis is often restricted to a particular region of interest that contains both LV and RV, as shown in Figure 9.2.

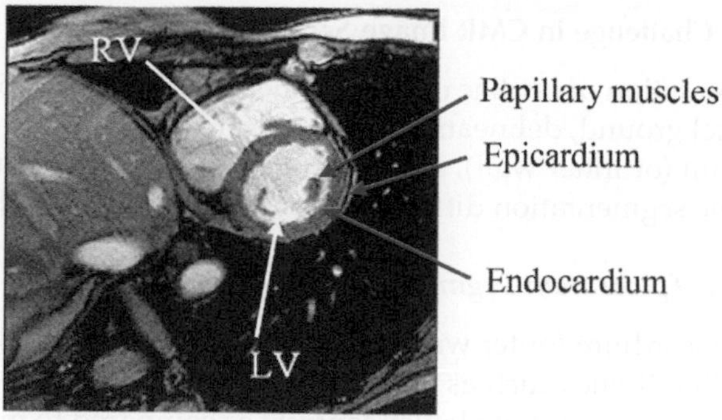

FIGURE 9.2
Short axis CMR image of the heart, left ventricle (LV) and right ventricle (RV) (http://education.rad.msu.edu/Courses/CHM_domain/Cardiovascular/CV_Imaging/Images/breathhold.htm).

For a typical CMR image, as seen in Figure 9.2, the blood pool appears bright, while myocardium and the background appear dark due to the use of balanced fast field echo sequences [5]. These differences will introduce variability in the multi-dimensional matrix used to store CMR images. In addition, as shown in Figure 9.3, CMR images often exhibit a great level of variability, in terms of gray levels and/or structure of LV (or RV) shapes. The gray level, resulting in changes in pixel values, can also change due to the use of different CMR scans or different balance fast field echo sequences. Further, blurry boundaries can also be observed on some parts of the CMR images, mostly resulting from the blood flow and the effects of partial volume, aggravated by respiration motion artefacts. Lastly, the shapes of LV and RV can change over time as seen in Figure 9.3. For accurate image segmentation, it is necessary to account for these variabilities.

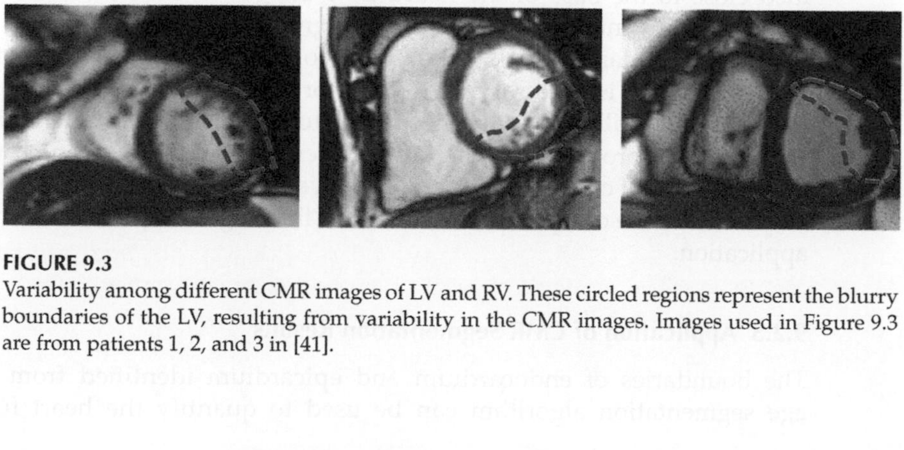

FIGURE 9.3
Variability among different CMR images of LV and RV. These circled regions represent the blurry boundaries of the LV, resulting from variability in the CMR images. Images used in Figure 9.3 are from patients 1, 2, and 3 in [41].

9.2.2 Challenge in CMR Image Segmentation

Segmentation of cardiac chambers includes identification of LV and RV from the background, delineation of the epicardium (or outer wall) from the endocardium (or inner wall), as seen in Figure 9.2 Each of the segmentations has specific segmentation difficulties as described below [5].

9.2.2.1 Epicardium Segmentation

The epicardium (outer wall) is in the middle of the myocardium and the surrounding tissues such as fat and lung, which may have different pixel value profiles and may show lower contrast as compared to myocardium. Segmentation of epicardium is difficult, especially for the RV due to the reduced thickness.

9.2.2.2 Endocardium Segmentation

Endocardium surrounds the LV cavity. As shown in Figure 9.2 and 9.3, CMR images can provide good contrast between myocardium and the blood flow. However, there still some segmentation difficulties, which may result from the gray level inhomogeneities in the blood flow, such as the presence of papillary muscles and trabeculations inside the heart chambers, as seen in Figure 9.2. These may introduce uncertainty, when separating the LV cavity from the background and the endocardium. Since the identification of the endocardial wall can be used to estimate the ventricular volume, some image analysis works in the literature focus only on the endocardium segmentation.

9.2.2.3 Segmentation in the Presence of Uncertainty

The accuracy of segmentation also depends on the resolution of images. However, the resolution of CMR is often not high enough to separate the size of small structures. In addition, the shapes of ventricles can be strongly modified close to the base of the heart. Low image resolution and changes in the shapes of ventricles may introduce significant variations in pixel value along the boundary of cardiac chambers. To improve the robustness of image segmentation, it is necessary to account for these variations for quantitative analysis. This will lead to the notion of stochastic image segmentation [13, 14, 20], which provides a probabilistic description of the segmented volume and the shape of cardiac chambers. However, stochastic image segmentation may increase the computational cost, thus limiting its application in medical application.

9.2.3 Application of CMR Segmentation Results

The boundaries of endocardium and epicardium identified from an image segmentation algorithm can be used to quantify the heart function

Estimation of the LV and RV mass and volume are two areas of special interests. The volume can be estimated from the boundaries of the endocardium, while the mass can be estimated from the integration of both endocardial and epicardial surfaces [21]. The segmentation results also allow one to track endocardial and epicardial wall motion, as well as myocardium thickness. It should be noted that intramyocardial motion cannot be approximated from standard CMR images, due to the aperture issues. Tracking intramyocardial motion requires more information such as dedicated modalities from tagged CMR images [22].

9.3 Level Set Method for Image Segmentation

While many image segmentation algorithms are available in the literature, we only focus on the level set based method, since it does not heavily rely on the edge detection. The level set-based image segmentation was initially developed in previous studies [23, 24]. For a given image U_0, the idea is to identify a curve $C \subset \mathbb{R}^n$ with a zero level set of a higher dimensional function ϕ as:

$$C = \{x \in \mathbb{R}^n : \phi(t, x) = 0\} \tag{9.1}$$

where C can be progressively calculated for a given image, which can separate the objects from the background at any given time $t > 0$. It is possible to describe the evolution of the curve C by solving the level set function as [25]:

$$\phi_t + F|\nabla\phi| = 0 \tag{9.2}$$

where F denotes the speed in the normal direction. Generally, (9.2) can be solved with numerical methods. For example, based on the Hamilton-Jacobi equation, front propagation with curvature dependent speed was developed by discretizing (9.2) [26]. To overcome the convergence issues with simple finite difference techniques, efficient methods such as Narrow Band were developed, which solve (9.2) in the vicinity of the zero level set ϕ other than a matrix defined by U_0. It is important to note that signed distance functions, i.e., functions satisfy $|\nabla\phi| = 1$, are often used as level set functions, due to numerical calculation reasons. However, the level set function may lose this attribute during the evolution of the curve, thus re-initialization of the signed distance function is often done during the identification of C [27]. For this purpose, the evolution of the curve can be calculated as [25]:

$$\phi_t = sign(\phi)(1 - |\nabla\phi|) \tag{9.3}$$

Based on the definition of level set function, a closed initial curve C_0 can be firstly placed in a bounded domain subjected to the constraints of the image, in order to segment the object from the background. Then, level set functions can be used to adjust the curve to the edges iteratively. Such an approach can ensure that the segmentation results have a closed contour.

In the following sections, three widely used level set-based image segmentation methods will be briefly discussed, i.e., gradient-based segmentation [28], geodesic active contours [29], and active contours with edges (Chan-Vese) algorithm [17].

9.3.1 Gradient-Based Segmentation

For level set function-based segmentation as shown in (9.2), a concrete approach is to define a speed F that depends on characteristic of a given image U_0. The most popular way is to set F as: $F = F(\nabla U_0)$, which can ensure the evolution of curve C stops at the edge in the image. As discussed in [28], the speed in the normal direction F can be defined as:

$$F := g_u := \frac{1}{1 + |\nabla G_\sigma * U_0|}(1 - \eta\kappa) \tag{9.4}$$

where U_0 is the image, G_σ is a Gaussian smoothing function with a width of σ, κ is the curvature of the level set function ϕ, and η ($\eta > 0$) is a scaling parameter that can control the influence of the curvature smoothing term on the segmentation. When the gradient of pixel values separating the object from the background is high, the gradient-based method can provide accurate image segmentation results. Figure 9.4 shows the segmentation results with the gradient-based method for algorithm clarification.

For the gradient-based segmentation, it is possible that the zero level set can cross the edge, since the speed g_u in (9.4) is positive even in the vicinity of

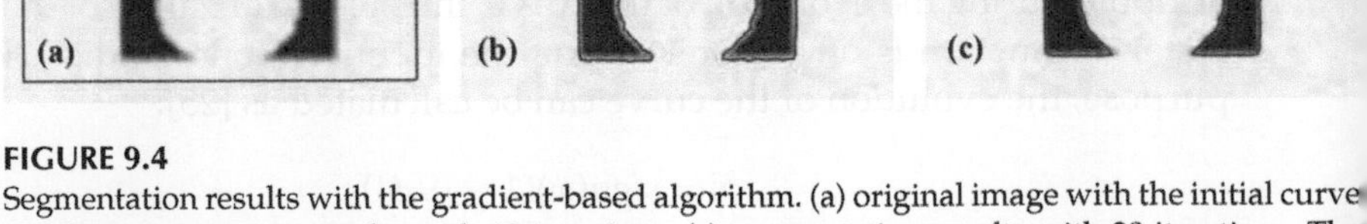

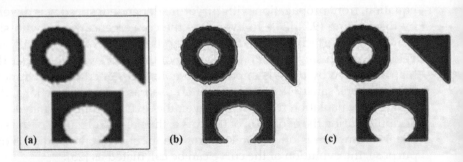

FIGURE 9.4
Segmentation results with the gradient-based algorithm. (a) original image with the initial curve C_0, (b) segmentation results with 10 iterations, (c) segmentation results with 20 iterations. The number of iterations increases from (a) to (c), and the boundary can be accurately approximated with 20 iterations. The image used for the algorithm demonstration is from reference [17].

the boundary [28]. Thus, a stop criterion has to be appropriately determined, which can avoid over-segmentation by checking the difference between the level set function values of subsequent time steps. In addition, it is also possible to find the zero level set at the boundary by using complicated methods, such as the geodesic active algorithm in next section, which can provide a convergent solution of segmentation.

9.3.2 Geodesic Active Contours

The geodesic active contours-based image segmentation was developed in the work of Caselles et al [29]. The key idea is to minimize an energy function E, which depends on the curve C and the parametrization of $C(q)$ as [29]:

$$E(C) = \alpha \int_0^1 |C'(q)|^2 dq + \beta \int_0^1 g(|\nabla U_0(C(q))|)^2 dq \tag{9.5}$$

where g is an edge (boundary) indicator, i.e., a decreasing function approaches to zero, α and β are two positive coefficients that penalize the contribution of each term on the energy function E. As discussed in [29], the energy function E can be minimized by using a level set representation of the curve C and by calculating the Euler-Lagrange equations of E. This will produce a level set equation, for which an additional term is used to force the zero-level set to stay inside regions with a high gradient. The formulation of the level set function can be described as:

$$E\phi_t = -\alpha \nabla g \cdot \nabla \phi - \beta g |\nabla \phi| + \eta \kappa |\nabla \phi| \tag{9.6}$$

where α, β, and η are tuning parameters for segmentation. For a given initial closed curve C_0, (9.2) can be optimized to evolve the boundary of object in an image. Figure 9.5 shows the segmentation results with the geodesic active contours method for algorithm clarification.

9.3.3 Chan-Vese Segmentation

The methods described above use the image gradient to terminate the curve evolution for image segmentation, which can only accurately identify objects with edges defined by gradient [17]. In addition, due to measurement noise and uncertainty, the curve may pass through the edge, which may produce inaccurate segmentation results. Based on the Mumford-Shah techniques [30], an active contours without edges model (or Chan-Vese model) was developed, which does not use the gradient as a stopping criterion [17]. The Chan-Vese model and active contour without edges will be interchangeably used hereafter in this chapter.

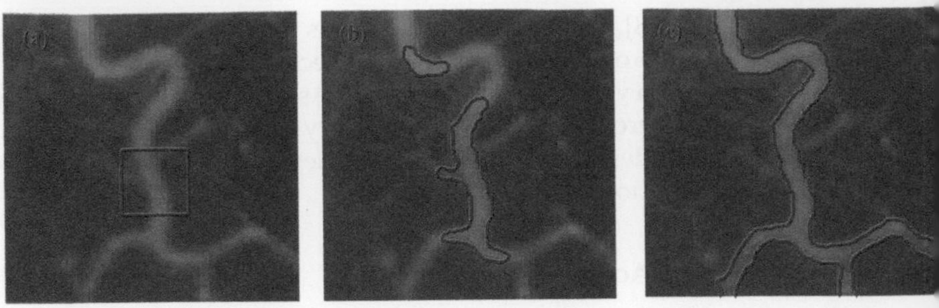

FIGURE 9.5
Segmentation results with the geodesic active algorithm. (a) original image with the initial curve C_0, (b) segmentation results with 20 iterations, (c) segmentation results with 120 iterations. The number of iterations increases from (a) to (c), and the boundary can be accurately approximated within 100 iterations. The image used for the algorithm demonstration is from reference [27].

The key idea behind the active contours without edges model is to seek a best approximation of a curve C for a given image u by minimizing an energy function defined as [15], [17]:

$$
\begin{aligned}
arg \min_{m_1, m_1, C} J &= \mu_1 L(C) + \mu_2 A(C) \\
&+ \lambda_1 \int_{inside(C)} |U_0(x,y) - m_1(C)|^2 dxdy \\
&+ \lambda_2 \int_{outside(C)} |U_0(x,y) - m_2(C)|^2 dxdy
\end{aligned}
\quad (9.7
$$

where μ_1, μ_2, λ_1, and λ_2 are positive tuning parameters; m_1 and m_2, depending on the evolving curve C, represent the mean values of pixel values inside C and outside C, respectively. The coordinates (e.g., Ω), defining the domain of image U_0, are described by the x-axis and y-axis. The first term in (9.7 controls the regularity of curve C by penalizing its length. The second term penalizes the enclosed area using a curve C, which can control the size of the segmented objects. The last two terms in (9.7) penalize the discrepancy between pixel values within and outside the curve C in terms of the mean of pixel values.

The minimization of (9.7) can be solved with a level set formulation by using the Euler-Lagrange equation [24]. The unknown curve C can be replaced by an unknown level set function Z defined in the x-y-plane, subjected to the constraints of the image. That is, the minimization of (9.7) can be represented as the evaluation of a level set function Z other than manipulating C. Then the curve C can be determined by using the geometric locus of the points in $Z(x, y) = 0$. Suppose that the level set function Z is smooth, the active contour without edges (Chan-Vese) function in (9.7) can be re-written in terms of the level set function Z as [15], [17]:

$$\begin{aligned} arg \min_{m_1,m_1,C} J = \mu_1 &\int_\Omega \delta_\varepsilon(Z(x,y))|\nabla Z(x,y)|^2 dxdy \\ &+ \mu_2 \int_\Omega H_\varepsilon(Z(x,y))dxdy \\ &+ \lambda_1 \int_\Omega |U_0(x,y) - m_1(Z)|^2 H_\varepsilon(Z(x,y))dxdy \\ &+ \lambda_2 \int_\Omega |U_0(x,y) - m_2(Z)|^2 (1 - H_\varepsilon(Z(x,y)))dxdy \end{aligned} \tag{9.8}$$

where H_ε is a modified Heaviside function, and δ_ε is a regularized Dirac δ-function determined by the derivative of H_ε. The mean values in (9.8), m_1 and m_2, depending on the evolving level set function Z, are calculated with the intensities of the image u within and outside Z as [15], [17]:

$$m_1(Z) = average\ (U_0) \qquad in \quad \{Z \geq 0\} \tag{9.9}$$

$$m_2(Z) = average\ (U_0) \qquad in \quad \{Z < 0\} \tag{9.10}$$

In order to obtain a global minimization of J with respect to Z, a modified Heaviside function H_ε can be used, which is defined as follows [17]:

$$H_\varepsilon = \frac{1}{2}\left(1 + \frac{2}{\pi}\arctan\left(\frac{Z(x,y)}{\varepsilon}\right)\right) \tag{9.11}$$

The optimization of (9.8) can be solved by alternatively updating the mean values of m_1, m_2, and Z. For a fixed Z, the values of m_1 and m_2 can be calculated by averaging the regions enclosed by Z as [15], [17]:

$$m_1 = \frac{\int_\Omega U_0(x,y)H_\varepsilon(Z(x,y))dxdy}{\int_\Omega H_\varepsilon(Z(x,y))dxdy} \tag{9.12}$$

$$m_2 = \frac{\int_\Omega U_0(x,y)(1 - H_\varepsilon(Z(x,y)))dxdy}{\int_\Omega (1 - H_\varepsilon(Z(x,y)))dxdy} \tag{9.13}$$

For fixed m_1 and m_2, a gradient descent equation can be further formulated with the level set function Z as [15], [17]:

$$\begin{aligned} \frac{\partial Z}{\partial t} = \delta_\varepsilon(Z)[\mu_1 div\left(\frac{\nabla Z}{|\nabla Z|}\right) - \mu_2 div\left(\frac{\nabla Z}{|\nabla Z|}\right) \\ -\lambda_1(U_0 - m_1(Z))^2 + \lambda_2(U_0 - m_2(Z))^2 + r(Z_t) \end{aligned} \tag{9.14}$$

$$Z(0,x,y) = Z_0(x,y) \qquad in \quad \Omega \tag{9.15}$$

$$\frac{\delta_\varepsilon(Z)}{|\nabla Z|}\frac{\partial Z}{\partial \vec{e}} = 0 \qquad on \quad \partial\Omega \tag{9.16}$$

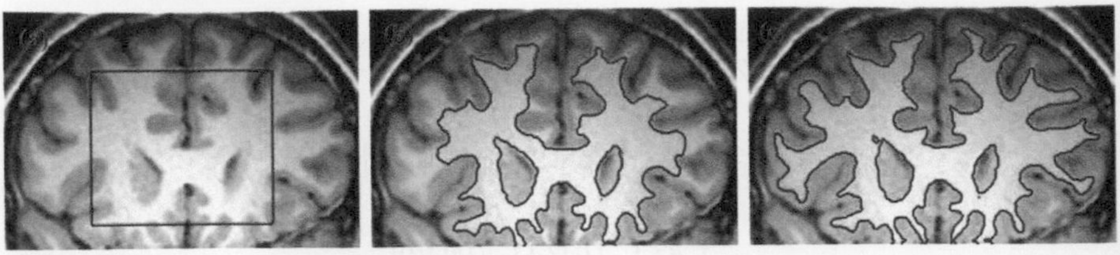

FIGURE 9.6
Segmentation results with the active contours without edges (Chan-Vese model). (a) original image with the initial curve C_0, (b) segmentation results with 20 iterations, (c) segmentation results with 300 iterations. The number of iterations increases from (a) to (c), and the boundary can be accurately approximated with 260 iterations. The image used for the algorithm demonstration is from reference [27].

where $\vec{e}$ is the outward normal with respect to the boundary $\partial\Omega$. As compared to the original Chan-Vese model, a level regularization term r can be used to ensure the convergence of Z [22] and [27], which can be defined as:

$$r(Z_t) = \int_{\Omega} \frac{1}{2} (|\nabla Z_t(x, y| - 1)^2 dxdy \tag{9.17}$$

where the subscript t represents that the regularization r is evaluated and updated with respect to the evolution of Z at each time instant t. It is important to note that the minimization of (9.13) can be solved until convergence and the time t is an artificial time defined to iteratively solve Z. As compared to the gradient and the geodesic active contours-based methods, the active contours without edges (Chan-Vese model) can ignore edges of objects completely. Therefore, it can be integrated with uncertainty analysis technique for stochastic image segmentation, which will be discussed in the later part of this chapter. For algorithm illustration, Figure 9.6 shows the segmentation results with the Chan-Vese model for a given image.

9.4 Stochastic Image Segmentation

All the aforementioned techniques can provide accurate segmentation results for various types of images. However, most of these approaches have drawbacks in terms of robustness in the presence of measurement noise and uncertainty in pixel values of images. Thus, stochastic image analysis is introduced in this section to account for uncertainty. Following this, the notion of stochastic image is combined with the level set function-based segmentation, i.e., the active contours without edges in the previous section, which leads to a stochastic image segmentation problem.

9.4.1 Generalized Polynomial Chaos Expansion

The concept of stochastic images was first introduced in [13, 20], which can take into account the uncertainty and errors in pixel values of images. Following this notion, pixel values of images are described with random variables that have a predefined probability density function (PDF). Further, generalized polynomial chaos (gPC) expansion will be used to approximate the PDF. The gPC expansion was developed from polynomial chaos expansion, which was initially introduced to approximate Gaussian random variables in [31]. The gPC can represent various distributions using orthogonal polynomials of random variables that follow different distributions [16].

Based on the gPC expansion, pixel values U in a given image U_0 can be approximated with finite second order moments as [13] and [15]:

$$U(\omega) = \sum_{i=0}^{\infty} u_i \Phi_i(\xi(\omega)) \tag{9.18}$$

where U denotes the pixel values in U_0, and $\xi = \{\xi_1, \cdots, \xi_n\}$ is a set of independent, identically distributed (*iid*) random variables defined by a random event ω, for which n is a fixed number of *iid* random variables. In addition, $\{\Phi_i(\xi)\}$ are multi-dimensional orthogonal polynomial basis functions of ξ, and $\{u_i\}$ are the gPC coefficients for each polynomial basis function. For practical applications, approximation in (9.18) is often truncated into a finite number of terms as below [15]:

$$U(\omega) = \sum_{i=0}^{p} u_i \Phi_i(\xi(\omega)) \tag{9.19}$$

where p is the number of terms that can be used to approximate the distribution of pixel values. In the case of multi-dimensional random variables, i.e., $n > 1$ in (9.18), the orthogonal polynomial basis functions $\{\Phi_i(\xi)\}$ can be defined as products between polynomials. For brevity this is not shown here, but the details can be found in the Appendix.

The explicit gPC approximation of pixel values in (9.19) can be used to propagate uncertainty onto the evolution of the level set function Z, defined in the previous section. For clarification, let's assume the evolution of Z in (9.14) ~ (9.16) can be described as [13] and [15]:

$$Z_t = f(U_0, Z_0, t) \tag{9.20}$$

where f represents the image segmentation operator (algorithm) such as the Chan-Vese model in the previous section, and Z_0 defines an initial level set function that can segment objects from the image background with f. To quantify the effect of uncertainty in pixel values on the evolution of level set function Z, a gPC approximation of Z in each time interval t can be defined as follows [13]:

$$Z_t(\omega) = \sum_{i=0}^{P} \zeta_{i,t} \Phi_i(\xi(\omega)) \tag{9.21}$$

where $\{\zeta_{i,t}\}$ are the gPC coefficients used to approximate the level set function at time t, and P is the total number of required terms. The number of terms, P in (9.21), depends on the number of the *iid* random variables (n) and the maximum gPC approximation degrees, i.e., p in (9.18), which can be determined as follows [16]:

$$P = \frac{(p+n)!}{p!n!} - 1 \tag{9.22}$$

As seen in (9.22), P grows significantly when the number of random variables n and the degree of approximation p in (9.18) increases, which may further increase the computational time. To reduce the computational burden and ensure the convergence of gPC approximation, polynomial basis functions $\{\Phi_i(\xi)\}$ should be appropriately selected with respect to the corresponding PDFs of random variables ξ. For example, Hermite polynomial basis function can be used for normally distributed ξ, whereas Legendre polynomial basis functions are the best choice for uniformly distributed random variables ξ [16, 32, 33].

9.4.2 GPC-Based Image Segmentation

Using the gPC approximation of the pixel values in (9.19), the formulation of the stochastic level set function-based image segmentation can be derived by replacing all quantities in (9.14) with the corresponding gPC approximations. Substituting the gPC approximations in (9.19) and (9.21) into (9.20) can result in the following segmentation problem [13] and [15]:

$$Z_t(\omega) \approx f(U(\omega), Z_0(\omega), t) \tag{9.23}$$

$$\sum_{i=0}^{P} \zeta_{i,t}\Phi_i(\xi(\omega)) \approx f\left(\sum_{i=0}^{p} u_i\Phi_i(\xi(\omega)), \sum_{i=0}^{P} \zeta_{i,0}\Phi_i(\xi(\omega)), t\right) \tag{9.24}$$

where $\{\zeta_{i,0}\}$ are the gPC coefficients of the level set function at $t = 0$, which is used as initial values to numerically solve the boundaries at each time instant t ($t > 0$). It should be noted that the approximately equal sign is used in (9.23) and (9.24) due to the truncations in (9.19) and (9.21). In addition, the gPC coefficients $\{u_i\}$ can be estimated from pixel values of images, but $\{\zeta_{i,t}\}$ have to be calculated. Using Galerkin projection, it is possible to calculate $\{\zeta_{i,t}\}$ by projecting both sides of (9.24) onto each of the polynomial basis function $\{\Phi_i(\xi)\}$ as [13] and [15]:

$$\langle Z_t, \Phi_i(\xi) \rangle = \langle f(U(\omega), Z_0(\omega), t), \Phi_i(\xi) \rangle \tag{9.25}$$

where $\langle \cdot \rangle$ represents the inner product between two vectors that can be defined as follows [15]:

$$\langle \vartheta_1, \vartheta_2 \rangle = \int \vartheta_1 \vartheta_1 W(\xi) d\xi \tag{9.26}$$

where $\{\vartheta_i\}(i = 1, 2)$ represents two vectors, and the integration in (9.26) can be calculated over the entire domain defined by the random variables ξ. In (9.26), $W(\xi)$ is a weighting function, which can be chosen corresponding to the polynomial basis function $\{\Phi_i(\xi)\}$ of ξ so that the integral in (9.26) is either 1 or 0.

Once the gPC coefficients $\{\zeta_{i,t}\}$ in (9.24) are available, it is possible to analytically compute the mean value, variance, and other higher order statistical moments of the level set function Z. For example, the mean and the variance at a particular time can be calculated as [13], [15], and [16]:

$$E(Z_t) = E\left[\sum_{i=0}^{P} \zeta_{i,t}\Phi_i\right] = \zeta_{0,t}E[\Phi_i] + \sum_{i=0}^{P} E[\Phi_i] = \zeta_{0,t} \tag{9.27}$$

$$\begin{aligned} V(Z_t) &= E\left[(\zeta_t - E(\zeta_t))^2\right] = E\left[\left(\sum_{i=0}^{P} \zeta_{i,t}\Phi_i - \zeta_{0,t}\right)^2\right] \\ &= E\left[\left(\sum_{i=1}^{P} \zeta_{i,t}\Phi_i\right)^2\right] = \sum_{i=0}^{P} (\zeta_{i,t})^2 E[\Phi_i]^2 \end{aligned} \tag{9.28}$$

The availability of analytical formulae enables the rapid calculations of the mean and the variance of the level set function Z as described in (9.27) and (9.28), which is the main rationale for using the gPC approximations. The gPC-based stochastic image segmentation can account for the variabilities in pixel values, while progressively updating the level set function. As seen in (9.21), the first coefficient $\{\zeta_{0,t}\}$, representing the mean value of the stochastic level set function, can be used to identify the edge that separates the object from the background, while the higher order coefficients can be used to estimate the distribution of curvature along the object boundary.

Substituting (9.19) and (9.21) into the image segmentation operator, such as the Chan-Vese model in (9.14), a stochastic image segmentation model can be derived as [15]:

$$\begin{aligned} \frac{\partial Z(\xi)}{\partial t} = \delta_\varepsilon(Z(\xi)) \Bigg[&\mu_1 div\left(\frac{\nabla Z(\xi)}{|\nabla Z(\xi)|}\right) - \mu_2 \\ &-\lambda_1(U_0 - m_1(Z(\xi)))^2 + \lambda_2(U_0 - m_2(Z(\xi)))^2 \Bigg] + r(Z_t(\xi)) \end{aligned} \tag{9.29}$$

where $Z(\xi)$ is the gPC approximation of the unknown level set function in (9.21), $\delta_\varepsilon(Z(\xi))$ is the derivative of a stochastic Heaviside function $H_\varepsilon(Z(\xi))$, which can be defined as [15]:

$$H_\varepsilon(Z(\xi)) = \frac{1}{2}\left(1 + \frac{2}{\pi}\arctan\left(\frac{Z(\xi)}{\varepsilon}\right)\right) \tag{9.30}$$

Similar to the deterministic level set function in (9.14), two mean values are used in (9.29), i.e., $m_1(Z(\xi))$ and $m_2(Z(\xi))$, which can be calculated by averaging pixel values that are found to be inside and outside the mean value of the level set function $Z(\xi)$ as [15]:

$$m_1(Z(\xi)) = average\ (U_0(\xi)) \quad in\ \{\zeta_{0,t} \geq 0\} \tag{9.31}$$

$$m_2(Z(\xi)) = average\ (U_0(\xi)) \quad in\ \{\zeta_{0,t} < 0\} \tag{9.32}$$

where $\zeta_{0,t}$ is the mean value of the gPC approximation of $Z(\xi)$, i.e., the first term in (9.21), which is iteratively updated at each time t.

9.4.3 Numerical Calculations

Further, we integrate the gPC approximation of uncertainty in pixel values with the Chan-Vese model for image segmentation. Following the gPC approximation, Galerkin projection can be used to solve the gPC coefficients of level set function by substituting (9.19) and (9.21) into (9.29) and by solving the partial differential equations through numerical discretization. The minimization of Chan-Vese model can be solved using different optimization techniques, such as semi-implicit gradient descent method [18], topological derivative [34], and multigrid method [35]. For brevity, the details of each optimization technique are not discussed for brevity.

Suppose the pixel values U of an image U_0 can be sampled on a regular grid $\Omega = \{0, \ldots, N\} \times \{0, \ldots, N\}$. The evolution of the level set function Z at each grid can be discretized in Ω as [13]:

$$\frac{\partial z_{i,j}(\xi)}{\partial t} = \delta_\varepsilon\left(z_{i,j}(\xi)\right)\left[\mu_1\left(\nabla_x^- \frac{\nabla_x^+ z_{i,j}(\xi)}{\sqrt{\left(\nabla_x^+ z_{i,j}(\xi)\right)^2 + \left(\nabla_y^0 z_{i,j}(\xi)\right)^2 + \varepsilon^2}} + \nabla_y^- \frac{\nabla_y^+ z_{i,j}(\xi)}{\sqrt{\left(\nabla_x^0 z_{i,j}(\xi)\right)^2 + \left(\nabla_y^+ z_{i,j}(\xi)\right)^2 + \varepsilon^2}}\right) - \mu_2 - \lambda_1(U_{i,j} - m_1(Z(\xi)))^2 + \lambda_2(U_{i,j} - m_2(Z(\xi)))^2\right] + r\left(z_{i,j}^t(\xi)\right) \tag{9.33}$$

where $Z(\xi) = \{z_{i,j}(\xi)\}$, $(i,\ j = 1, \cdots, N-1)$, ∇_x^+ and ∇_x^- are the forward difference and the backward difference in the x dimension, respectively, $\nabla_x^0 = (\nabla_x^+ + \nabla_x^+)/2$ is the central difference. Similar definitions are used in the y dimension, i.e., ∇_y^+, ∇_y^- are the forward difference and backward different in the

y dimension, respectively, and $\nabla_y^0 = (\nabla_y^+ + \nabla_y^+)/2$ represents the central difference. In addition, a small positive number $\varepsilon = 10^{-6}$ is used to prevent a division by zero in (9.33). For simplicity, it is assumed that [13]:

$$A_{i,j} = \frac{\mu_1}{\sqrt{\left(\nabla_x^+ z_{i,j}(\xi)\right)^2 + \left(\nabla_y^0 z_{i,j}(\xi)\right)^2 + \varepsilon^2}} \tag{9.34}$$

$$B_{i,j} = \frac{\mu_1}{\sqrt{\left(\nabla_x^0 z_{i,j}(\xi)\right)^2 + \left(\nabla_y^+ z_{i,j}(\xi)\right)^2 + \varepsilon^2}} \tag{9.35}$$

then the discretization can be re-written as [13] and [15]:

$$\begin{aligned}\frac{\partial z_{i,j}}{\partial t} &= \delta_\varepsilon(z_{i,j})\big[(A_{i,j}(z_{i+1,j} - z_{i,j}) - A_{i-1,j}(z_{i,j} - z_{i-1,j}))\\ &\quad + (B_{i,j}(z_{i,j+1} - z_{i,j}) - A_{i,j-1}(z_{i,j} - z_{i,j-1}))\\ &\quad - \mu_2(U_{i,j} - m_1(Z))^2 + \lambda_2(U_{i,j} - m_2(Z))^2\big] + r(z_{i,j|t}(\xi))\end{aligned} \tag{9.36}$$

where $z_{i,j}$ other than $z_{i,j}(\xi)$ is used in (9.36) for simplicity. It should be noted that, on the right-hand side, the first two terms can discretize the curvature as [13] and [15]:

$$\begin{aligned}div\left(\frac{\nabla Z(\xi)}{|\nabla Z(\xi)|}\right) &= \partial_x\left(\frac{\partial_x Z}{\sqrt{(\partial_x Z)^2 + (\partial_y Z)^2}}\right) + \partial_y\left(\frac{\partial_y Z}{\sqrt{(\partial_y Z)^2 + (\partial_y Z)^2}}\right)\\ &\approx \nabla_x^- \frac{\nabla_x^+ Z}{\sqrt{\left(\nabla_x^+ Z\right)^2 + \left(\nabla_y^0 Z\right)^2 + \varepsilon^2}} + \nabla_y^- \frac{\nabla_y^+ Z}{\sqrt{\left(\nabla_x^0 Z\right)^2 + \left(\nabla_y^+ Z\right)^2 + \varepsilon^2}}\end{aligned} \tag{9.37}$$

where a mix of the forward, backward, and central differences is used for better discretization [18]. In addition, the time is discretized with a semi-implicit Gauss-Seidel method [36], which only needs to store one copy of the Z matrix at a particular time instant, and values of $\{z_{i,j}\}$ at each grid can be updated as they are calculated [18]. The values of $\{z_{i,j}\}$, $\{z_{i-1,j}\}$, and $\{z_{i,j-1}\}$ are updated at time instant $t+1$ and all others at time t as [13] and [15]:

$$\begin{aligned}\frac{z_{i,j}^{t+1} - z_{i,j}^t}{dt} &= \delta_\varepsilon\left(z_{i,j}^t\right)\big[(A_{i,j} z_{i+1,j}^t + A_{i-1,j} z_{i-1,j}^{t+1} + B_{i,j} z_{i,j+1}^t + B_{i,j-1} z_{i,j-1}^{t+1})\\ &\quad - (A_{i,j} + A_{i-1,j} + B_{i,j} + B_{i,j-1}) z_{i,j}^{t+1} - \mu_2\\ &\quad - \lambda_1(U_{i,j} - m_1(Z))^2 + \lambda_2(U_{i,j} - m_2(Z))^2\big] + r(z_{i,j|t}(\xi))\end{aligned} \tag{9.38}$$

where $\{z_{i,j}\}$ at time instant $t+1$ can be solved with Gauss-Seidel method from left to right and from top to bottom as [13] and [15]:

$$\begin{aligned} z_{i,j}^{t+1} \leftarrow & \left[z_{i,j}^{t} + dt\, \delta_{\varepsilon}\left(z_{i,j}^{t}\right)\left(A_{i,j}z_{i+1,j}^{t} + A_{i-1,j}z_{i-1,j}^{t+1} + B_{i,j}z_{i,j+1}^{t} + B_{i,j-1}z_{i,j-1}^{t+1}\right)\right. \\ & - \mu_2 - \lambda_1(U_{i,j} - m_1(Z))^2 + \lambda_2(U_{i,j} - m_2(Z))^2 \\ & \left. + r(z_{i,j|t}(\xi))\right] / \left[1 + dt\delta_{\varepsilon}\left(z_{i,j}^{t}\right)(A_{i,j} + A_{i-1,j} + B_{i,j} + B_{i,j-1})\right] \end{aligned} \tag{9.39}$$

where the coefficients A and B can be calculated using the value at time instants t and $t+1$ as:

$$A_{i,j} = \frac{\mu_1}{\sqrt{\left(z_{i+1,j}^{t} - z_{i,j}^{t}\right)^2 + \left(\left(z_{i,j+1}^{t} - z_{i,j-1}^{t+1}\right)/2\right)^2 + \varepsilon^2}} \tag{9.40}$$

$$B_{i,j} = \frac{\mu_1}{\sqrt{\left(\left(z_{i+1,j}^{t} - z_{i-1,j}^{t+1}\right)/2\right)^2 + \left(z_{i,j}^{t} - z_{i+1,j}^{t}\right)^2 + \varepsilon^2}} \tag{9.41}$$

Additionally, boundary conditions can be enforced by duplicating pixel values near the boundary of the image U_0 as [15]:

$$z_{-1,j} = z_{0,j}, z_{M,j} = z_{M-1,j}, z_{i,-1} = z_{i,0}, z_{i,M} = z_{i,M-1} \tag{9.42}$$

Since the pixel values are approximated with gPC as shown in (9.19), the level set function $z_{i,j}(\xi)$ at each grid point has a gPC approximation as defined in (9.21). Following the Galerkin projection and using orthogonality properties, each equation above, e.g., (9.33) to (9.39), can be transformed into a family of coupled deterministic equations. For example, (9.33) can be re-written as (9.43) by multiplying both sides of (9.33) with polynomial basis functions $\Phi_i(\xi)$ and by performing a Galerkin projection.

$$\begin{aligned} \sum_{i=0}^{P} \frac{\partial z_{i,j}}{\partial t}\left\langle \Phi_i^2 \right\rangle = \sum_{j=0}^{P}\sum_{i=0}^{P} \Bigg\{ \delta_{\varepsilon}(z_{i,j}) \Bigg[\mu_1 \Bigg(& \nabla_x^{-} \frac{\nabla_x^{+} z_{i,j}}{\sqrt{\left(\nabla_x^{+} z_{i,j}\right)^2 + \left(\nabla_y^{0} z_{i,j}\right)^2 + \varepsilon^2}} \\ & + \nabla_y^{-} \frac{\nabla_y^{+} z_{i,j}}{\sqrt{\left(\nabla_x^{0} z_{i,j}\right)^2 + \left(\nabla_y^{+} z_{i,j}\right)^2 + \varepsilon^2}} \Bigg) - \mu_2 \\ & -\lambda_1\left(U_{i,j} - m_1(Z)\right)^2 + \lambda_2\left(U_{i,j} - m_2(Z)\right)^2 \Bigg] + r\left(z_{i,j}^{t}\right) \Bigg\} e_{i,j} \end{aligned} \tag{9.43}$$

where $e_{i,j} = \langle \Phi_i, \Phi_j \rangle$, and its result is either 1 or 0. It should be noted that the finite difference method requires calculating the gPC coefficients of Z at each grid point, which is not a trivial task. The commonly used basic operations of gPC variables can be found in previously reported work [37]. In addition, in order to improve the computational efficiency, a stochastic lookup table for typical calculations of polynomial chaos variables, such as multiplication and quotient of two random variables, can be generated offline [13].

To terminate the evolution of the level set function Z, one approach is to stop when the difference between Z_{t+1} and Z_t is below a predefined tolerance value. For example, the default value is set to 10^{-3} in this chapter. It is worth mentioning that the computational cost depends on the number of pixels in an image, the time interval, and the initialization. The discussion of computational efficiency can be found in [17]. In addition, it is important to note that the stochastic formulation of (9.43) may be solved using sampling-based approaches such as Monte Carlo simulations. However, such calculations can be computationally prohibitive, since a large number of samples are required to obtain accurate results as reported previously [13].

9.5 Results and Discussion

9.5.1 Formulation of gPC Models for Pixel Values

The key idea in this chapter is to distinguish the cardiac chambers from the background of CMR images, while providing a probabilistic description of the identified boundary. The pixel values of CMR images can be efficiently approximated with a gPC model, which can be propagated onto the Chan-Vese model-based segmentation algorithm to evaluate the effect of uncertainty in pixel values on segmentation results. Generally, the probability density function (PDF) of pixel values can be calibrated with imaging data. However, this is less efficient, since each CMR image may have significantly different pixel values due to the heterogeneity in patients and cardiac structures. In addition, CMR images usually contain many regions (cardiac chambers) of different pixel value intensities. One solution of the multi-region segmentation problem is to simultaneously evolve a few level set functions [38]. However, the computational cost of multi-level set functions is high, and it is possible that two curves can overlap with others at some pixel values during the evolution.

To overcome these challenges, we propose an iterative segmentation algorithm and calibrate the PDF profile of pixel values for each individual image. Following this idea, a two-step stochastic image segmentation method can be developed as: (*i*) *deterministic segmentation*: using the active contours without edges method (Chan-Vese model) to identify the boundary of cardiac

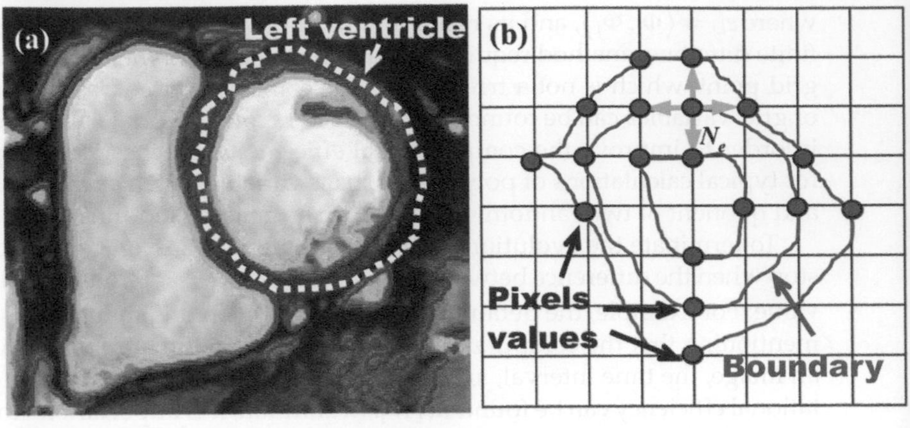

FIGURE 9.7
Schematic for generating an immediate neighborhood along the boundary of the left and right ventricles [41].

chambers, and (*ii*) *stochastic segmentation*: the gPC-based segmentation in immediate neighborhoods along the boundary of cardiac chambers. Figure 9.7 shows the schematic of the two-step image segmentation algorithm.

As seen in Figure 9.7 (a), two curves (in red) in the yellow circled region represents the immediate neighborhood of the left ventricle (LV) in the given image, which can be generated per the following procedures: (*i*) Set a value N_e as shown in Figure 9.7 (b), which defines the number of pixel values in the neighborhood region of each pixel along the boundary of the LV (blue line) identified from the deterministic segmentation step, i.e., the Chan-Vese model described in Section 9.3.3; (*ii*) Connect all pixel values along the boundary of LV in order to build an immediate neighborhood region. i.e., enclosed area with red lines in Figure 9.7 (b). The mean and variance of all the pixel values in the immediate neighborhood will be used to calibrate a gPC model as defined in (9.19) to identify gPC coefficients of $\{u_i\}$. Following this, the gPC model can be adjusted for each individual neighborhood in a given CMR image. For simplicity, it is assumed that pixel values in the neighborhood region only depend on one random variable, i.e., $\xi = \xi_1$ in (9.19). Then, the mean and variance of pixel values in the neighborhood can be calibrated from an optimization problem defined as follows:

$$\min_{\kappa} J = \sum_{i=1}^{n} (\nu_{1,i} - \vartheta_{1,i})^2 + \sum_{i=1}^{n} (\nu_{2,i} - \vartheta_{2,i})^2 \tag{9.44}$$

where κ is the decision variables, consisting of the mean and variance of the pixel values in a neighborhood of interest, n is the total number of pixel values in the neighborhood, $\nu_{1,i}$ and $\nu_{1,i}$ are the mean and variance that can be estimated with the gPC coefficients as shown in (9.19). The terms $\vartheta_{1,i}$ and $\vartheta_{1,i}$

are the mean and variance of pixel values that can be numerically estimated with pixels found to be inside the neighborhood region.

In summary, the two-step image segmentation algorithm in this chapter involves initialization, model calibration, and segmentation. It should be noted that the accuracy of the two-step image segmentation can be affected by the accuracy of the gPC approximation of pixel values. As seen in (9.19), the gPC expansion is determined by the polynomial basis functions and the number of required terms, i.e., p in (9.19). Therefore, an appropriate polynomial basis function should be chosen based on the statistical distribution of pixel values in a neighborhood region along the boundary. Meanwhile, the orthogonality of polynomial basis functions should be ensured. Figure 9.8 shows segmentation results, using the deterministic (Chan-Vese) algorithm and the PDF profiles of pixel values in the neighborhood regions, which are generated given $N_e = 1$.

As shown in Figure 9.8, the red lines describe the boundary that can separate the cardiac regions from the CMR image background. The boundary corresponds to pixel values, for which $Z \approx 0$ in (9.14). It is important to note that the Chan-Vese segmentation algorithms can segment the left ventricle (LV) and the right ventricle (RV) from the background simultaneously. Since the LV usually appears as a circular region, a special mathematical treatment for

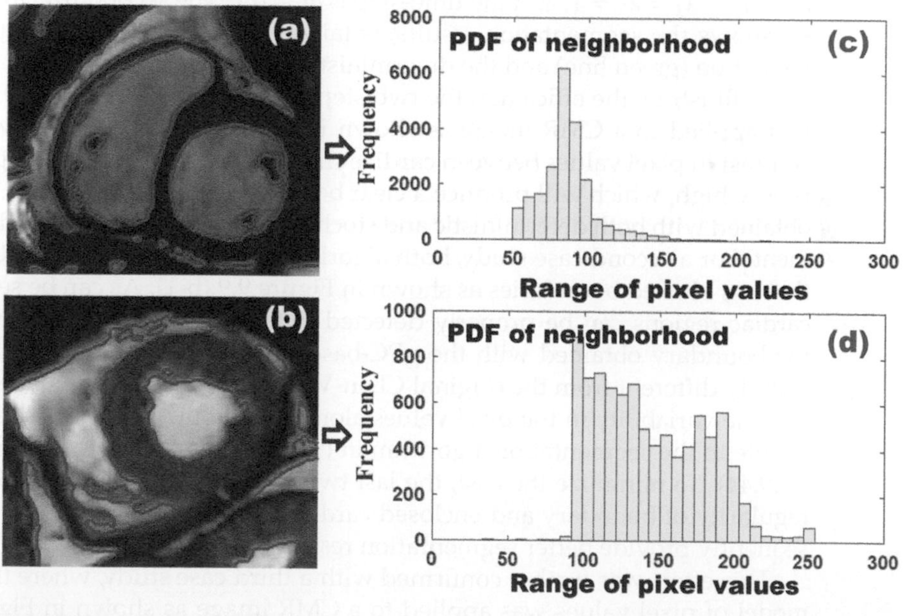

FIGURE 9.8
Illustration of segmentation with the Chan-Vese model and the PDF profiles of pixel values in the neighborhood region of cardiac chambers. Images used for algorithm illustration are from reference [41].

estimating the shape information of ventricles, i.e., center point and radius of a circle, can be used to distinguish the LV from the RV. However, details are not discussed in this chapter for brevity. The procedures can be found in [39].

For clarification, the PDF profile of pixel values in the neighborhood regions of LV is estimated using a binning algorithm, as shown in Figures 9.8 (c) and (d). Each bin shows the number of pixel that exhibits values within a particular range of pixel values. As shown in Figures 9.8 (c) and (d), it was found that the pixel values in different neighborhood regions of the LV follow different distributions, i.e., different PDF profiles, which are not standard distributions in the Wiener-Askey scheme [16]. Similar results can be observed for the neighborhood regions of the RVs, which is not shown in this chapter for brevity. In order to efficient quantify the PDF profile of pixel values in the immediate neighborhood regions and ensure the orthogonality of polynomial basis functions for non-standard distributions, the Gram-Schmidt polynomial basis functions [40] are used to capture variability in pixel values. The formulation of Gram-Schmidt polynomial basis function can be found in [40].

9.5.2 Stochastic Image Segmentation with gPC and Chan-Vese Models

For three given CMR images as shown in the first row of Figure 9.9, parameters used for the stochastic image segmentation in (9.43) are chosen as: $\mu_1 = \mu_2 = \lambda_1 = \lambda_1 = 1$, and the time-step is $dt = 0.1$. The second row in Figure 9.9 shows the segmentation results, obtained with both the stochastic segmentation (green line) and the deterministic methods (red line).

To illustrate the efficiency, the two-step image segmentation algorithm is first applied to a CMR image as shown in Figure 9.9 (a-1). As shown, the contrast in pixel values between cardiac chambers and the CMR background is very high, which will produce a clear boundary. The segmentation results obtained with both deterministic and stochastic methods are in a good agreement. For a second case study, both algorithms are applied to a CMR image that has blurred boundaries as shown in Figure 9.9 (b-1). As can be seen, the cardiac regions can be properly detected with both approaches. However the boundary obtained with the gPC-based stochastic Chan-Vese model is slightly different from the original Chan-Vese model. The probable reason is that the variability in the pixel values along and on the boundaries can contribute to the segmentation algorithm in (9.43), due to the model calibration in (9.44). To minimize the cost, the last two terms in (9.43) will penalize the regularity of boundary and enclosed cardiac chamber area, which will consequently provide better segmentation results.

This effect was further confirmed with a third case study, where the gPC model of pixel values was applied to a CMR image as shown in Figure 9.9 (c-1). As compared to previous case study, the gPC model of pixel value was calibrated with pixel values in the neighborhood of all cardiac chambers. Compared to the deterministic Chan-Vese model, the gPC-based stochastic method can provide a better segmentation result because of the gPC mode

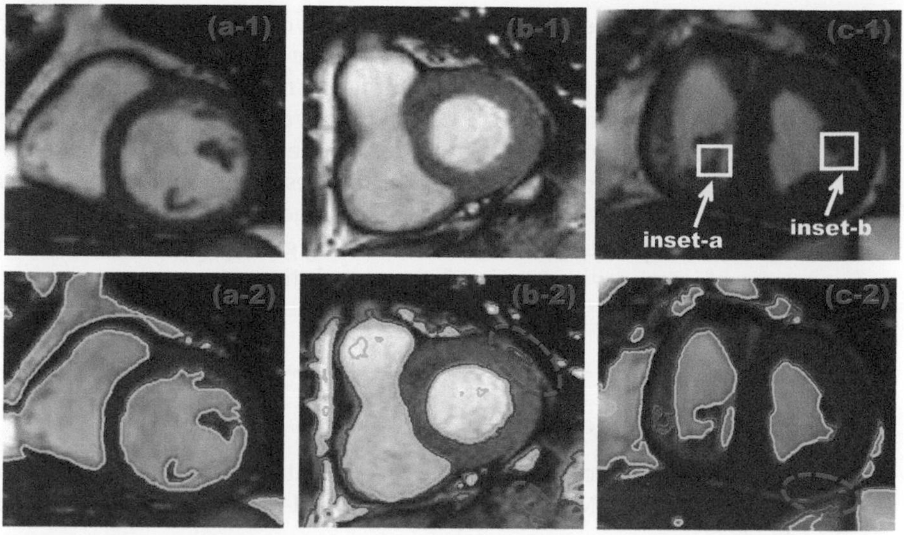

FIGURE 9.9
Comparison of the two-step stochastic image segmentation and the deterministic image segmentation algorithm: deterministic (red contours) vs. stochastic (green contours) [41].

calibration. For example, the stochastic method can eliminate artifacts that are not cardiac chambers as seen in Figure 9.9 (c-2).

It should be noted that only a geometric locus of the zero value of a level set function Z is shown in the aforementioned case studies for brevity. As discussed in Section 9.2, the higher order gPC coefficients in (9.28) can provide a probabilistic quantity of segmentation. This is very useful to evaluate the confidence interval along the boundary of segmentation. For example, the average of variances calculated with the higher order gPC coefficients of Z in (9.28) for two insets in Figure 9.9 (c-1) are 0.1 and 0.08, respectively. This can provide a probabilistic description of the segmentation near the boundary, which can be refered back to the PDF profiles approximated to evaluate the reliability of segmentation.

9.6 Conclusion

In this work, an automated stochastic image segmentation algorithm is developed to segment cardiac chambers from the background of CMRI images. A generalized polynomial chaos (gPC) expansion is combined with a level set function to evolve the boundary in a stochastic way. The current design takes the uncertainties in the pixel values into account and quantifies and propagates variabilities of pixel values onto image segmentation procedures. The method does not require prior information, since the calibration of the gPC model is based on a pre-processing procedure, i.e., deterministic segmentation and an extension method to build an immediate neighborhood in each image. Using pixel values inside the neighborhood, the model calibration of gPC model is applied to each cardiac chamber. The probabilistic descriptions of heart boundaries enable reliable and robust segmentation. The fast estimation of pixel values using gPC model greatly reduces the computational cost; thus showing great potentials for dealing with a mass of images with varying image resolutions.

9.7 Acknowledgement

The financial support in this work from Natural Science Foundation (NSF) (CMMI-1727487, CMMI-1728338, and CMMI-1646664) is gratefully acknowledged.

References

1. C. Petitjean and J.-N. Dacher, "A review of segmentation methods in short axis cardiac MR images," *Medical Image Anlysis*, vol. 2, no. 169–184, p. 15, 2011.
2. M. R. M. Jongbloed, M. J. Schalij, K. Zeppenfled, P. V. Oemrawsingh, E. E. Wall and J. J. Bax, "Clinical applications of intracardiac echocardiography in interventional preocedures," *Heart*, vol. 91, no. 7, pp. 981–990, 2005.
3. T. Gerber, B. Kantor and E. Williamson, Computed tomography of the cardiovascular system, Boca Raton, FL: Taylor & Francis Group, LLC, 2007.
4. M. Dewey, E. Zimmermann, F. Deissenrieder, M. Laule, H. Dubel, P. Schlattmann, F. Knebel, W. Rutsch and B. Hamm, "Noninvasive Coronary Angiography by 320-Row Computed Tomography With Lower Radiation Exposure and Maintained Diagnostic Accuracy," *Circulation*, vol. 120, no. 10, pp. 867–875, 2009.
5. C. Petitjean and J.-N. Dacher, "A review of segmentation methods in short axis cardiac MR images," *Medical Image Analysis*, vol. 15, pp. 169–184, 2011.
6. D. Mahapatra, "Cardiac image segmentation from cine cardiac MRI using graph cuts and shape priors," *Journal of Digital Imaging*, vol. 26, pp. 721–730, 2013.
7. T. Donnell, G. Funka-Lea, H. Tek, M.-P. Jolly, M. Rasch and R. Setser, "Comprehensive cardiovascular image analysis using MR and CT at Siemens Corporate Research," *International Journal of Computer Vision*, vol. 70, no. 2, pp. 165–178, 2006.
8. J. Woo, P. Slomka, J. Kou and B.-W. Hong, "Multiphase segmentation using animplicit dual shape prior: application to detection of left ventricle in cardiac MRI," *Computer Vision and Image Understanding*, vol. 117, pp. 1084–1094, 2013.
9. X. Zhuang, K. S. Rhode and R. S. Razavi, "A registration-based propagation framework for automatic whole heart segmentation of cardiac MRI," *IEEE Transactions on Medical Imaging*, vol. 29, no. 9, pp. 1612–1625, 2010.

10. P. Kalshetti, M. Bundele, P. Rahangdale, D. Jangra, C. Chattopadhyay, G. Harit and A. Elhence, "An interactive medical image segmentation framework using iterative refinement," *Computers in Biology and Medicine*, vol. 83, pp. 22–33, 2017.
11. T. F. Chan and J. Shen, Image Processing and Analysis: Variational, PDE, Wavelet, and Stochastic Methods, Philadelphia, PA: The Society for Industrial and Applied Mathematics, 2005.
12. A. Ziadi, X. Maldague, L. Saucier, C. Duchesne and R. Gosselin, "Visible and near- infrared light transmission: a hybrid imaging method for non-destructive meat quality evaluation," *Infrared Physics & Technology*, vol. 55, no. 5, pp. 412–420, 2012.
13. T. Patz and T. Preusser, "Segmentation of stochastic images using level set propagation with uncertain speed," *Journal of Mathematical Imaging and Vision*, vol. 48, no. 3, pp. 467–487, 2014.
14. T. Preusser, H. Scharr, K. Krajsek and R. M. Kirby, "Building blocks for computer vision with stochastic partial differential equations," *International Journal of Computer Vision*, vol. 80, no. 3, pp. 375–405, 2008.
15. Y. Du, H. Budman and T. Duever, "Classification of normal and apoptotic cells from fluorescence microscopy images using generalized polynomial chaos and level set function," *Microscopy and Microanalysis*, vol. 22, no. 3, pp. 475–486, 2016.
16. D. Xiu, Numerical methods for stochastic computations: a spectral method approach, Princeton, New Jersey: Princeton University Press, 2010.
17. T. Chan and L. Vese, "Active contours without edges," *IEEE Transactions on Image Processing*, vol. 10, no. 2, pp. 266–278, 2001.
18. P. Getreuer, "Chan-Vese segmentation," *Image Processing On Line*, vol. 2, pp. 214–224, 2012.
19. S. Shors, C. Fung, C. Francois, P. Finn and D. Fieno, "Accurate quantification of right ventricular mass at MR imaging by using cine true fast imaging with steady state precession: study in dogs," *Radiology*, vol. 230, no. 2, pp. 383–388, 2004.
20. T. F. Chan and J. Shen, Image processing and analysis variational, PDE, Wavelet, and stochastic methods, Philadelphia, PA: The Society for Industrial and Applied Mathematics, 2005.
21. J. Caudron, J. Fares, F. Bauer and J. N. Dacher, "Left ventricular diastolic function assessment by cardiac MRI," *Radio Graphics*, vol. 31, no. 1, pp. 259–261, 2010.
22. N. Rougon, C. Petitjean, P. Cluzel, F. Preteux and P. Grenier, "A non rigid registration approach for quantifying myocardial contraction in tagged MRI using generalized information measures," *Medical Image Analysis*, vol. 9, no. 4, pp. 353–375, 2005.
23. A. Dervieus and F. Thomasset, "A finite element method for simulation of a Rayleigh- Taylor instability," *Approximation Methods for Navier-Stokes Problems. Lecture notes in Mathematics*, vol. 771, pp. 145–158, 1980.
24. S. Osher and J. A. Sethian, "Fronts propagating with curvature dependent speed: algorithm based on Hamilton-Jacobi formulations," *Journal of Computational Physics*, vol. 79, no. 1, pp. 12–49, 1998.
25. J. A. Sethian, Level set methods and fast marching methods, Cambridge, UK: Cambridge University Press, 1999.
26. S. Osher and J. A. Sethian, "Fronts propagating with curvature dependent speed: algorithms based on Hamilton-Jacobi formulation," *Journal of Computational Physics*, vol. 79, no. 1, pp. 12–49, 1998.

27. C. Li, C. Y. Kao, J. C. Gore and Z. Ding, "Minimization of region scalable fitting energy for image segmentation," *IEEE Transactions on Image Processing*, vol. 17, no. 10, pp. 1940–1949, 2008.
28. R. Malladi, J. A. Sethian and B. C. Vemuri, "Evolutionary fronts for topology independent shape modeling and recovery," in *Proceeding of the Third European Conference on Computer Vision*, Stockholm, Sweden, 1994.
29. V. Caselles, R. Kimmel and G. Sapiro, "Geodesic active contours," *International Journal of Computer Vision*, vol. 22, no. 1, pp. 61–79, 1997.
30. D. Mumford and J. Shah, "Optimal approximation by piecewise smooth functions and associated variational problems," *Communications on Pure and Applied Mathematics*, vol. 42, pp. 577–685, 1989.
31. N. Wiener, "The homogeneous chaos," *American Journal of Mathematics*, vol. 60, no. 4, pp. 897–936, 1938.
32. R. Ghanem and P. Spanos, Stochastic Finite Elements - A Spectral Approach, Mineola, New York, USA: Dover Publications, INC, 1991.
33. Y. Du, H. Budman and T. Duever, "Fault detection and diagnosis with parametric uncertainty using generalized polynomial chaos," *Computers and Chemical Engineering*, vol. 76, pp. 63–75, 2015.
34. L. He and S. Osher, "Solving the Chan-Vese Model by a multiphase level set algorithm based on the topological derivative," in *International Conference on Scale Space and Variational Methods in Computer Vision*, Ischia, Italy, 2007.
35. N. Badshah and K. Chen, "Multigrid method for the Chan-Vese model in variational segmentation," *Communications in Computational Physics*, vol. 4, no. 2, pp 294–316, 2008.
36. G. Aubert and L. A. Vese, "A variational method in image recovery," *SIAM Journal of Numerical Analysis*, vol. 34, no. 5, pp. 1948–1979, 1997.
37. B. Debsschere, H. Najm, P. Pebay, O. Knio, R. Ghanem and O. Le Maitre, "Numerical challenges in the use of polynomial chaos representations for stochastic processes," *SIAM Journal of Scientific Computation*, vol. 26, no. 2, pp. 698–719, 2004.
38. L. A. Vese and T. F. Chan, "A multiphase level set framework for image segmentation using the Mumford and Shah model," *International Journal of Computer Vision*, vol. 50, no. 3, pp. 271–293, 2002.
39. Y. Du, H. Budman and T. Duever, "Segmentation and quantitative analysis of apoptosis of Chinese Hamster Ovary cells from fluorescence microscopy images," *Microscopy and Miscroanalysis*, vol. 23, no. 3, pp. 569–583, 2017.
40. Y. Du, H. Budman and T. Duever, "Parameter estimation for an inverse nonlinear stochastic problem: reactivity ratio studies in copolymerization," *Macromolecular Theory and Simulations*, vol. 26, no. 2, pp. 1–15, 2017.
41. Jordan, M. Ringenberg, Computerized 3D modeling and simulations of patient specific cardiac anatomy fUom segmented MRI, Ph.D. Dissertation, The University of Toledo, December 2014.

Appendix

As discussed in Section 9.4.1, random variables such as the level set function can be approximated by a truncated gPC approximation as shown in (9.21). As seen in the gPC approximation, the level set function is related to: (*i*)

TABLE 9.1

One-Dimensional Polynomial Chaos Basis Functions and Their Corresponding Variance

i	P*	i^{th} Polynomial Basis Function Φ_i	$\langle \Phi_i^2 \rangle$
0	0	1	1
1	1	ξ_1	1
2	2	$\xi_1^2 - 1$	2
3	3	$\xi_1^3 - 3\xi_1$	6
4	4	$\xi_1^4 - 6\xi_1^2 + 3$	24

*As defined in (9.21), P is the order of homogenous polynomial chaos.

stochastic space defined by random variables $\boldsymbol{\xi} = \{\xi_i\}$ $(i = 1, \cdots, n)$, where ξ_i is the ith random variables with a prior known distribution, (*ii*) gPC coefficients; and (*iii*) polynomial chaos basis functions $\{\Phi_i\}$. For normally distributed variables, Tables 9.1 to Table 9.3 shows the polynomial basis functions for one-, two-, and three-dimensional polynomial chaos basis functions and their corresponding variances. More details can be found in Chapter 2 of [32].

TABLE 9.2

Two-Dimensional Polynomial Chaos Basis Functions and Their Corresponding Variance

i	P*	i^{th} Polynomial Basis Function Φ_i	$\langle \Phi_i^2 \rangle$
0	0	1	1
1	1	ξ_1	1
2		ξ_2	1
3		$\xi_1^2 - 1$	2
4	2	$\xi_1\xi_2$	1
5		$\xi_1^2 - 1$	2
6		$\xi_1^3 - 3\xi_1$	6
7	3	$\xi_1^2\xi_2 - \xi_2$	2
8		$\xi_1\xi_2^2 - \xi_1$	2
9		$\xi_2^3 - 3\xi_2$	6
10		$\xi_1^4 - 6\xi_1^2 + 3$	24
11		$\xi_1^3 - 3\xi_1\xi_2$	6
12	4	$\xi_1^2\xi_2^2 - \xi_1^2 - \xi_2^2 + 1$	4
13		$\xi_1\xi_2^3 - 3\xi_1\xi_2$	6
14		$\xi_2^4 - 6\xi_2^2 + 3$	24

TABLE 9.3

Three-Dimensional Polynomial Chaos Basis Functions and Their Corresponding Variance

i	P^*	i^{th} **Polynomial Basis Function** Φ_i	$\langle\Phi_i^2\rangle$
0	0	1	1
1		ξ_1	1
2	1	ξ_2	1
3		ξ_3	1
4		$\xi_1^2 - 1$	2
5		$\xi_1\xi_2$	1
6		$\xi_1\xi_3$	1
7	2	$\xi_1^2 - 1$	2
8		$\xi_2\xi_3$	1
9		$\xi_3^2 - 1$	2
10		$\xi_1^3 - 3\xi_1$	6
11		$\xi_1^2\xi_2 - \xi_2$	2
12		$\xi_1^2\xi_3 - \xi_3$	2
13		$\xi_1\xi_2^2 - \xi_1$	2
14	3	$\xi_1\xi_2\xi_3$	1
15		$\xi_1\xi_3^2 - \xi_1$	2
16		$\xi_2^3 - 3\xi_2$	6
17		$\xi_2^2\xi_3 - \xi_3$	2
18		$\xi_2\xi_3^2 - \xi_2$	2
19		$\xi_3^3 - 3\xi_3$	6
20		$\xi_1^4 - 6\xi_1^2 + 3$	24
21		$\xi_1^3\xi_2 - 3\xi_1\xi_2$	6
22		$\xi_1^3\xi_3 - 3\xi_1\xi_3$	6
23		$\xi_1^2\xi_2^2 - \xi_1^2 - \xi_2^2 + 1$	4
24		$\xi_1^2\xi_2\xi_3 - 3\xi_1\xi_3$	2
25		$\xi_1^2\xi_3^2 - \xi_3^2 - \xi_1^2 + 1$	4
26		$\xi_1\xi_2^3 - 3\xi_1\xi_2$	6
27	4	$\xi_1\xi_2^2\xi_3 - \xi_1\xi_3$	2
28		$\xi_1\xi_2\xi_3^2 - \xi_1\xi_2$	2
29		$\xi_1\xi_3^3 - 3\xi_1\xi_3$	6
30		$\xi_2^4 - 6\xi_2^2 + 3$	2
31		$\xi_2^3\xi_3 - 3\xi_2\xi_3$	6
32		$\xi_2^2\xi_3^2 - \xi_3^2 - \xi_2^2 + 1$	4
33		$\xi_2\xi_2^3 - 3\xi_2\xi_3$	6
34		$\xi_3^4 - 6\xi_3^2 + 3$	24

10

Medical Image Segmentation Approach That Uses Level Sets with Statistical Shape Priors

Ahmed ElTanboly, Mohammed Ghazal, Hassan Hajjdiab, Ali Mahmoud, Ahmed Shalaby, Jasjit S. Suri, Robert Keynton, and Ayman El-Baz

CONTENTS

10.1 Introduction

The level set method is a simple and versatile method for computing and analyzing the motion of an interface contour Γ in two or three dimensions [1]. That interface bounds a connected, or possibly a multiply connected, region. The goal is to compute and analyze the subsequent motion of this evolving curve/surface under a velocity field. This velocity can depend on position, time, geometry of the interface (e.g., its normal or its mean curvature), and external physics. The interface is captured for a later time as the zero level set of a smooth (at least Lipschitz continuous) function $\phi(\mathbf{x}, t)$. Such level set function ϕ is defined as positive inside the region, negative outside, and zero on Γ. The original idea behind the level set method was a simple one. Given an interface contour Γ in 2-D/3-D, bounding a (perhaps multiply connected) open region, we wish to analyze and compute its subsequent motion under a velocity field.

A deformable model is a curve in a 2-D digital image or a surface in a 3-D volume that evolves to outline a desired object. The evolution is controlled by internal and external forces combined, together with user defined constraints, into internal and external energy terms, respectively. Kass et al. [2] first introduced such models, that gave rise to one of the most dynamic and successful research areas in edge detection, image segmentation, shape modeling, and visual tracking. By representation and implementation, deformable models are broadly categorized into parametric and geometric classes. El-Baz et al. [3] proposed the stochastic force and has been embedded in the geometric deformable models (level sets). In this chapter, the main focus is to discuss the geometric deformable models and how to deform it under a particular stochastic force till it captures the object properties of interest.

The performance of the deformable models depends on proper initialization, efficiency of the energy minimization process, and the adequate selection of force functions and energy functionals. Amini et al. [4] pointed to these shortcomings of the minimization process in [2] and improved it by representing a snake as a linked chain of control points and using discrete dynamic programming to minimize the total energy related to the chain. This approach allows for rigid constraints on the energy function and more minimization stability. However, its control parameters must be adjusted very carefully and the process is time consuming. Another advanced greedy algorithm proposed by Williams and Shah [5] has linear time complexity both in the number of control points and in the number of their neighbors taken into account for energy minimization. It is much more stable and is simultaneously more than an order of magnitude and faster than previous techniques. Wong et al. [6] developed a more flexible segmented snake. Their model is able to handle regions with relatively sharp corners due to a recursive split and merge procedure dividing a boundary into segments to approximate them locally. An alternative flexible snake model in [7] is based on B–spline representation and multiple stages energy minimization.

In spite of good segmentation results for objects of relatively simple shapes, the above conventional deformable models have serious drawbacks. Most of them are slow compared to other segmentation techniques, and the model evolution frequently stops well before approaching a complicated object boundary with concavities. Also, to initialize the model, typically a closed curve has to be interactively drawn near the desired boundary, and this manual step hinders its use in many applications [8].

Leventon et al. [9] used prior shape with deformable models in order to control the evolution of the active contours. They obtained their shape model by applying the principal component analysis (PCA) to the training shape signed distance maps. Shen and Davatzikos [10] used attribute vectors with the deformable models which identify the surrounding geometry of th model points during the deformation. Based on [9], Tsai et al. [11] presented a deformable model based segmentation technique in which the segmenting curve is represented implicitly using a parametric model. This eliminates the need of obtaining correspondence between points at the time of training and hence more robustness to variations in the segmenting curve. The implicit shape is parametrically represented using the mean and eigen shapes resulting from the PCA of the signed distance maps of the training shapes. Later on, this method was extended by Tsai et al. [12] to handle the simultaneous segmentation of multiple objects by using multiple signed distance maps to implicitly represent the shapes. PCA is applied to these distance maps and co-variation between various shapes is acquired. This time, the cost function involved in the segmentation is based on mutual information. However inconsistent modeling can occur due to the non-closure of distance functions with linear operation. This issue was addressed by Pohl et al. [13] where they embedded the signed distance maps into the logarithm of the odds linear space. Also for segmentation based on level sets, Yang and Duncan [14] performed 3–D segmentation using joint prior shape and intensity model making use of the dependency between shape and intensity of objects, where they developed a maximum a posteriori (MAP) model using the joint information. Huang et al. [15] presented a problem of energy minimization that combines both segmentation and registration. A level set of a distance function of a higher dimensionality embeds either the evolving surface or curve which is iteratively registered using the shape model. Rousson et al. [16] employed distance functions to build a shape model using shapes in the training dataset in order to be used for a 3–D level set shape based segmentation technique.

This chapter proposes a novel and promising level set based technique for segmentation and that is dependent on the information from both the shape and the intensity. The information about the former is extracted from a training set of co-aligned shapes. The value of the gray level intensity is used to form the probability density functions (PDFs) of the object and the background. The mentioned functions are found using our novel approach which is named as the modified expectation maximization (EM). The modified EM uses a linear combination of Gaussians (LCDG) that have negative and positive components to estimate the density function. Using the estimated PDFs in a variational manner lead to accurate and fast segmentation.

10.1.1 Basic Notations

- $\mathbf{x} = (x_1, x_2, \ldots, x_n) \in \mathbb{R}^n$ denotes a point in $\mathbb{R}^n$. In $\mathbb{R}^2$, $\mathbf{x} = (x, y)$ and in $\mathbb{R}^3$, $\mathbf{x} = (x, y, z)$.
- $\phi(\mathbf{x}, t)$ denotes the level set function, implicitly represents the interface to be captured for all later time t.

- $\Gamma = \{\mathbf{x} : \phi(\mathbf{x}, t) = 0\}$ denotes the captured interface contour representing the zero level of ϕ (i.e. points where ϕ vanishes).
- $R = \{(x, y) : x = 0, 1, 2, \ldots, X-1; y = 0, 1, 2, \ldots, Y-1\}$ be the finite arithmetic lattice supporting digital images and their region maps.
- $g = \{g_{x,y} : (x, y) \in R, g_{x,y} \in \{0, 1, 2, \ldots, q-1\}\}$ be a grayscale digital image taking q different values from a finite set $\{0, 1, 2, \ldots, q-1\}$.
- $m = \{m_{x,y} : (x, y) \in R, m_{x,y} \in \{ob, bg\}\}$ a region map taking labels from a binary set. Each label $m_{x,y}$ indicates whether the pixel (x, y) is in the image g belongs to an object (ob) or a background (bg).

10.2 Evolutionary Curve/Surface Based on Level Set Model

Shape delineation is the primary task in shape analysis. Such representation is essential in the computer vision field and in a number of medical imaging applications, such as registration and segmentation. There are several shape representation techniques explained in [17–19]. Despite the fact that some of those methods are powerful enough to acquire local deformations, they need a large number of parameters in order to handle significant shape deformations. Thus, an emerging way to represent shapes is derived using level sets [20]. Such representation is invariant to translation and rotation. Given a curve/surface Γ that determines boundaries of a specific 2-D/3-D region Ω, we may be able to propose the level set function form. Generally, for each 3-D image voxel (x, y, z) or simply for 2-D image pixel (x, y), we define the following level set function:

$$\phi(x,y,z) = \begin{cases} 0, & (x,y,z) \in \partial\Omega = \Gamma, \\ d((x,y,z),\Gamma), & (x,y,z) \in \Omega, \\ -d((x,y,z),\Gamma), & \text{Otherwise.} \end{cases} \tag{10.1}$$

where $d((x, y, z), \Gamma)$ stands for the shortest Euclidean distance between the image voxel (x, y, z) and the contour surface Γ. Such representation is capable of handling local invisible deformations and geometrical features of the shape that also can be derived consequently using this representation.

In describing the level set formally as in [21, 22], the evolving contour is a propagating front embedded as the zero level of an implicit scalar function $\phi(\mathbf{x}, t)$, with $\mathbf{x}$ details into (x, y) for 2-D plane (simple representation) or (x, y, z) for 3-D space (general representation). The continuous change of $\phi(\mathbf{x}, t)$ with time can be described by the level set partial differential equation (PDE):

$$\frac{\partial\phi(\mathbf{x},t)}{\partial t} + F_N(\mathbf{x})|\nabla\phi(\mathbf{x},t)| = 0, \tag{10.2}$$

where the original velocity vector $\overrightarrow{F(\mathbf{x})}$ can be written as $\overrightarrow{F(\mathbf{x})} = F_N\hat{u}_n + F_T\hat{u}_t$ describing the evolving action with the normal component F_N responsible only for the deformation process while the tangential component F_T has no deformation effect. In Eq.(10.2), $\nabla = (\frac{\partial}{\partial x}, \frac{\partial}{\partial y}, \frac{\partial}{\partial z})$. The function $\phi(\mathbf{x}, t)$ deforms sequentially according to $F_N(\mathbf{x})$, and the location of the 2-D/3-D propagating front is given at each time step by setting $\phi(\mathbf{x}, t) = 0$. Practically, instead of analytically solving Eq.(10.2) for $\phi(\mathbf{x}, t)$, we numerically use the first difference formula for time derivative to get the value $\phi(\mathbf{x}, t_{n+1})$ at time step $n + 1$ which is computed from $\phi(\mathbf{x}, t_n)$ at step n using the difference relation:

$$\phi(\mathbf{x}, t_{n+1}) = \phi(\mathbf{x}, t_n) - \Delta t F |\nabla\phi(\mathbf{x}, t_n)|. \tag{10.3}$$

The selection of the speed function $F_N(\mathbf{x})$ plays the principal role in the evolution process. Among multiple formulations introduced in [23,24], we have chosen according to simplicity and ease of implementation, the following formulation:

$$F_N(\mathbf{x}) = \nu - \epsilon k(\mathbf{x}), \tag{10.4}$$

where ν takes -1 or 1 for the expanding or contracting front respectively, ϵ is a smoothing parameter which is always small relative to 1, and $k(x, y, z)$ is the local curvature of the propagating front. The latter parameter acts as a regularization term.

The term ($\nu = \pm 1$) within Eq. (10.4) determines the direction of the front propagation. multiple approaches were introduced to make all fronts either expanding or contracting (see for example, [25]) for the sake of evolving in both directions and avoiding overlap between regions. The problem can be rephrased as classification of each point at the evolving front. With the assumption that the initial shape lies entirely inside the main object (final deformation target), if the point belongs to the associated class (object), the front expands; otherwise it contracts.

10.2.1 PDE System

Considering the 3-D as the general space, the term *voxel* will be generally used to indicate location (x, y, z) with the normal component F_N of velocity function recalled the *speed* function and simply written as, F(x, y, z). The classification procedure is based on Bayesian decision [26] at voxel (x, y, z) in the front. The term (ν) is replaced by the function for each point $\nu(x, y, z)$ so the velocity function is defined as:

$$F(x, y, z) = \nu(x, y, z) - \epsilon k(x, y, z). \tag{10.5}$$

where

$$\nu(x, y, z) = \begin{cases} -1 & \text{if } p_g(q|1)p_{sh}(d|1) > p_g(q|2)p_{sh}(d|2) \\ 1 & \text{otherwise.} \end{cases} \tag{10.6}$$

The terms p_g and p_{sh} represent the intensity and shape models, respectively. Next two sections (10.3 and 10.4) describe the mathematical formulation and more information about how they are computed are introduced.

Now, using the derivative of the Heaviside step function ($\delta_\alpha(.)$) [27], we put the Eq. (10.2) in the more general form as follows :

$$\frac{\partial\phi(x,y,z,t)}{\partial t} = \delta_{\alpha(x,y,z)}(\phi(x,y,z))(\epsilon k(x,y,z) - \nu(x,y,z))|\nabla\phi(x,y,z)|. \quad (10.7)$$

The function $\delta_\alpha(.)$ picks the narrow band points around the front while the parameter α controls the width of this narrow band.

10.3 Statistical Intensity Model

In this chapter a robust algorithm called a modified EM algorithm is introduced that approximates the empirical PDF of scalar data with an LCDG including negative and positive components. Because of these two components, the LCDG approximates the inter-class transitions more accurately than a conventional mixture of only positive Gaussians.

This approach is suitable for estimating the marginal density for the intensity gray level distribution $p_g(q)$ in each region in the given image. In the following section we will describe this model for estimating the distribution $p_g(q)$ in each region.

To accurately identify the model, the marginal gray level probability is approximated density in each region with a LCDG having $C_{p,i}$ positive and $C_{n,i}$ negative components:

$$p_g(q|i) = \sum_{r=1}^{C_{p,i}} w_{p,i,r}\varphi(q|\theta_{p,i,r}) - \sum_{l=1}^{C_{n,i}} w_{n,i,l}\varphi(q|\theta_{n,i,l}); \quad (10.8)$$

with $\int_{-\infty}^{\infty} p_g(q|i)dq = 1$. Here, q is the intensity gray level, and $\varphi(q|\theta)$ is a Gaussian density having a shorthand notation $\theta = (\mu, \sigma^2)$ for its mean, μ and variance, σ^2. In contrast to more conventional normal mixture models the components have only one obvious constraint in line with Eq. (10.8) $\sum_{r=1}^{C_{p,i}} w_{p,i,r} - \sum_{l=1}^{C_{n,i}} w_{n,i,l} = 1$. Those weights are not the prior probabilities, and the LCDG of Eq. (10.8) is considered as a functional form of the approximation of a probability density depending on two parameters namely, (w, θ) of each component.

The mixture of K LCDGs, $p(q) = \sum_{i=1}^{K} w_i p(q|i)$, has the same form but with a larger number of components, e.g., $C_\mathrm{p} = \sum_{i=1}^{K} C_{\mathrm{p},i}$ and $C_\mathrm{n} = \sum_{i=1}^{K} C_{\mathrm{n},i}$ if all the values $\theta_{\mathrm{p},i,r}$ and $\theta_{\mathrm{n},i,l}$ differ for the individual models:

$$p_g(q) = \sum_{r=1}^{C_\mathrm{p}} w_{\mathrm{p},r}\varphi(q|\theta_{\mathrm{p},r}) - \sum_{l=1}^{C_\mathrm{n}} w_{\mathrm{n},l}\varphi(q|\theta_{\mathrm{n},l}). \tag{10.9}$$

To identify this model in the unsupervised manner, the mixed empirical distribution of the intensity gray levels over the image has to be represented initially by a joint LCDG of Eq. (10.9) and then split into separate LCDG-models per each class $i = 1, \ldots, K$.

Under the fixed number of the positive and negative components, C, the model parameters $\mathbf{w} = \{w_c; c = 1, \ldots, C\}$ and $\boldsymbol{\Theta} = \{\theta_c : c = 1, \ldots, C\}$ maximizing the image likelihood can be found using an EM algorithm introduced in [28].

The modified EM algorithm is sensitive to both its initial state specified by the numbers of negative and positive Gaussians, along with the initial parameters (mean and variance) of each component. To find an initial LCDG-approximation close to the empirical distribution, we developed a sequential initializing EM-based algorithm detailed in [29].

Since the EM algorithm converges to a local maximum of the likelihood function, it may be repeated iteratively with different initial parameter values for choosing the model giving the best approximation. In principle, this process can be repeated several times in order to approximate more closely the residual absolute deviations between $f(q)$ and $p_g(q)$. Since each Gaussian in the latter model impacts all the values of the mixture density $p(q)$, the iterations should be ended when the approximation quality begins to decrease.

The final mixed LCDG-model $p_g(q)$ has to be split into K LCDG-submodels, one per class, by associating each subordinate component with a particular dominant term in such a way as to minimize the expected misclassification rate. To illustrate the association principle, let us consider the bi-modal case with the two dominant Gaussians having the mean values μ_1 and μ_2; $0 < \mu_1 < \mu_2 < Q$. Let all the subordinate components be ordered by their mean values, too. Then let those with the mean values smaller than μ_1 and greater than μ_2 relate to the first and second class, respectively. The components having the mean values in the range $[\mu_1, \mu_2]$ are associated with the classes by simple thresholding such that the means below the threshold, t, belong to the components associated with the first class. The desired threshold minimizes the classification error $e(t)$:

$$e(t) = \int_{-\infty}^{t} p_g(q|2)dq + \int_{t}^{\infty} p_g(q|1)dq. \tag{10.10}$$

10.4 Statistical Shape Model

To enhance the segmentation accuracy, expected shapes of goal objects are constrained with a probabilistic shape prior. A training set of images, collected for different subjects, are co-aligned by rigid, affine 2-D transformations maximizing their mutual information (MI) [30]. The shape prior is a spatially variant independent random field of region labels:

$$P_{sh}(m) = \prod_{(x,y)\in R} p_{sh:x,y}(m_{x,y}) \tag{10.11}$$

for the co-aligned, manually segmented training images, specified by a pixel-wise empirical object and background probabilities [$p_{sh:x,y}(ob)$ and $p_{sh:x,y}(bg) = 1 - p_{sh:x,y}(ob)$, respectively].

Shape model is basically an average shape obtained from the images in the dataset. The steps to construct this average shape is as follows: first, manually segment the objects of interest from the database as shown in Figure 10.1

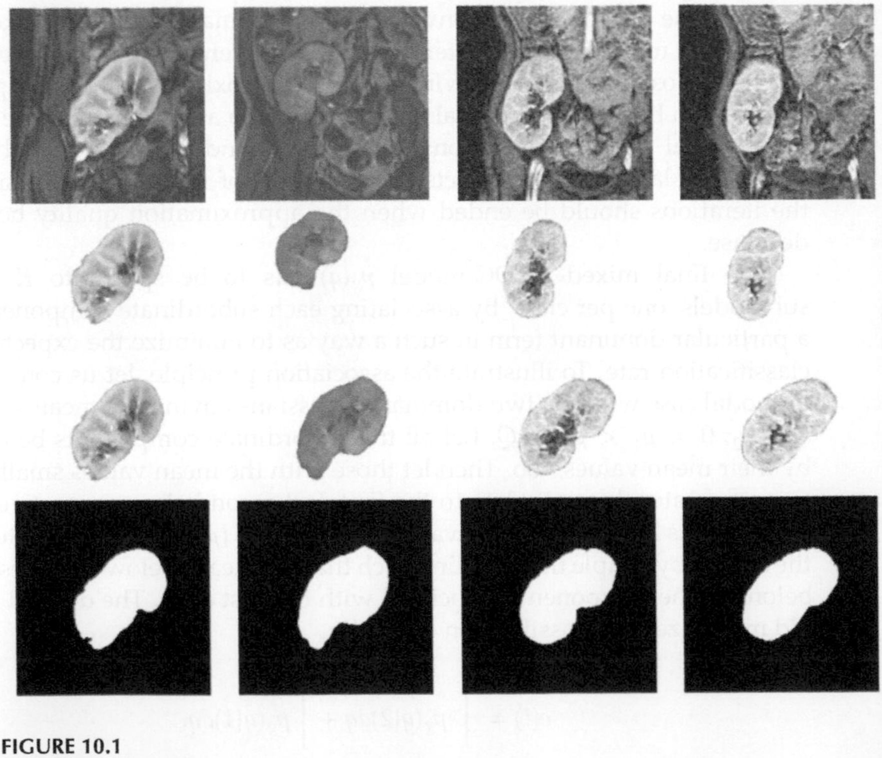

FIGURE 10.1
Steps of shape reconstruction using CT images for kidney.

first two rows, then align the images in the training datasets using 2-D rigid registration [30, 31], shown in Figure 10.1 third row, then convert aligned images obtained from the pervious step as to binary images as shown in Figure 10.1 last row, and finally calculate the p_{sh} according to Eq. 10.11. The similar shapes are overlapped more significantly after the alignment, i.e decreasing variabilities between shapes.

10.5 Experimental Results

In the following subsections, various 2-D and 3-D datasets are used to evaluate the performance and illustrate the results of the proposed segmentation approach. Quantitatively, Dice similarity coefficient (DSC) is used to evaluate the performance of our segmentation. The DSC measures the concordance among two enclosed curves/volumes as follows:

$$DSC\,\% = 100\,\frac{2TP}{FP + 2TP + FN}$$

where *FP*, *FN*, *TN* and *TP* denote the counts of false positive, false negative, true negative and true positive respectively. Namely, *FP* is the number of the background pixels/voxels that are misclassified, *FN* is the number of the object pixels/voxels that are misclassified, *TN* is the number of the background pixels/voxels that are correctly classified, and *TP* is the number of the object pixels/voxels that are correctly classified, as illustrated in Figure 10.2.

10.5.1 Segmentation of 2-D Objects

The first example is a starfish segmentation, where the starfish is separated from the background surrounding it. Such images contain two dominant objects only. The first one is the starfish which is brighter and the second is the background which is darker, thus $K = 2$. The initialization which is based on the sequential EM is illustrated in Figure 10.3.a.

The results for our proposed approach for segmentation is shown in Figure 10.3 where the DSC with the ground truth is 98.6% after multiplication of the aligned starfish image and the inverse transformation used in the rigid registration. Moreover, additional results are provided in Figure 10.4 using various real images of starfish.

For more examples for the segmentation of 2-D clinical medical images, Figure 10.5 represents the results of a human kidney segmentation in diffusion weighted-magnetic resonance imaging (DW-MRI) using the proposed method.

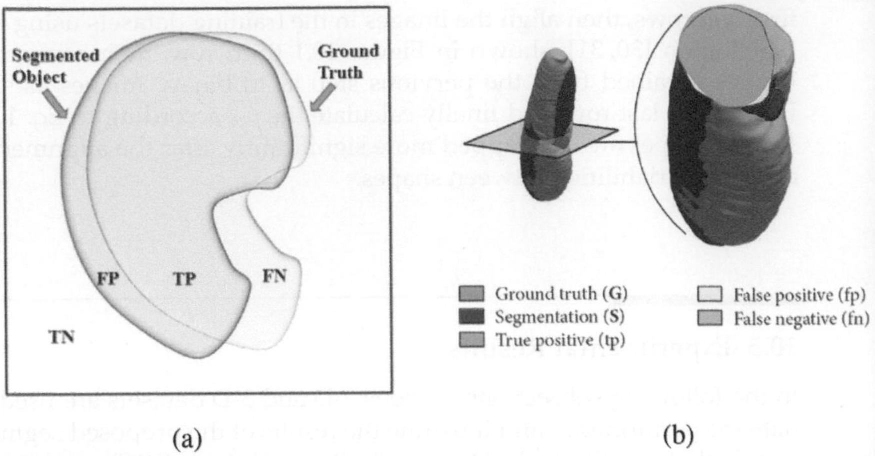

FIGURE 10.2
Illustration of the Dice similarity coefficient (DSC) measurements for segmentation evaluation between the ground truth G and model segmentation S for (a) 2-D objects, and (b) 3-D objects.

10.5.2 Segmentation of 3-D Objects

In this section, our proposed approach for segmentation is tested on 3-D datasets in order to see how robust it is. Figure 10.6 demonstrates an example for the projections of final 3-D segmentation results in sagittal, coronal and axil views for different examples of CT spine clinical datasets. The average overall DSC of the 3-D spine datasets of 40 subjects is 94.12%. This indicates the high accuracy of the proposed approach.

On the other hand, we tested our approach on 3-D kidney CT scans for 60 subjects. The average overall DSC of the segmented kidney reaches 96.98%

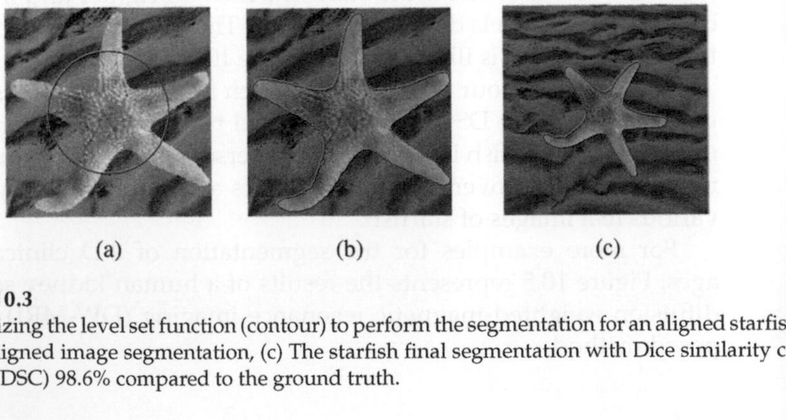

FIGURE 10.3
(a) Initializing the level set function (contour) to perform the segmentation for an aligned starfish (b) The aligned image segmentation, (c) The starfish final segmentation with Dice similarity coefficient (DSC) 98.6% compared to the ground truth.

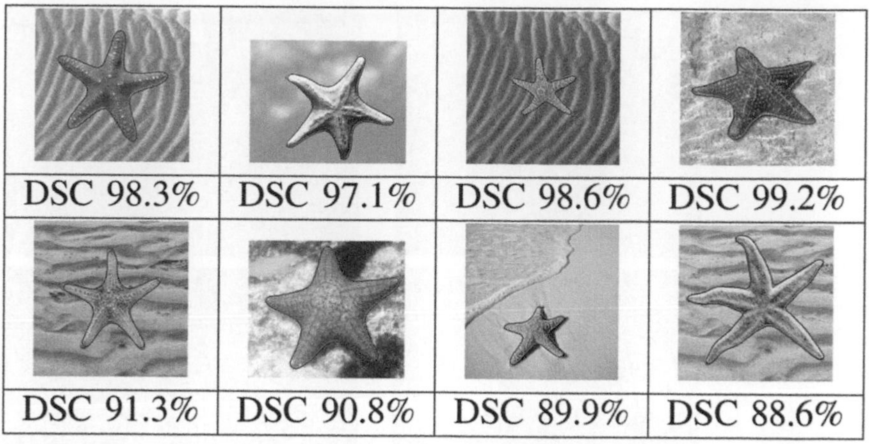

FIGURE 10.4
Additional results using starfish images that have different appearance and deformations.

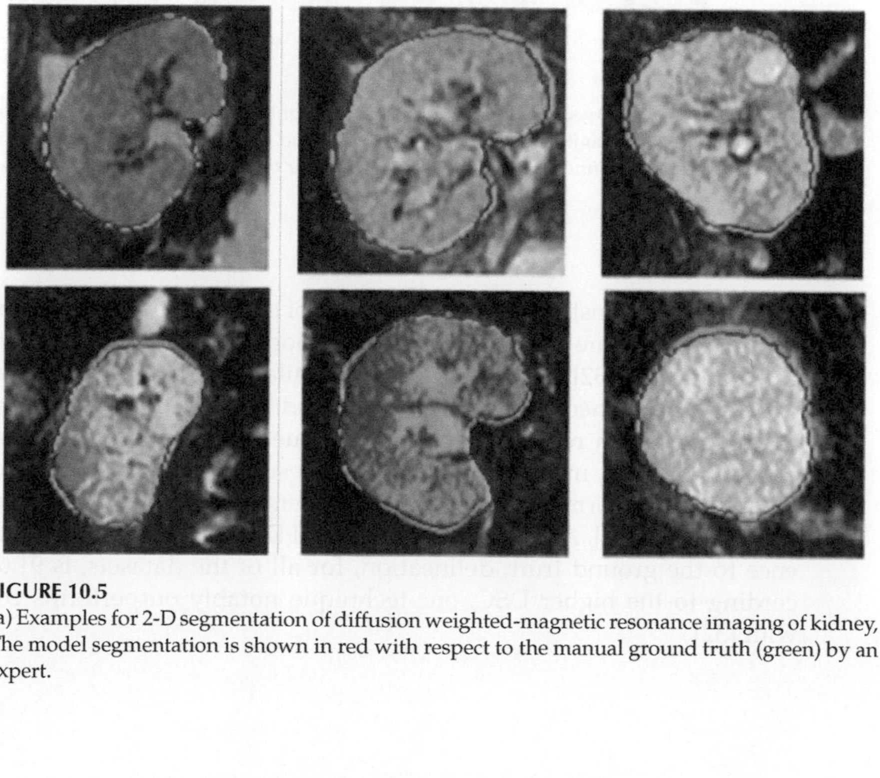

FIGURE 10.5
(a) Examples for 2-D segmentation of diffusion weighted-magnetic resonance imaging of kidney, The model segmentation is shown in red with respect to the manual ground truth (green) by an expert.

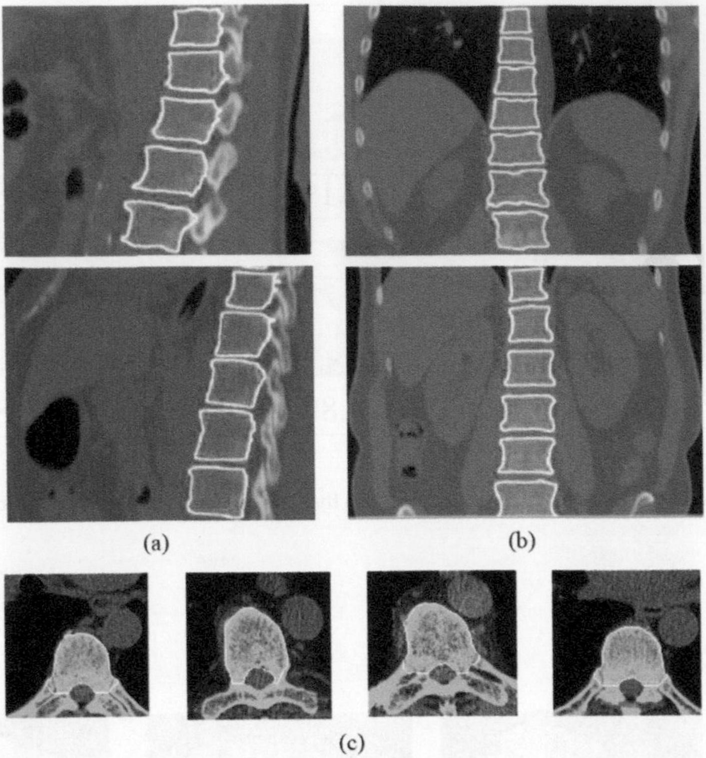

FIGURE 10.6
Projections of our 3-D segmentation method for different examples of vertebral bodies from our clinical datasets: (a) Sagittal view, (b) Coronal view, and (c) Axial view. The red color represents the contour of the ground truths while the yellow color represents the contour of the segmented regions.

In order to demonstrate the high accuracy of our kidney segmentation framework, we compare it with the segmentation approach that was presented by Zhang et al. [32], which has a freely available software package and thus avoids re-implementing an existing method. Figure 10.7 demonstrates sample segmentation results comparing our method versus the approach proposed in [32] on multiple subjects. The results in Figure 10.7 indicate the reliability in determining the kidney borders of our technique compared to the other one [32]. Additionally, the overall DSC of their method, with reference to the ground truth delineation, for all of the datasets, is 91.60%. According to the higher DSC, our technique notably outperforms compared with [32].

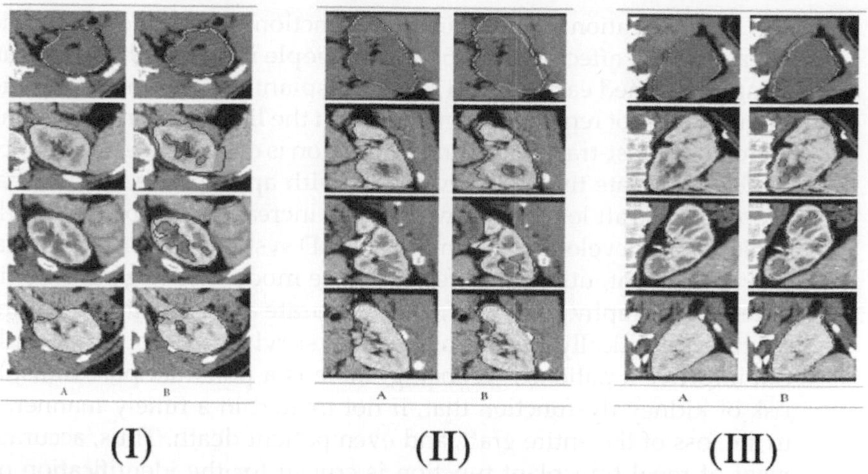

FIGURE 10.7
Comparing segmentation results of our approach (A) and the approach of Zhang et al. [32] (B): (I) Axial view, (II) Sagittal view, and (III) Coronal view. The segmentation is done at different contrast enhancement phases for multiple subjects. The red contours refer to model segmentation while the green ones refer to the ground truth.

10.6 Conclusion and Future Work

In this chapter, we proposed an approach for segmentation that is dependent on both the shape and the gray level intensity information. The density distribution of the input image gray values is estimated using the modified EM algorithm we introduced. This density distribution is enclosed in the PDE that governs the level set function evolution. A key step in the proposed approach, is the registration between the object to segment and the average shape, either 2–D or 3–D. In contrast to other approaches, energy minimization is not needed in our segmentation approach, which helps in staying away from the local minimum problem. We tested our approach with various image types and the results we obtained are promising. Moreover, our approach works well in segmenting noisy and inhomogeneous anatomical structures. In addition, the invariance of our approach to scaling, rotation and translation gives it significant robustness and accuracy. Accordingly, our segmentation approach can be used in various computer vision and medical imaging applications. For future work, we will investigate using our approach for 2–D and 3–D segmentation of colored objects.

This work could also be applied to various other applications in medical imaging, such as the kidney, the heart, the prostate, the lung, and the retina.

One application is renal transplant functional assessment. Chronic kidney disease (CKD) affects about 26 million people in U.S. with 17,000 transplants being performed each year. In renal transplant patients, acute rejection is the leading cause of renal dysfunction. Given the limited number of donors, routine clinical post-transplantation evaluation is of immense importance to help clinicians initiate timely interventions with appropriate treatment and thus prevent the graft loss. In recent years an increased area of research has been dedicated to developing noninvasive CAD systems for renal transplant function assessment, utilizing different image modalities (e.g., ultrasound, computed tomography (CT), MRI, etc.). Accurate assessment of renal transplant function is critically important for graft survival. Although transplantation can improve a patient's wellbeing, there is a potential post-transplantation risk of kidney dysfunction that, if not treated in a timely manner, can lead to the loss of the entire graft, and even patient death. Thus, accurate assessment of renal transplant function is crucial for the identification of proper treatment. In recent years, an area of increased research has been in developing non-invasive image-based CAD systems for the assessment of renal transplant function. In particular, dynamic and diffusion MRI-based systems have been clinically used to assess transplanted kidneys with the advantage of providing information on each kidney separately. For more details about renal transplant functional assessment, please read [33–50, 50–58].

This work also has important application to the heart. The clinical assessment of myocardial perfusion plays a major role in the diagnosis, management, and prognosis of ischemic heart disease patients. Thus, there have been ongoing efforts to develop automated systems for accurate analysis of myocardial perfusion using first-pass images [59–75].

Another application for this work could be the detection of retinal abnormalities. The majority of ophthalmologists depend on visual interpretation for the identification of diseases types. However, inaccurate diagnosis will affect the treatment procedure which may lead to fatal results. Hence, there is a crucial need for computer automated diagnosis systems that yield highly accurate results. Optical coherence tomography (OCT) has become a powerful modality for the non-invasive diagnosis of various retinal abnormalities such as glaucoma, diabetic macular edema, and macular degeneration. The problem with diabetic retinopathy (DR) is that the patient is not aware of the disease until changes in the retina have progressed to a level to which treatment tends to be less effective. Therefore, automated early detection could limit the severity of the disease and assist ophthalmologists in investigating and treating it more efficiently [76, 77].

Abnormalities of the lung could also be another promising area of research and a related application to this work. Radiation-induced lung injury is the main side effect of radiation therapy for lung cancer patients. Although higher radiation doses increase the radiation therapy effectiveness for tumor control, this can lead to lung injury as a greater quantity of normal lung tissues is included in the treated area. Almost one-third of patients who undergo radiation therapy develop lung injury following radiation treatment. The severity of radiation-induced lung injury ranges from ground-glass opacities and consolidation at the early phase, to fibrosis and traction bronchiectasis in the late phase. Early detection of lung injury will thus help to improve management of the treatment [78–121].

This work can also be applied to other brain abnormalities, such as Dyslexia and autism. Dyslexia is one of the most complicated developmental brain disorders affecting children's learning abilities. Dyslexia leads to the failure to develop age-appropriate reading skills in spite of a normal intelligence level and adequate reading instructions. Neuropathological studies have revealed an abnormal anatomy of some structures, such as the Corpus Callosum in dyslexic brains. There has been a lot of work in the literature that aims at developing CAD systems for diagnosing this condition along with other brain disorders [122–143].

For the vascular system [144], this work could also be applied for the extraction of blood vessels e.g., from phase contrast (PC) magnetic resonance angiography (MRA). Accurate cerebrovascular segmentation using non-invasive MRA is crucial for the early diagnosis and timely treatment of intracranial vascular diseases [127, 128, 145, 146].

References

1. S. Osher and R. P. Fedkiw, "Level set methods: an overview and some recent results," *Journal of Computational Physics*, vol. 169, no. 2, pp. 463–502, 2001.
2. M. Kass, A. Witkin, and D. Terzopoulos, "Snakes: Active contour models," *International Journal of Computer Vision*, vol. 1, no. 4, pp. 321–331, 1988.
3. A. S. El-Baz, A. A. Farag, H. A. El Munim, and S. E. Yuksel, "Level set segmentation using statistical shape priors," in *Computer Vision and Pattern Recognition Workshop, 2006. CVPRW'06. Conference on*. IEEE, 2006, pp. 78–78.
4. A. A. Amini, T. E. Weymouth, and R. C. Jain, "Using dynamic programming for solving variational problems in vision," *IEEE Transactions on Pattern Analysis and Machine Intelligence*, vol. 12, no. 9, pp. 855–867, 1990.
5. D. J. Williams and M. Shah, "A fast algorithm for active contours and curvature estimation," *CVGIP: Image Understanding*, vol. 55, no. 1, pp. 14–26, 1992.
6. Y. Wong, P. C. Yuen, and C. S. Tong, "Segmented snake for contour detection," *Pattern Recognition*, vol. 31, no. 11, pp. 1669–1679, 1998.
7. M. Wang, J. Evans, L. Hassebrook, and C. Knapp, "A multistage, optimal active contour model," *IEEE Transactions on Image Processing*, vol. 5, no. 11, pp. 1586–1591, 1996.
8. A. S. El-Baz, "Novel stochastic models for medical image analysis," Ph.D. dissertation, J.B. Speed School of Engineering, University of Louisville, 2006.
9. M. E. Leventon, W. E. L. Grimson, and O. Faugeras, "Statistical shape influence in geodesic active contours," in *Computer Vision and Pattern Recognition, 2000. Proceedings. IEEE Conference on*, vol. 1. IEEE, 2000, pp. 316–323.

10. D. Shen and C. Davatzikos, "An adaptive-focus deformable model using statistical and geometric information," *IEEE Transactions on Pattern Analysis and Machine Intelligence*, vol. 22, no. 8, pp. 906–913, 2000.
11. A. Tsai, A. Yezzi, W. Wells, C. Tempany, D. Tucker, A. Fan, W. E. Grimson, and A. Willsky, "A shape-based approach to the segmentation of medical imagery using level sets," *IEEE Transactions on Medical Imaging*, vol. 22, no. 2, pp. 137–154, 2003.
12. A. Tsai, W. Wells, C. Tempany, E. Grimson, and A. Willsky, "Mutual information in coupled multi-shape model for medical image segmentation," *Medical Image Analysis*, vol. 8, no. 4, pp. 429–445, 2004.
13. K. Pohl, J. Fisher, M. Shenton, R. McCarley, W. Grimson, R. Kikinis, and W. Wells, "Logarithm odds maps for shape representation," *Medical Image Computing and Computer-Assisted Intervention–MICCAI 2006*, pp. 955–963, 2006.
14. J. Yang and J. S. Duncan, "3d image segmentation of deformable objects with joint shape-intensity prior models using level sets," *Medical Image Analysis*, vol. 8, no. 3, pp. 285–294, 2004.
15. X. Huang, D. Metaxas, and T. Chen, "Metamorphs: Deformable shape and texture models," in *Computer Vision and Pattern Recognition, 2004. CVPR 2004. Proceedings of the 2004 IEEE Computer Society Conference on*, vol. 1. IEEE, 2004, pp. I–I.
16. M. Rousson, N. Paragios, and R. Deriche, "Implicit active shape models for 3d segmentation in mr imaging," in *International Conference on Medical Image Computing and Computer-Assisted Intervention*. Springer, 2004, pp. 209–216.
17. M. E. Leventon, "Statistical models in medical image analysis," Ph.D. dissertation, Citeseer, 2000.
18. T. B. Sebastian, P. N. Klein, and B. B. Kimia, "Recognition of shapes by editing shock graphs." in *ICCV*, vol. 1, 2001, pp. 755–762.
19. K. Siddiqi, A. Shokoufandeh, S. Dickenson, and S. W. Zucker, "Shock graphs and shape matching," in *Computer Vision, 1998. Sixth International Conference on*. IEEE, 1998, pp. 222–229.
20. S. Osher and J. A. Sethian, "Fronts propagating with curvature-dependent speed: algorithms based on hamilton-jacobi formulations," *Journal of Computational Physics*, vol. 79, no. 1, pp. 12–49, 1988.
21. J. A. Sethian, *Level set methods and fast marching methods: evolving interfaces in computational geometry, fluid mechanics, computer vision, and materials science*. Cambridge University Press, 1999, vol. 3.
22. R. Malladi, J. A. Sethian, and B. C. Vemuri, "Shape modeling with front propagation: A level set approach," *IEEE Transactions on Pattern Analysis and Machine Intelligence*, vol. 17, no. 2, pp. 158–175, 1995.
23. J. Gomes and O. Faugeras, "Reconciling distance functions and level sets," in *Biomedical Imaging, 2002. 5th IEEE EMBS International Summer School on*. IEEE, 2002, pp. 15–pp.
24. N. Paragios and R. Deriche, "Unifying boundary and region-based information for geodesic active tracking," in *Computer Vision and Pattern Recognition, 1999. IEEE Computer Society Conference on.*, vol. 2. IEEE, 1999, pp. 300–305.
25. X. Zeng, L. H. Staib, R. T. Schultz, H. Tagare, L. Win, and J. S. Duncan, "A new approach to 3d sulcal ribbon finding from mr images," in *International Conference on Medical Image Computing and Computer-Assisted Intervention*. Springer, 1999, pp. 148–157.

26. R. O. Duda, P. E. Hart, and D. G. Stork, *Pattern classification.* John Wiley & Sons, 2012.
27. C. Samson, L. Blanc-Féraud, G. Aubert, and J. Zerubia, "Multiphase evolution and variational image classification," Ph.D. dissertation, INRIA, 1999.
28. T. K. Moon, "The expectation-maximization algorithm," *IEEE Signal Processing Magazine*, vol. 13, no. 6, pp. 47–60, Nov 1996.
29. G. Gimel'farb, A. A. Farag, and A. El-Baz, "Expectation-maximization for a linear combination of gaussians," in *Proceedings of the 17th International Conference on Pattern Recognition, 2004. ICPR 2004.*, vol. 3, Aug 2004, pp. 422–425 Vol. 3.
30. P. Viola and W. M. Wells, "Alignment by maximization of mutual information," in *Computer Vision, 1995. Proceedings., Fifth International Conference on.* IEEE, 1995, pp. 16–23.
31. S. Ourselin, A. Roche, S. Prima, and N. Ayache, "Block matching: A general framework to improve robustness of rigid registration of medical images," in *International Conference on Medical Image Computing And Computer-Assisted Intervention.* Springer, 2000, pp. 557–566.
32. Y. Zhang, B. J. Matuszewski, L.-K. Shark, and C. J. Moore, "Medical image segmentation using new hybrid level-set method," in *BioMedical Visualization, 2008. MEDIVIS'08. Fifth International Conference.* IEEE, 2008, pp. 71–76.
33. A. M. Ali, A. A. Farag, and A. El-Baz, "Graph cuts framework for kidney segmentation with prior shape constraints," in *Proceedings of International Conference on Medical Image Computing and Computer-Assisted Intervention, (MICCAI'07)*, vol. 1, Brisbane, Australia, October 29–November 2, 2007, pp. 384–392.
34. A. S. Chowdhury, R. Roy, S. Bose, F. K. A. Elnakib, and A. El-Baz, "Non-rigid biomedical image registration using graph cuts with a novel data term," in *Proceedings of IEEE International Symposium on Biomedical Imaging: From Nano to Macro, (ISBI'12)*, Barcelona, Spain, May 2–5, 2012, pp. 446–449.
35. A. El-Baz, A. A. Farag, S. E. Yuksel, M. E. El-Ghar, T. A. Eldiasty, and M. A. Ghoneim, "Application of deformable models for the detection of acute renal rejection," in *Deformable models.* Springer, New York, NY, 2007, pp. 293–333.
36. A. El-Baz, A. Farag, R. Fahmi, S. Yuksel, M. A. El-Ghar, and T. Eldiasty, "Image analysis of renal DCE MRI for the detection of acute renal rejection," in *Proceedings of IAPR International Conference on Pattern Recognition (ICPR'06)*, Hong Kong, August 20–24, 2006, pp. 822–825.
37. A. El-Baz, A. Farag, R. Fahmi, S. Yuksel, W. Miller, M. A. El-Ghar, T. El-Diasty, and M. Ghoneim, "A new CAD system for the evaluation of kidney diseases using DCE-MRI," in *Proceedings of International Conference on Medical Image Computing and Computer-Assisted Intervention, (MICCAI'08)*, Copenhagen, Denmark, October 1–6, 2006, pp. 446–453.
38. A. El-Baz, G. Gimel'farb, and M. A. El-Ghar, "A novel image analysis approach for accurate identification of acute renal rejection," in *Proceedings of IEEE International Conference on Image Processing, (ICIP'08)*, San Diego, California, USA, October 12–15, 2008, pp. 1812–1815.
39. ——, "Image analysis approach for identification of renal transplant rejection," in *Proceedings of IAPR International Conference on Pattern Recognition, (ICPR'08)*, Tampa, Florida, USA, December 8–11, 2008, pp. 1–4.
40. ——, "New motion correction models for automatic identification of renal transplant rejection," in *Proceedings of International Conference on Medical Image*

Computing and Computer-Assisted Intervention, (MICCAI'07), Brisbane, Australia, October 29–November 2, 2007, pp. 235–243.

41. A. Farag, A. El-Baz, S. Yuksel, M. A. El-Ghar, and T. Eldiasty, "A framework for the detection of acute rejection with Dynamic Contrast Enhanced Magnetic Resonance Imaging," in *Proceedings of IEEE International Symposium on Biomedical Imaging: From Nano to Macro, (ISBI'06)*, Arlington, Virginia, USA, April 6–9, 2006, pp. 418–421.
42. F. Khalifa, G. M. Beache, M. A. El-Ghar, T. El-Diasty, G. Gimel'farb, M. Kong, and A. El-Baz, "Dynamic contrast-enhanced MRI-based early detection of acute renal transplant rejection," *IEEE Transactions on Medical Imaging*, vol. 32, no. 10, pp. 1910–1927, 2013.
43. F. Khalifa, A. El-Baz, G. Gimel'farb, and M. A. El-Ghar, "Non-invasive image-based approach for early detection of acute renal rejection," in *Proceedings of International Conference Medical Image Computing and Computer-Assisted Intervention, (MICCAI'10)*, Beijing, China, September 20–24, 2010, pp. 10–18.
44. F. Khalifa, A. El-Baz, G. Gimel'farb, R. Ouseph, and M. A. El-Ghar, "Shape-appearance guided level-set deformable model for image segmentation," in *Proceedings of IAPR International Conference on Pattern Recognition, (ICPR'10)*, Istanbul, Turkey, August 23–26, 2010, pp. 4581–4584.
45. F. Khalifa, M. A. El-Ghar, B. Abdollahi, H. Frieboes, T. El-Diasty, and A. El-Baz, "A comprehensive non-invasive framework for automated evaluation of acute renal transplant rejection using DCE-MRI," *NMR in Biomedicine*, vol. 26, no. 11, pp. 1460–1470, 2013.
46. F. Khalifa, M. A. El-Ghar, B. Abdollahi, H. B. Frieboes, T. El-Diasty, and A. El-Baz, "Dynamic contrast-enhanced MRI-based early detection of acute renal transplant rejection," in *2014 Annual Scientific Meeting and Educational Course Brochure of the Society of Abdominal Radiology, (SAR'14)*, Boca Raton, Florida, March 23–28, 2014, p. CID: 1855912.
47. F. Khalifa, A. Elnakib, G. M. Beache, G. Gimel'farb, M. A. El-Ghar, G. Sokhadze, S. Manning, P. McClure, and A. El-Baz, "3D kidney segmentation from CT images using a level set approach guided by a novel stochastic speed function," in *Proceedings of International Conference Medical Image Computing and Computer-Assisted Intervention, (MICCAI'11)*, Toronto, Canada, September 18–22, 2011, pp. 587–594.
48. F. Khalifa, G. Gimel'farb, M. A. El-Ghar, G. Sokhadze, S. Manning, P. McClure, R. Ouseph, and A. El-Baz, "A new deformable model-based segmentation approach for accurate extraction of the kidney from abdominal CT images," in *Proceedings of IEEE International Conference on Image Processing, (ICIP'11)*, Brussels, Belgium, September 11–14, 2011, pp. 3393–3396.
49. M. Mostapha, F. Khalifa, A. Alansary, A. Soliman, J. Suri, and A. El-Baz, "Computer-aided diagnosis systems for acute renal transplant rejection: Challenges and methodologies," in *Abdomen and Thoracic Imaging*, A. El-Baz and L. saba J. Suri, Eds. Springer, 2014, pp. 1–35.
50. M. Shehata, F. Khalifa, E. Hollis, A. Soliman, E. Hosseini-Asl, M. A. El-Ghar, M. El-Baz, A. C. Dwyer, A. El-Baz, and R. Keynton, "A new non-invasive approach for early classification of renal rejection types using diffusion-weighted mri," in *IEEE International Conference on Image Processing (ICIP), 2016*. IEEE, 2016, pp. 136–140.

51. F. Khalifa, A. Soliman, A. Takieldeen, M. Shehata, M. Mostapha, A. Shaffie, R. Ouseph, A. Elmaghraby, and A. El-Baz, "Kidney segmentation from CT images using a 3D NMF-guided active contour model," in *IEEE 13th International Symposium on Biomedical Imaging (ISBI), 2016*. IEEE, 2016, pp. 432–435.
52. M. Shehata, F. Khalifa, A. Soliman, A. Takieldeen, M. A. El-Ghar, A. Shaffie, A. C. Dwyer, R. Ouseph, A. El-Baz, and R. Keynton, "3d diffusion mri-based cad system for early diagnosis of acute renal rejection," in *Biomedical Imaging (ISBI), 2016 IEEE 13th International Symposium on*. IEEE, 2016, pp. 1177–1180.
53. M. Shehata, F. Khalifa, A. Soliman, R. Alrefai, M. A. El-Ghar, A. C. Dwyer, R. Ouseph, and A. El-Baz, "A level set-based framework for 3d kidney segmentation from diffusion mr images," in *IEEE International Conference on Image Processing (ICIP), 2015*. IEEE, 2015, pp. 4441–4445.
54. M. Shehata, F. Khalifa, A. Soliman, M. A. El-Ghar, A. C. Dwyer, G. Gimel'farb, R. Keynton, and A. El-Baz, "A promising non-invasive cad system for kidney function assessment," in *International Conference on Medical Image Computing and Computer-Assisted Intervention*. Springer, 2016, pp. 613–621.
55. F. Khalifa, A. Soliman, A. Elmaghraby, G. Gimel'farb, and A. El-Baz, "3d kidney segmentation from abdominal images using spatial-appearance models," *Computational and mathematical methods in medicine*, vol. 2017, pp. 1–10, 2017.
56. E. Hollis, M. Shehata, F. Khalifa, M. A. El-Ghar, T. El-Diasty, and A. El-Baz, "Towards non-invasive diagnostic techniques for early detection of acute renal transplant rejection: A review," *The Egyptian Journal of Radiology and Nuclear Medicine*, vol. 48, no. 1, pp. 257–269, 2016.
57. M. Shehata, F. Khalifa, A. Soliman, M. A. El-Ghar, A. C. Dwyer, and A. El-Baz, "Assessment of renal transplant using image and clinical-based biomarkers," in *Proceedings of 13th Annual Scientific Meeting of American Society for Diagnostics and Interventional Nephrology (ASDIN'17), New Orleans, LA, USA, February 10-12, 2017*, 2017.
58. ——, "Early assessment of acute renal rejection," in *Proceedings of 12th Annual Scientific Meeting of American Society for Diagnostics and Interventional Nephrology (ASDIN'16), Pheonix, AZ, USA, February 19-21, 2016*, 2017.
59. F. Khalifa, G. Beache, A. El-Baz, and G. Gimel'farb, "Deformable model guided by stochastic speed with application in cine images segmentation," in *Proceedings of IEEE International Conference on Image Processing, (ICIP'10)*, Hong Kong, September 26–29, 2010, pp. 1725–1728.
60. F. Khalifa, G. M. Beache, A. Elnakib, H. Sliman, G. Gimel'farb, K. C. Welch, and A. El-Baz, "A new shape-based framework for the left ventricle wall segmentation from cardiac first-pass perfusion MRI," in *Proceedings of IEEE International Symposium on Biomedical Imaging: From Nano to Macro, (ISBI'13)*, San Francisco, CA, April 7–11, 2013, pp. 41–44.
61. ——, "A new nonrigid registration framework for improved visualization of transmural perfusion gradients on cardiac first–pass perfusion MRI," in *Proceedings of IEEE International Symposium on Biomedical Imaging: From Nano to Macro, (ISBI'12)*, Barcelona, Spain, May 2–5, 2012, pp. 828–831.
62. F. Khalifa, G. M. Beache, A. Firjani, K. C. Welch, G. Gimel'farb, and A. El-Baz, "A new nonrigid registration approach for motion correction of cardiac first-pass perfusion MRI," in *Proceedings of IEEE International Conference on Image Processing, (ICIP'12)*, Lake Buena Vista, Florida, September 30–October 3, 2012, pp. 1665–1668.

63. F. Khalifa, G. M. Beache, G. Gimel'farb, and A. El-Baz, "A novel CAD system for analyzing cardiac first-pass MR images," in *Proceedings of IAPR International Conference on Pattern Recognition (ICPR'12)*, Tsukuba Science City, Japan, November 11–15, 2012, pp. 77–80.
64. ——, "A novel approach for accurate estimation of left ventricle global indexes from short-axis cine MRI," in *Proceedings of IEEE International Conference on Image Processing, (ICIP'11)*, Brussels, Belgium, September 11–14, 2011, pp. 2645–2649.
65. F. Khalifa, G. M. Beache, G. Gimel'farb, G. A. Giridharan, and A. El-Baz, "A new image-based framework for analyzing cine images," in *Handbook of Multi Modality State-of-the-Art Medical Image Segmentation and Registration Methodologies*, A. El-Baz, U. R. Acharya, M. Mirmedhdi, and J. S. Suri, Eds. Springer, New York, 2011, vol. 2, ch. 3, pp. 69–98.
66. ——, "Accurate automatic analysis of cardiac cine images," *IEEE Transactions on Biomedical Engineering*, vol. 59, no. 2, pp. 445–455, 2012.
67. F. Khalifa, G. M. Beache, M. Nitzken, G. Gimel'farb, G. A. Giridharan, and A. El-Baz, "Automatic analysis of left ventricle wall thickness using short-axis cine CMR images," in *Proceedings of IEEE International Symposium on Biomedical Imaging: From Nano to Macro, (ISBI'11)*, Chicago, Illinois, March 30–April 2, 2011, pp. 1306–1309.
68. M. Nitzken, G. Beache, A. Elnakib, F. Khalifa, G. Gimel'farb, and A. El-Baz, "Accurate modeling of tagged cmr 3D image appearance characteristics to improve cardiac cycle strain estimation," in *Image Processing (ICIP), 2012 19th IEEE International Conference on*. Orlando, Florida, USA: IEEE, Sep. 2012, pp. 521–524.
69. ——, "Improving full-cardiac cycle strain estimation from tagged cmr by accurate modeling of 3D image appearance characteristics," in *Biomedical Imaging (ISBI), 2012 9th IEEE International Symposium on*. Barcelona, Spain: IEEE, May 2012, pp. 462–465, (Selected for oral presentation).
70. M. J. Nitzken, A. S. El-Baz, and G. M. Beache, "Markov-gibbs random field model for improved full-cardiac cycle strain estimation from tagged cmr," *Journal of Cardiovascular Magnetic Resonance*, vol. 14, no. 1, pp. 1–2, 2012.
71. H. Sliman, A. Elnakib, G. Beache, A. Elmaghraby, and A. El-Baz, "Assessment of myocardial function from cine cardiac MRI using a novel 4D tracking approach," *J Comput Sci Syst Biol*, vol. 7, pp. 169–173, 2014.
72. H. Sliman, A. Elnakib, G. M. Beache, A. Soliman, F. Khalifa, G. Gimel'farb, A. Elmaghraby, and A. El-Baz, "A novel 4D PDE-based approach for accurate assessment of myocardium function using cine cardiac magnetic resonance images," in *Proceedings of IEEE International Conference on Image Processing (ICIP'14)*, Paris, France, October 27–30, 2014, pp. 3537–3541.
73. H. Sliman, F. Khalifa, A. Elnakib, G. M. Beache, A. Elmaghraby, and A. El-Baz, "A new segmentation-based tracking framework for extracting the left ventricle cavity from cine cardiac MRI," in *Proceedings of IEEE International Conference on Image Processing, (ICIP'13)*, Melbourne, Australia, September 15–18, 2013, pp. 685–689.
74. H. Sliman, F. Khalifa, A. Elnakib, A. Soliman, G. M. Beache, A. Elmaghraby, G. Gimel'farb, and A. El-Baz, "Myocardial borders segmentation from cine MR images using bi-directional coupled parametric deformable models," *Medical Physics*, vol. 40, no. 9, pp. 1–13, 2013.
75. H. Sliman, F. Khalifa, A. Elnakib, A. Soliman, G. M. Beache, G. Gimel'farb, A. Emam, A. Elmaghraby, and A. El-Baz, "Accurate segmentation framework

for the left ventricle wall from cardiac cine MRI," in *Proceedings of International Symposium on Computational Models for Life Science, (CMLS'13)*, vol. 1559, Sydney, Australia, November 27–29, 2013, pp. 287–296.

76. N. Eladawi, M. Elmogy, M. Ghazal, O. Helmy, A. Aboelfetouh, A. Riad, S. Schaal, and A. El-Baz, "Classification of retinal diseases based on oct images," *Front Biosci (Landmark Ed)*, vol. 23, pp. 247–264, 2018.
77. A. ElTanboly, M. Ismail, A. Shalaby, A. Switala, A. El-Baz, S. Schaal, G. Gimel'farb, and M. El-Azab, "A computer-aided diagnostic system for detecting diabetic retinopathy in optical coherence tomography images," *Medical Physics*, vol. 44, no. 3, pp. 914–923, 2017.
78. B. Abdollahi, A. C. Civelek, X.-F. Li, J. Suri, and A. El-Baz, "PET/CT nodule segmentation and diagnosis: A survey," in *Multi Detector CT Imaging*, L. Saba and J. S. Suri, Eds. Taylor , Francis, 2014, ch. 30, pp. 639–651.
79. B. Abdollahi, A. El-Baz, and A. A. Amini, "A multi-scale non-linear vessel enhancement technique," in *Engineering in Medicine and Biology Society, EMBC, 2011 Annual International Conference of the IEEE*. IEEE, 2011, pp. 3925–3929.
80. B. Abdollahi, A. Soliman, A. Civelek, X.-F. Li, G. Gimel'farb, and A. El-Baz, "A novel gaussian scale space-based joint MGRF framework for precise lung segmentation," in *Proceedings of IEEE International Conference on Image Processing, (ICIP'12)*. IEEE, 2012, pp. 2029–2032.
81. B. Abdollahi, A. Soliman, A. Civelek, X.-F. Li, G. Gimel'farb, and A. El-Baz, "A novel 3D joint MGRF framework for precise lung segmentation," in *Machine Learning in Medical Imaging*. Springer, 2012, pp. 86–93.
82. A. M. Ali, A. S. El-Baz, and A. A. Farag, "A novel framework for accurate lung segmentation using graph cuts," in *Proceedings of IEEE International Symposium on Biomedical Imaging: From Nano to Macro, (ISBI'07)*. IEEE, 2007, pp. 908–911.
83. A. El-Baz, G. M. Beache, G. Gimel'farb, K. Suzuki, and K. Okada, "Lung imaging data analysis," *International journal of biomedical imaging*, vol. 2013, pp. 1–2, 2013.
84. A. El-Baz, G. M. Beache, G. Gimel'farb, K. Suzuki, K. Okada, A. Elnakib, A. Soliman, and B. Abdollahi, "Computer-aided diagnosis systems for lung cancer: Challenges and methodologies," *International Journal of Biomedical Imaging*, vol. 2013, pp. 1–46, 2013.
85. A. El-Baz, A. Elnakib, M. Abou El-Ghar, G. Gimel'farb, R. Falk, and A. Farag, "Automatic detection of 2D and 3D lung nodules in chest spiral CT scans," *International Journal of Biomedical Imaging*, vol. 2013, pp. 1–11, 2013.
86. A. El-Baz, A. A. Farag, R. Falk, and R. La Rocca, "A unified approach for detection, visualization, and identification of lung abnormalities in chest spiral CT scans," in *International Congress Series*, vol. 1256. Elsevier, 2003, pp. 998–1004.
87. ——, "Detection, visualization and identification of lung abnormalities in chest spiral CT scan: Phase-I," in *Proceedings of International conference on Biomedical Engineering, Cairo, Egypt*, vol. 12, no. 1, 2002.
88. A. El-Baz, A. Farag, G. Gimel'farb, R. Falk, M. A. El-Ghar, and T. Eldiasty, "A framework for automatic segmentation of lung nodules from low dose chest CT scans," in *Proceedings of International Conference on Pattern Recognition, (ICPR'06)*, vol. 3. IEEE, 2006, pp. 611–614.
89. A. El-Baz, A. Farag, G. Gimel'farb, R. Falk, and M. A. El-Ghar, "A novel level set-based computer-aided detection system for automatic detection of lung nodules in low dose chest computed tomography scans," *Lung Imaging and Computer Aided Diagnosis*, vol. 10, pp. 221–238, 2011.

90. A. El-Baz, G. Gimel'farb, M. Abou El-Ghar, and R. Falk, "Appearance-based diagnostic system for early assessment of malignant lung nodules," in *Proceedings of IEEE International Conference on Image Processing, (ICIP'12)*. IEEE, 2012, pp. 533–536.
91. A. El-Baz, G. Gimel'farb, and R. Falk, "A novel 3D framework for automatic lung segmentation from low dose CT images," in *Lung Imaging and Computer Aided Diagnosis*, A. El-Baz and J. S. Suri, Eds. Taylor , Francis, 2011, ch. 1, pp. 1–16.
92. A. El-Baz, G. Gimel'farb, R. Falk, and M. El-Ghar, "Appearance analysis for diagnosing malignant lung nodules," in *Proceedings of IEEE International Symposium on Biomedical Imaging: From Nano to Macro (ISBI'10)*. IEEE, 2010, pp. 193–196.
93. A. El-Baz, G. Gimel'farb, R. Falk, and M. A. El-Ghar, "A novel level set-based CAD system for automatic detection of lung nodules in low dose chest CT scans," in *Lung Imaging and Computer Aided Diagnosis*, A. El-Baz and J. S. Suri, Eds. Taylor , Francis, 2011, vol. 1, ch. 10, pp. 221–238.
94. ——, "A new approach for automatic analysis of 3D low dose CT images for accurate monitoring the detected lung nodules," in *Proceedings of International Conference on Pattern Recognition, (ICPR'08)*. IEEE, 2008, pp. 1–4.
95. ——, "A novel approach for automatic follow-up of detected lung nodules," in *Proceedings of IEEE International Conference on Image Processing, (ICIP'07)*, vol. 5. IEEE, 2007, pp. V–501.
96. ——, "A new CAD system for early diagnosis of detected lung nodules," in *Image Processing, 2007. ICIP 2007. IEEE International Conference on*, vol. 2. IEEE, 2007, pp. II–461.
97. A. El-Baz, G. Gimel'farb, R. Falk, M. A. El-Ghar, and H. Refaie, "Promising results for early diagnosis of lung cancer," in *Proceedings of IEEE International Symposium on Biomedical Imaging: From Nano to Macro, (ISBI'08)*. IEEE, 2008, pp. 1151–1154.
98. A. El-Baz, G. L. Gimel'farb, R. Falk, M. Abou El-Ghar, T. Holland, and T. Shaffer, "A new stochastic framework for accurate lung segmentation," in *Proceedings of Medical Image Computing and Computer-Assisted Intervention, (MICCAI'08)*, 2008, pp. 322–330.
99. A. El-Baz, G. L. Gimel'farb, R. Falk, D. Heredis, and M. Abou El-Ghar, "A novel approach for accurate estimation of the growth rate of the detected lung nodules," in *Proceedings of International Workshop on Pulmonary Image Analysis*, 2008, pp. 33–42.
100. A. El-Baz, G. L. Gimel'farb, R. Falk, T. Holland, and T. Shaffer, "A framework for unsupervised segmentation of lung tissues from low dose computed tomography images," in *Proceedings of British Machine Vision, (BMVC'08)*, 2008, pp. 1–10.
101. A. El-Baz, G. Gimel'farb, R. Falk, and M. A. El-Ghar, "3D MGRF-based appearance modeling for robust segmentation of pulmonary nodules in 3D LDCT chest images," in *Lung Imaging and Computer Aided Diagnosis*. 2011, ch. 3, pp. 51–63.
102. ——, "Automatic analysis of 3D low dose CT images for early diagnosis of lung cancer," *Pattern Recognition*, vol. 42, no. 6, pp. 1041–1051, 2009.
103. A. El-Baz, G. Gimel'farb, R. Falk, M. A. El-Ghar, S. Rainey, D. Heredia, and T. Shaffer, "Toward early diagnosis of lung cancer," in *Proceedings of Medical Image Computing and Computer-Assisted Intervention, (MICCAI'09)*. Springer, 2009, pp. 682–689.

104. A. El-Baz, G. Gimel'farb, R. Falk, M. A. El-Ghar, and J. Suri, "Appearance analysis for the early assessment of detected lung nodules," in *Lung Imaging and Computer Aided Diagnosis*. 2011, ch. 17, pp. 395–404.
105. A. El-Baz, F. Khalifa, A. Elnakib, M. Nitkzen, A. Soliman, P. McClure, G. Gimel'farb, and M. A. El-Ghar, "A novel approach for global lung registration using 3D Markov Gibbs appearance model," in *Proceedings of International Conference Medical Image Computing and Computer-Assisted Intervention, (MICCAI'12)*, Nice, France, October 1–5, 2012, pp. 114–121.
106. A. El-Baz, M. Nitzken, A. Elnakib, F. Khalifa, G. Gimel'farb, R. Falk, and M. A. El-Ghar, "3D shape analysis for early diagnosis of malignant lung nodules," in *Proceedings of International Conference Medical Image Computing and Computer-Assisted Intervention, (MICCAI'11)*, Toronto, Canada, September 18–22, 2011, pp. 175–182.
107. A. El-Baz, M. Nitzken, G. Gimel'farb, E. Van Bogaert, R. Falk, M. A. El-Ghar, and J. Suri, "Three-dimensional shape analysis using spherical harmonics for early assessment of detected lung nodules," in *Lung Imaging and Computer Aided Diagnosis*. 2011, ch. 19, pp. 421–438.
108. A. El-Baz, M. Nitzken, F. Khalifa, A. Elnakib, G. Gimel'farb, R. Falk, and M. A. El-Ghar, "3D shape analysis for early diagnosis of malignant lung nodules," in *Proceedings of International Conference on Information Processing in Medical Imaging, (IPMI'11)*, Monastery Irsee, Germany (Bavaria), July 3–8, 2011, pp. 772–783.
109. A. El-Baz, M. Nitzken, E. Vanbogaert, G. Gimel'Farb, R. Falk, and M. Abo El-Ghar, "A novel shape-based diagnostic approach for early diagnosis of lung nodules," in *Biomedical Imaging: From Nano to Macro, 2011 IEEE International Symposium on*. IEEE, 2011, pp. 137–140.
110. A. El-Baz, P. Sethu, G. Gimel'farb, F. Khalifa, A. Elnakib, R. Falk, and M. A. El-Ghar, "Elastic phantoms generated by microfluidics technology: Validation of an imaged-based approach for accurate measurement of the growth rate of lung nodules," *Biotechnology Journal*, vol. 6, no. 2, pp. 195–203, 2011.
111. ——, "A new validation approach for the growth rate measurement using elastic phantoms generated by state-of-the-art microfluidics technology," in *Proceedings of IEEE International Conference on Image Processing, (ICIP'10)*, Hong Kong, September 26–29, 2010, pp. 4381–4383.
112. A. El-Baz, P. Sethu, G. Gimel'farb, F. Khalifa, A. Elnakib, R. Falk, and M. A. E.-G. J. Suri, "Validation of a new imaged-based approach for the accurate estimating of the growth rate of detected lung nodules using real CT images and elastic phantoms generated by state-of-the-art microfluidics technology," in *Handbook of Lung Imaging and Computer Aided Diagnosis*, A. El-Baz and J. S. Suri, Eds. Taylor & Francis, New York, 2011, vol. 1, ch. 18, pp. 405–420.
113. A. El-Baz, A. Soliman, P. McClure, G. Gimel'farb, M. A. El-Ghar, and R. Falk, "Early assessment of malignant lung nodules based on the spatial analysis of detected lung nodules," in *Proceedings of IEEE International Symposium on Biomedical Imaging: From Nano to Macro, (ISBI'12)*. IEEE, 2012, pp. 1463–1466.
114. A. El-Baz, S. E. Yuksel, S. Elshazly, and A. A. Farag, "Non-rigid registration techniques for automatic follow-up of lung nodules," in *Proceedings of Computer Assisted Radiology and Surgery, (CARS'05)*, vol. 1281. Elsevier, 2005, pp. 1115–1120.
115. A. S. El-Baz and J. S. Suri, *Lung Imaging and Computer Aided Diagnosis*. CRC Press, 2011.

116. A. oliman, F. Khalifa, A. Shaffie, N. Liu, N. Dunlap, B. Wang, A. Elmaghraby, G. Gimel'farb, and A. El-Baz, "Image-based cad system for accurate identification of lung injury," in *Proceedings of IEEE International Conference on Image Processing, (ICIP'16)*. IEEE, 2016, pp. 121–125.
117. A. Soliman, F. Khalifa, N. Dunlap, B. Wang, M. El-Ghar, and A. El-Baz, "An iso-surfaces based local deformation handling framework of lung tissues," in *Biomedical Imaging (ISBI), 2016 IEEE 13th International Symposium on*. IEEE, 2016, pp. 1253–1259.
118. A. Soliman, F. Khalifa, A. Shaffie, N. Dunlap, B. Wang, A. Elmaghraby, and A. El-Baz, "Detection of lung injury using 4d-ct chest images," in *Biomedical Imaging (ISBI), 2016 IEEE 13th International Symposium on*. IEEE, 2016, pp. 1274–1277.
119. A. Soliman, F. Khalifa, A. Shaffie, N. Dunlap, B. Wang, A. Elmaghraby, G. Gimel'farb, M. Ghazal, and A. El-Baz, "A comprehensive framework for early assessment of lung injury," in *Image Processing (ICIP), 2017 IEEE International Conference on*. IEEE, 2017, pp. 3275–3279.
120. A. Shaffie, A. Soliman, M. Ghazal, F. Taher, N. Dunlap, B. Wang, A. Elmaghraby, G. Gimel'farb, and A. El-Baz, "A new framework for incorporating appearance and shape features of lung nodules for precise diagnosis of lung cancer," in *Image Processing (ICIP), 2017 IEEE International Conference on*. IEEE, 2017, pp. 1372–1376.
121. A. Soliman, F. Khalifa, A. Shaffie, N. Liu, N. Dunlap, B. Wang, A. Elmaghraby, G. Gimel'farb, and A. El-Baz, "Image-based cad system for accurate identification of lung injury," in *Image Processing (ICIP), 2016 IEEE International Conference on*. IEEE, 2016, pp. 121–125.
122. B. Dombroski, M. Nitzken, A. Elnakib, F. Khalifa, A. El-Baz, and M. F. Casanova, "Cortical surface complexity in a population-based normative sample," *Translational Neuroscience*, vol. 5, no. 1, pp. 17–24, 2014.
123. A. El-Baz, M. Casanova, G. Gimel'farb, M. Mott, and A. Switala, "An MRI-based diagnostic framework for early diagnosis of dyslexia," *International Journal of Computer Assisted Radiology and Surgery*, vol. 3, no. 3-4, pp. 181–189, 2008.
124. A. El-Baz, M. Casanova, G. Gimel'farb, M. Mott, A. Switala, E. Vanbogaert, and R. McCracken, "A new CAD system for early diagnosis of dyslexic brains," in *Proc. International Conference on Image Processing (ICIP'2008)*. IEEE, 2008, pp. 1820–1823.
125. A. El-Baz, M. F. Casanova, G. Gimel'farb, M. Mott, and A. E. Switwala, "A new image analysis approach for automatic classification of autistic brains," in *Proc. IEEE International Symposium on Biomedical Imaging: From Nano to Macro (ISBI'2007)*. IEEE, 2007, pp. 352–355.
126. A. El-Baz, A. Elnakib, F. Khalifa, M. A. El-Ghar, P. McClure, A. Soliman, and G. Gimel'farb, "Precise segmentation of 3-D magnetic resonance angiography," *IEEE Transactions on Biomedical Engineering*, vol. 59, no. 7, pp. 2019–2029, 2012.
127. A. El-Baz, A. Farag, G. Gimel'farb, M. A. El-Ghar, and T. Eldiasty, "Probabilistic modeling of blood vessels for segmenting mra images," in *18th International Conference on Pattern Recognition (ICPR'06)*, vol. 3. IEEE, 2006, pp. 917–920.
128. A. El-Baz, A. A. Farag, G. Gimel'farb, M. A. El-Ghar, and T. Eldiasty, "A new adaptive probabilistic model of blood vessels for segmenting mra images," in *Medical Image Computing and Computer-Assisted Intervention–MICCAI 2006*, vol. 4191. Springer, 2006, pp. 799–806.
129. A. El-Baz, A. A. Farag, G. Gimel'farb, and S. G. Hushek, "Automatic cerebrovascular segmentation by accurate probabilistic modeling of tof-mra

images," in *Medical Image Computing and Computer-Assisted Intervention–MICCAI 2005*. Springer, 2005, pp. 34–42.
130. A. El-Baz, A. Farag, A. Elnakib, M. F. Casanova, G. Gimel'farb, A. E. Switala, D. Jordan, and S. Rainey, "Accurate automated detection of autism related corpus callosum abnormalities," *Journal of Medical Systems*, vol. 35, no. 5, pp. 929–939, 2011.
131. A. El-Baz, A. Farag, and G. Gimel'farb, "Cerebrovascular segmentation by accurate probabilistic modeling of tof-mra images," in *Image Analysis*, vol. 3540. Springer, 2005, pp. 1128–1137.
132. A. El-Baz, G. Gimel'farb, R. Falk, M. A. El-Ghar, V. Kumar, and D. Heredia, "A novel 3D joint Markov-gibbs model for extracting blood vessels from PC–mra images," in *Medical Image Computing and Computer-Assisted Intervention–MICCAI 2009*, vol. 5762. Springer, 2009, pp. 943–950.
133. A. Elnakib, A. El-Baz, M. F. Casanova, G. Gimel'farb, and A. E. Switala, "Image-based detection of corpus callosum variability for more accurate discrimination between dyslexic and normal brains," in *Proc. IEEE International Symposium on Biomedical Imaging: From Nano to Macro (ISBI'2010)*. IEEE, 2010, pp. 109–112.
134. A. Elnakib, M. F. Casanova, G. Gimel'farb, A. E. Switala, and A. El-Baz, "Autism diagnostics by centerline-based shape analysis of the corpus callosum," in *Proc. IEEE International Symposium on Biomedical Imaging: From Nano to Macro (ISBI'2011)*. IEEE, 2011, pp. 1843–1846.
135. A. Elnakib, M. Nitzken, M. Casanova, H. Park, G. Gimel'farb, and A. El-Baz, "Quantification of age-related brain cortex change using 3D shape analysis," in *Pattern Recognition (ICPR), 2012 21st International Conference on*. IEEE, 2012, pp. 41–44.
136. M. Mostapha, A. Soliman, F. Khalifa, A. Elnakib, A. Alansary, M. Nitzken, M. F. Casanova, and A. El-Baz, "A statistical framework for the classification of infant dt images," in *Image Processing (ICIP), 2014 IEEE International Conference on*. IEEE, 2014, pp. 2222–2226.
137. M. Nitzken, M. Casanova, G. Gimel'farb, A. Elnakib, F. Khalifa, A. Switala, and A. El-Baz, "3D shape analysis of the brain cortex with application to dyslexia," in *Image Processing (ICIP), 2011 18th IEEE International Conference on*. Brussels, Belgium: IEEE, Sep. 2011, pp. 2657–2660, (Selected for oral presentation. Oral acceptance rate is 10 percent and the overall acceptance rate is 35 percent).
138. F. E.-Z. A. El-Gamal, M. M. Elmogy, M. Ghazal, A. Atwan, G. N. Barnes, M. F. Casanova, R. Keynton, and A. S. El-Baz, "A novel cad system for local and global early diagnosis of alzheimer's disease based on pib-pet scans," in *2017 IEEE International Conference on Image Processing (ICIP)*. IEEE, 2017, pp. 3270–3274.
139. M. Ismail, A. Soliman, M. Ghazal, A. E. Switala, G. Gimel'farb, G. N. Barnes, A. Khalil, and A. El-Baz, "A fast stochastic framework for automatic mr brain images segmentation," 2017.
140. M. M. Ismail, R. S. Keynton, M. M. Mostapha, A. H. ElTanboly, M. F. Casanova, G. L. Gimel'farb, and A. El-Baz, "Studying autism spectrum disorder with structural and diffusion magnetic resonance imaging: a survey," *Frontiers in Human Neuroscience*, vol. 10, p. 211, 2016.
141. A. Alansary, M. Ismail, A. Soliman, F. Khalifa, M. Nitzken, A. Elnakib, M. Mostapha, A. Black, K. Stinebruner, M. F. Casanova *et al.*, "Infant brain extraction in t1-weighted mr images using bet and refinement using lcdg and

mgrf models," *IEEE Journal of Biomedical and Health Informatics*, vol. 20, no. 3, pp. 925–935, 2016.

142. M. Ismail, A. Soliman, A. ElTanboly, A. Switala, M. Mahmoud, F. Khalifa, G. Gimel'farb, M. F. Casanova, R. Keynton, and A. El-Baz, "Detection of white matter abnormalities in mr brain images for diagnosis of autism in children," pp. 6–9, 2016.
143. M. Ismail, M. Mostapha, A. Soliman, M. Nitzken, F. Khalifa, A. Elnakib, G. Gimel'farb, M. Casanova, and A. El-Baz, "Segmentation of infant brain mr images based on adaptive shape prior and higher-order mgrf," pp. 4327–4331, 2015.
144. A. Mahmoud, A. El-Barkouky, H. Farag, J. Graham, and A. Farag, "A non-invasive method for measuring blood flow rate in superficial veins from a single thermal image," in *Proceedings of the IEEE Conference on Computer Vision and Pattern Recognition Workshops*, 2013, pp. 354–359.
145. A. El-baz, A. Shalaby, F. Taher, M. El-Baz, M. Ghazal, M. A. El-Ghar, A. Takieldeen, and J. Suri, "Probabilistic modeling of blood vessels for segmenting magnetic resonance angiography images," 2017, vol. 5, no. 3.
146. A. S. Chowdhury, A. K. Rudra, M. Sen, A. Elnakib, and A. El-Baz, "Cerebral white matter segmentation from MRI using probabilistic graph cuts and geometric shape priors." in *ICIP*, 2010, pp. 3649–3652.

11

Level Set Method in Medical Imaging Segmentation

Jiangxiong Fang

CONTENTS

11.1 Introduction

As a central problem in the field of medical image processing, image segmentation has been the subjects of a considerable number of studies. It plays an important role in numerous useful applications since it facilitates the extraction of information and interpretation of image contents, e.g. image object extraction [1], biomedical image processing [2], scene interpretation [3], video image analysis [4]. However, it remains a difficult problem since it is highly ill-posed. There are many advanced approaches for medical image segmentation, e.g. clustering, histogram-based, region-growing, graph cut and mean shift. In recent years, active contour methods have been extensively applied to image segmentation [5]. The basic idea [6] in active contour models is to evolve a curve to constraints from a given image. For instance, starting with a curve around the object to be detected, the curve moves toward its interior normal under some constraints from the image, and has to stop on the boundary of the object. The active contour methods have several advantages over classical image segmentation methods. First, active contour models can achieve sub-pixel accuracy of object boundaries [6–8]. Second, active contour models can be easily formulated under a principled energy minimization framework, and allow incorporation of various prior knowledge, such as shape and intensity distribution, for robust image segmentation [9]. Third, they can provide smooth and closed contours as segmentation results, which are necessary and can be readily used for further applications, such as shape analysis and recognition.

The existing active contour models can be categorized into two classes: edge-based models [5] and region-based models [6]. Edge-based active contour models stop the evolving contours by applying image gradient. These models are composed of an edge-based stopping term and a force term to control the motion of the contour. The edge-based stopping term is used to stop the contour on the desired object boundary. The force term can decide the desired object boundary of the active contour. But the choice of force term is difficult. Whether the force is too large or small, the evolving contour may be not able to pass some narrow parts of the object.

Region-based models use a certain region descriptor to guide the motion of the active contour to identify each region of interest. The models tend to rely on intensity homogeneity in each of the regions to be segmented. Compared with edge-based models, region-based active contour models have several advantages. First, region-based segmentation offers closed contours automatically while edge-based methods need an extra propagation step to obtain complete region contours. Second, region-based models do not utilize the image gradient and therefore have better performance for the image with weak object boundaries. Third, they are less sensitive to the location of initial contours. The Chan-Vese (C-V) model is one of the most popular region-based active contour models [6]. In later work, Vese and Chan also proposed a multiphase level set formulation [9], in which multiple regions can be represented by multiple level set functions. Region-based approaches are more appealing than with edge-based approaches because they have less of a dependency on edge detection, which can be sensitive to noise and clutter. Considerable work on region-based active contour has already been done to improve theperformance of image segmentation. Thus, region-based methods can be categorized into local region and global region partitioning. Global region partitioning makes use of global optimality criteria and can produce more semantically meaningful results. Local region-based active contour models utilize the local image information to detect the object, which focus on a localized energy that is based on the piecewise constant model.

In the local region-based model, a natural framework [8] is presented to allow any region-based segmentation energy to be re-formulated in a local way. It describes the localization of three well-known energies and an in-depth study of the behaviors of these energies in response to the degree of localization given. In [11], a local region-based active contour model utilizing image local information is proposed. Local binary fitting energy with a kernel function enables the extraction of accurate local image information. As for the global region-based active contour model, a region-based model for variational image segmentation by minimizing a cost function was proposed. Chan and Vese minimized the energy functional using level set methods for both piecewise-constant [6] and piecewise-smooth [5] approximations of the image.

Whether local or global region-based segmentation formulations in most work are seldom to extend beyond the two-region case of foreground and background using the level set method. These models lead to ambiguities in segmentation when the interior of two or more curves overlap or have vacuums. Multiregion level set image segmentation [8] [14] based on intensity-based segmentation is proposed to solve these problems. In [8] and [14], it introduces a comparatively simple way to extend active contours to multiple regions keeping the familiar quality of the two-phase case. A strategy is presented to determine the optimum number of regions as well as initializations for the contours.

In the classical active contour models, two-region image segmentation via active contours and level sets is straightforward, while arbitrary fixed number multiregion segmentation is difficult because two or more closed curves unambiguously partitioning the image domain into disjoint regions may overlap, which leads to ambiguous segmentation. To solve these problems, in this chapter, we will introduce an efficient multiresolution level set image segmentation method with multiple regions. Then, statistical formulation for image segmentation and two-region level set models are described, including representation of a partition, multiregion segmentation functional, curve evolution equations, level set implement, and description of our proposed method.

11.2 Multiresolution Level Set Image Segmentation with Multiple Regions

11.2.1 Two-Region Active Contour Models

Let $\Omega \subset R^2$ be the image domain, and $I : \Omega \to R$ be a given gray level image. Quite early, the problem was formalized by Mumford-Shah as the minimization of a functional [15]: given an image $\boldsymbol{I}$ and want to find a contour Γ which segments the image into non-overlapping regions. They proposed energy functional as follows:

$$E^{MS}(u, \Gamma) = \int_{\Omega} (u - I)^2 dx + \lambda \int_{\Omega \backslash \Gamma} |\nabla u|^2 \, dx + \mu \int_{\Gamma} ds \tag{11.1}$$

Where the parameters satisfy $\lambda > 0$ and $\mu > 0$. Its first term in Eq. (11.1) ensures the solution $\boldsymbol{u}$ to stay close to the input image and the second term penalizes deviations from smoothness within regions separated from each other by a boundary contour Γ. The third term minimizes the total length of Γ. The minimization of Mumford–Shah functional $E^{MS}(u, \Gamma)$ results in an optimal contour Γ, which segments the given image $\boldsymbol{I}$, makes an image $\boldsymbol{u}$ approximate the original image $\boldsymbol{I}$ and is smooth within each of the connected components. In fact, it is difficult to minimize the functional due to the unknown contour and the non-convexity of the functional.

Chan and Vese [6] proposed an active contour approach to the Mumford–Shah problem for a two-phase case, which is based on a piecewise constant function. For an image on the image domain $I(x, y)$, they propose to minimize the following energy:

$$E^{MS}(\Gamma, c_1, c_2) = \lambda_1 \int_{Out(\Gamma)} |I - c_1|^2 \, dx + \lambda_2 \int_{In(\Gamma)} |I - c_2|^2 \, dx + \mu \int_{\Gamma} ds \tag{11.2}$$

Where $Out(\Gamma)$ and $In(\Gamma)$ represent the regions outside and inside the contour Γ, respectively; c_1 and c_2 are two constants that approximate the image intensity in $Out(\Gamma)$ and $In(\Gamma)$; λ_1, λ_2 and μ are three constants and larger than zero. This energy function $E^{MS}(\Gamma, c_1, c_2)$ can be represented by a level set formulation, and the energy minimization problem can be converted to solving a level set evolution equation.

From the energy function in Eq. (11.2), the optimal constants c_1 and c_2 that minimize the energy are the averages of the intensities in the entire regions $Out(\Gamma)$ and $In(\Gamma)$, respectively. Such optimal constants c_1 and c_2 can be far away from the original image data if the intensities within or $In(\Gamma)$ are not homogeneous. So the piecewise model [6] generally fails to segment images with intensity inhomogeneity. In order to overcome the limitation of the piecewise models with intensity inhomogeneity, Vese and Chan [9] proposed a multiphase level set framework using the Piecewise-Smooth (PS) model. The image is divided into 2^N regions by N zero level functions. However, the involved computation in PS model is expensive, which limits its applications in practice.

11.2.2 Multiregion Level Set Segmentation Method

11.2.2.1 Representation of a Partition

Let $\Omega \subset R^d$ be a given vector valued image, and $I : \Omega \rightarrow R^n$ be the image domain, and $d \geq 1$ is the dimension of the vector I. The image being partitioned into **N** regions is to find a partition $\{R_i\}_{i=1}^{N}$ from the image domain Ω so that each region is homogeneous with respect to some image characteristics in terms of region parametric models. That is to say, a family subsets of Ω are pairwise disjoint such that they can cover Ω. Here, a fixed but arbitrary number of regions are considered for segmentation into multiple regions.

We consider a family $\{\vec{\gamma}_i\}_{i=1}^{N}$: $[0,1] \rightarrow \Omega$ of plane curves parametrized by the arc parameter $s \in [0,1]$. Two-region segmentation via active contours and level sets problem is straightforward, while arbitrary fixed number multiregion segmentation is difficult. To guarantee an unambiguous segmentation, we use a representation of a partition of the image domain by the following explicit correspondence between the family of regions $\{R_{\vec{\gamma}_i}\}$ enclosed by the curves $\{\vec{\gamma}_i\}_{i=1}^{N-1}$. The regions of partition $\{R_i\}_{i=1}^{N}$ of the image domain Ω denotes similar to [1] as follows:

$$
\begin{aligned}
R_1 &= R_{\vec{\gamma}_1} \\
R_2 &= R_{\vec{\gamma}_1}^{c} \bigcap R_{\vec{\gamma}_2} \\
&\cdots\cdots \\
R_k &= R_{\vec{\gamma}_1}^{c} \bigcap R_{\vec{\gamma}_2}^{c} \bigcap \cdots \bigcap R_{\vec{\gamma}_k} \\
&\cdots\cdots \\
R_N &= R_{\vec{\gamma}_1}^{c} \bigcap R_{\vec{\gamma}_2}^{c} \bigcap \cdots \bigcap R_{\vec{\gamma}_{N-1}}
\end{aligned}
\tag{11.3}
$$

The family obtained by $\{\vec{\gamma}_i\}_{i=1}^{N-1}$ is a partition of the image domain. The partition representation is shown in Figure 11.1 with five regions divided by four curves.

11.2.2.2 Multiregion Fitting Energy

With representation of a partition of the image domain into **N** regions, $N-1$ contours $\{\vec{\gamma}_i\}_{i=1}^{N-1}$ are represented by the zero level set of $N-1$ Lipschitz function. We define the region-based energy functional with extension to two-region active contour models:

$$
\begin{aligned}
E^R\left(\{\vec{\gamma}_i\}_{i=1}^{N-1}, \{c_i\}_{i=1}^{N}\right) &= \lambda_1 \int_{R_1} \chi_{R_1} |I(x) - c_1|^2 \, dx + \lambda_2 \int_{R_2} \chi_{R_2} |I(x) - c_2|^2 \, dx + \cdots \\
&\quad + \lambda_k \int_{R_k} \chi_{R_k} |I(x) - c_k|^2 \, dx + \cdots + \lambda_N \int_{R_N} \chi_{R_N} |I(x) - c_N|^2 \, dx \\
&= \sum_{i=1}^{N} \lambda_i \int_{R_i} \chi_{R_i} |I(x) - c_i|^2 \, dx
\end{aligned}
\tag{11.4}
$$

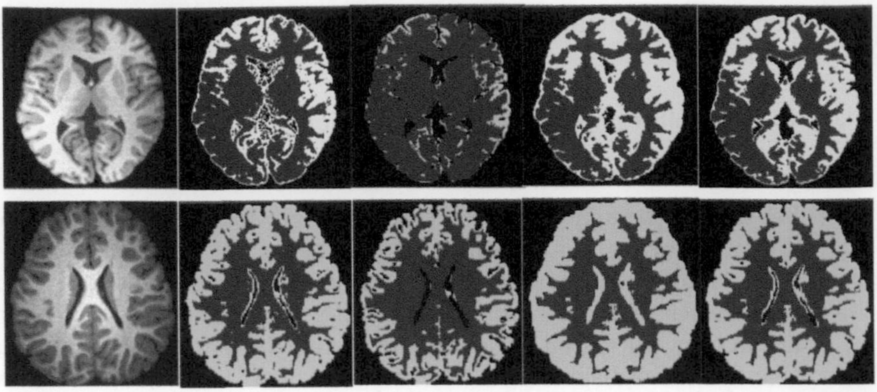

FIGURE 11.1
Comparison of different schemes for two brain MRI images. The left subfigure is of different input images. The remaining subfigures contain different segmentation results. From second to sixth column: ***Mean, Ker, Clust**, and Our proposed model, respectively.*

where the parameter $\chi_{R_i}, i = 1, \cdots, N$, is the characteristic function of *i–th* region and makes $\sum_{i=1}^{N} \chi_{R_i} = 1$, i.e. $\chi_{R_i} = 1$ if $x \in R_i$ and $\chi_{R_i} = 0$ if $x \in R_i^c$; c_i is the *i–th* region constants that approximate the *i–th* region intensity in the image $\boldsymbol{I}$; λ_i is positive constants. Here, let H be the Heaviside function, χ_{R_i} is represented as follows:

$$\begin{cases} \chi_{R_1} = \chi_{R_{\vec{\gamma}_1}} = \left[1 - H(\vec{\gamma}_0)\right] H(\vec{\gamma}_1) H(\vec{\gamma}_0) \equiv 0 \\ \chi_{R_2} = \chi_{R_{\vec{\gamma}_1^c}} \chi_{R_{\vec{\gamma}_2}} = \left[1 - H(\vec{\gamma}_0)\right] \left[1 - H(\vec{\gamma}_1)\right] H(\vec{\gamma}_2) \\ \qquad \vdots \\ \chi_{R_k} = \chi_{R_{\vec{\gamma}_1^c}} \chi_{R_{\vec{\gamma}_2^c}} \cdots \chi_{R_{\vec{\gamma}_{k-1}^c}} \chi_{R_{\vec{\gamma}_k}} = \prod_{i=0}^{k-1} \left[1 - H(\vec{\gamma}_i)\right] H(\vec{\gamma}_k) \\ \qquad \vdots \\ \chi_{R_{N-1}} = \chi_{R_{\vec{\gamma}_1^c}} \chi_{R_{\vec{\gamma}_2^c}} \cdots \chi_{R_{\vec{\gamma}_{N-2}^c}} \chi_{R_{\vec{\gamma}_{N-1}}} = \prod_{i=0}^{N-2} \left[1 - H(\vec{\gamma}_i)\right] H(\vec{\gamma}_{N-1}) \\ \chi_{R_N} = \chi_{R_{\vec{\gamma}_1^c}} \chi_{R_{\vec{\gamma}_2^c}} \cdots \chi_{R_{\vec{\gamma}_{N-2}^c}} \chi_{R_{\vec{\gamma}_{N-1}^c}} = \prod_{i=0}^{N-1} \left[1 - H(\vec{\gamma}_i)\right] \end{cases} . \tag{11.5}$$

From Eq. (11.5), it is clear

$$\chi_{R_1} + \chi_{R_2} + \cdots \chi_{R_k} + \cdots \chi_{R_{N-1}} + \chi_{R_N} = \chi_{R_{\vec{\gamma}_1}} + \chi_{R_{\vec{\gamma}_1^c}} \chi_{R_{\vec{\gamma}_2}} + \cdots + \chi_{R_{\vec{\gamma}_1^c}} \chi_{R_{\vec{\gamma}_2^c}} \cdots \chi_{R_{\vec{\gamma}_{k-1}^c}} \chi_{R_{\vec{\gamma}_k}} + \cdots + \chi_{R_{\vec{\gamma}_1^c}} \chi_{R_{\vec{\gamma}_2^c}} \cdots \chi_{R_{\vec{\gamma}_{N-2}^c}} \chi_{R_{\vec{\gamma}_{N-1}}} + \chi_{R_{\vec{\gamma}_1^c}} \chi_{R_{\vec{\gamma}_2^c}} \cdots \chi_{R_{\vec{\gamma}_{N-2}^c}} \chi_{R_{\vec{\gamma}_{N-1}^c}} = 1. \tag{11.6}$$

In practice, the Heaviside function $\boldsymbol{H}$ in Eq. (11.5) is approximated by a smooth function H_ε defined as:

$$H_\varepsilon(x) = \frac{1}{2}\left[1 + \frac{2}{\pi}\arctan\left(\frac{x}{\varepsilon}\right)\right]. \tag{11.7}$$

The derivative of H_ε is the following smooth function:

$$\delta_\varepsilon(x) = H_\varepsilon^{'}(x) = \frac{1}{\pi}\frac{\varepsilon}{\varepsilon^2 + x^2} \tag{11.8}$$

11.2.2.3 Curve Evolution Equations

To minimize the functional E^R in Eq. (11.4) with respect to the curves $\{\vec{\gamma}_i\}_{i=1}^{N-1}$, we considered it is performed by embedding by the family $\vec{\gamma}_i : [0,1] \rightarrow \Omega$, $i = 1, 2, \cdots, N-1$ of plane curves parameterized by arc parameter $s \in [0,1]$. The Euler-Lagrange descent equation corresponding to $\vec{\gamma}_i$ is obtained by embedding the curve into a family of one-parameter curves $\vec{\gamma}_i : [0,1] \times R^+ \rightarrow \Omega, i = 1, 2, \cdots, N-1$ by solving the evolution equations:

$$\frac{d\vec{\gamma}_i}{dt} = -\frac{\delta E^R}{\delta \vec{\gamma}_i}, i = 1, 2, \cdots, N-1 \tag{11.9}$$

The functional derivatives $\delta E^R / \delta \vec{\gamma}_i$ can be easily computed by suitably rewriting the area integrals appearing in the energy functional. Beginning with $\vec{\gamma}_1$, we can rewrite region-based energy functional Eq. (11.4) as follows:

$$E^R\left(\{\vec{\gamma}_i\}_{i=1}^{N-1}, \{c_i\}_{i=1}^{N}\right) = \lambda_1 \int_{R_1} \chi_{R_1} \left|I(x) - c_i\right|^2 dx + \int_{R_1^c} \Phi_1(x)dx \tag{11.10}$$

Where $\Phi_1(y)$ is defined as

$$\begin{aligned}\Phi_1(x) = &\lambda_2 \left|I(x) - c_2\right|^2 \chi_{R_{\vec{\gamma}_2}} + \lambda_3 \left|I(x) - c_3\right|^2 \chi_{R_{\vec{\gamma}_2^c}} \chi_{R_{\vec{\gamma}_3}} + \cdots \\ &+ \lambda_{N-1} \left|I(x) - c_{N-1}c\right|^2 \chi_{R_{\vec{\gamma}_2^c}} \cdots \chi_{R_{\vec{\gamma}_{N-2}^c}} \chi_{R_{\vec{\gamma}_{N-1}}} \\ &+ \lambda_N \left|I(x) - c_N\right|^2 \chi_{R_{\vec{\gamma}_2^c}} \cdots \chi_{R_{\vec{\gamma}_{N-2}^c}} \chi_{R_{\vec{\gamma}_{N-1}^c}}\end{aligned} \tag{11.11}$$

The functional derivative $\frac{\delta E^R}{\delta \vec{\gamma}_1}$ is computed and given the following evolution equation:

$$\frac{d\vec{\gamma}_1}{dt} = -\frac{\delta E^R}{\delta \vec{\gamma}_i} = -[\lambda_1 \left|I(x) - c_1\right|^2 - \Phi_1]\vec{n}_1 \tag{11.12}$$

Where $\vec{n}_1$ is the external unit normal of $\vec{\gamma}_1$. Proceeding similarly to compute the functional derivatives $\delta E^R / \delta \vec{\gamma}_i$ for all i, the minimization of the multi-region region-based energy functional is obtained and given the following evolution equations:

$$\begin{cases} \frac{d\vec{\gamma}_1}{dt} = -[\lambda_1 |I(x) - c_1|^2 - \Phi_1(\vec{\gamma}_1)]\vec{n}_1 \\ \frac{d\vec{\gamma}_2}{dt} = -[\lambda_2 |I(x) - c_2|^2 - \Phi_2(\vec{\gamma}_2)]\vec{n}_2 \\ \vdots \\ \frac{d\vec{\gamma}_k}{dt} = -[\lambda_k |I(x) - c_k|^2 - \Phi_k(\vec{\gamma}_k)]\vec{n}_k \\ \vdots \\ \frac{d\vec{\gamma}_{N-1}}{dt} = -[\lambda_{N-1} |I(x) - c_{N-1}|^2 - \Phi_{N-1}(\vec{\gamma}_{N-1})]\vec{n}_{N-1} \end{cases} \tag{11.13}$$

Where $\Phi_i(\vec{\gamma}_i)$ is defined as

$$\begin{aligned} \Phi_i(x) = {} & \lambda_{i+1} |I(x) - c_{i+1}|^2 \chi_{R_{\vec{\gamma}_{i+1}}} + \lambda_{i+2} |I(x) - c_{i+2}|^2 \chi_{R_{\vec{\gamma}^c_{i+1}}} \chi_{R_{\vec{\gamma}_{i+2}}} + \cdots \\ & + \lambda_{N-1} |I(x) - c_{N-1}|^2 \chi_{R_{\vec{\gamma}^c_{i+1}}} \cdots \chi_{R_{\vec{\gamma}^c_{N-2}}} \chi_{R_{\vec{\gamma}_{N-1}}} \\ & + \lambda_N |I(x) - c_N|^2 \chi_{R_{\vec{\gamma}^c_{i+1}}} \cdots \chi_{R_{\vec{\gamma}^c_{N-2}}} \chi_{R_{\vec{\gamma}^c_{N-1}}} \end{aligned} \tag{11.14}$$

In order to avoid the occurrence of small, isolated regions in the final segmentation, we add to a regularization term which is defined related to the length of the curve:

$$E^{\Gamma}\left(\{\vec{\gamma}_i\}_{i=1}^{N-1}\right) = \sum_{i=1}^{N-1} \int_{\vec{\gamma}_i} ds \tag{11.15}$$

The derivative of $E^{\Gamma}(\{\vec{\gamma}_i\}_{i=1}^{N-1})$ with respect to $\vec{\gamma}_i$ is:

$$\frac{\partial E^{\Gamma}\left(\{\vec{\gamma}_i\}_{i=1}^{N-1}\right)}{\partial \vec{\gamma}_i} = -\mu k_i \vec{n}_i \tag{11.16}$$

Where k_i is the mean curvature function of $\vec{\gamma}_i$;

To ensure the regularity of the level set function $\vec{\gamma}_i$, which can improve accurate computation and maintain stable level set evolution, we add the distance regularizing term in Li et al.'s variational level set formulation [16] to penalize the deviation of the level set function from a signed distance function:

$$\mathrm{P}\left(\{\vec{\gamma}_i\}_{i=1}^{N-1}\right) = \frac{1}{2} \sum_{i=1}^{N} \int_{\Omega} (|\nabla \vec{\gamma}_i| - 1)^2 dx \tag{11.17}$$

Which characterizes the deviation of the function from a signed distance function.

Thus, the energy functional is approximated with the term of multiregion fitting energy, a regularization term related to the length of curves, and the distance regularizing term:

$$E\left(\{\vec{\gamma}_i\}_{i=1}^{N-1},\{c_i\}_{i=1}^{N}\right) = E^R\left(\{\vec{\gamma}_i\}_{i=1}^{N-1},\{c_i\}_{i=1}^{N}\right) + \mu E^{\Gamma}\left(\{\vec{\gamma}_i\}_{i=1}^{N-1}\right) + v\mathrm{P}\left(\{\vec{\gamma}_i\}_{i=1}^{N-1}\right). \tag{11.18}$$

Where the parameters satisfy $\mu > 0$ and $v > 0$. Thus, compute the functional derivatives $\frac{\delta E}{\delta \gamma_i}$ for all i, the minimization of the energy functional is obtained and given the following evolution equations:

$$\begin{aligned}
\frac{d\vec{\gamma}_1}{dt} &= -[\lambda_1 \, |I(x) - c_1|^2 - \Phi_1(\vec{\gamma}_1) + \mu k_1]\vec{n}_1 + v\left(\nabla \vec{\gamma}_1^2 - k_1\right)\\
\frac{d\vec{\gamma}_2}{dt} &= -[\lambda_2 \, |I(x) - c_2|^2 - \Phi_2(\vec{\gamma}_2) + \mu k_2]\vec{n}_2 + v\left(\nabla \vec{\gamma}_2^2 - k_2\right)\\
&\vdots\\
\frac{d\vec{\gamma}_k}{dt} &= -[\lambda_k \, |I(x) - c_k|^2 - \Phi_k(\vec{\gamma}_k) + \mu k_k]\vec{n}_k + v\left(\nabla \vec{\gamma}_k^2 - k_k\right)\\
&\vdots\\
\frac{d\vec{\gamma}_{N-1}}{dt} &= -[\lambda_{N-1} \, |I(x) - c_{N-1}|^2 - \Phi_{N-1}(\vec{\gamma}_{N-1}) + \mu k_{N-1}]\vec{n}_{N-1} + v\left(\nabla \vec{\gamma}_{N-1}^2 - k_{N-1}\right)
\end{aligned} \tag{11.19}$$

11.2.2.4 Level Set Implementation

The system of curves evolution equations Eq. (11.19) can be implemented by discretizing the interval $[0, 1]$ on which the curves $\{\vec{\gamma}_i\}_{i=1}^{N-1}$ are defined. This leads to an explicit representation of each curve $\vec{\gamma}_i$. A better alternative is to represent the curve $\vec{\gamma}_i$ implicitly by the zero level set function. It is well-known that the level set method has advantages over an implicit representation and topology independence. The level sets representation allows topological changes in a natural way and can be implemented by stable numerical schemes. With level sets, the curve $\vec{\gamma}_i$ is represented implicitly by the zero level set function $u_i : R^2 \to R$, i.e., we define $\vec{\gamma}_i$ as the set:

$$\begin{cases} u_i(x,t) > 0 & x \in Inside(\vec{\gamma}_i) \\ u_i(x,t) = 0 & x \in \vec{\gamma}_i \\ u_i(x,t) < 0 & x \in Outside(\vec{\gamma}_i) \end{cases} \qquad \text{And} \quad \vec{n}_i = \frac{\vec{\nabla} u_i}{\|\vec{\nabla} u_i\|}. \tag{11.20}$$

For zero level set function, we have: $u_i(x, t) = 0$. This implies that:

$$\frac{du_i(x,t)}{dt} = \frac{\partial u_i}{\partial t}(x,t) + \vec{\nabla} u_i \cdot \frac{d\vec{\gamma}_i}{dt} = 0. \tag{11.21}$$

The level set evolution equations minimizing the functional (11.19) combing Eq. (11.8) are therefore given by the following system of coupled partial deferential equations:

$$\frac{d\vec{\gamma}_1}{dt} = -[\lambda_1 \, |I(x) - c_1|^2 - \Phi_1(\vec{\gamma}_1) + \mu k_1]\delta_\varepsilon(\vec{\gamma}_1) + v\big(\nabla \vec{\gamma}_1^2 - k_1\big)$$

$$\frac{d\vec{\gamma}_2}{dt} = -[\lambda_2 \, |I(x) - c_2|^2 - \Phi_2(\vec{\gamma}_2) + \mu k_2]\delta_\varepsilon(\vec{\gamma}_2) + v\big(\nabla \vec{\gamma}_2^2 - k_2\big)$$

$$\vdots$$

$$\frac{d\vec{\gamma}_k}{dt} = -[\lambda_k \, |I(x) - c_k|^2 - \Phi_k(\vec{\gamma}_k) + \mu k_k]\delta_\varepsilon(\vec{\gamma}_k) + v\big(\nabla \vec{\gamma}_k^2 - k_k\big) \tag{11.22}$$

$$\vdots$$

$$\frac{d\vec{\gamma}_{N-1}}{dt} = -[\lambda_{N-1} \, |I(x) - c_{N-1}|^2 - \Phi_{N-1}(\vec{\gamma}_{N-1}) + \mu k_{N-1}]\delta_\varepsilon(\vec{\gamma}_{N-1}) + v\big(\nabla \vec{\gamma}_{N-1}^2 - k_{N-1}\big)$$

where $\Phi_i(\vec{\gamma}_i)$ is given by

$$\begin{aligned}\Phi_i(x) = {} & \lambda_{i+1} \, |I(x) - c_{i+1}|^2 \chi_{u_{i+1}(x,t)>0} + \lambda_{i+2} \, |I(x) - c_{i+2}|^2 \chi_{u_{j+1}(x,t)<0}\chi_{u_{i+2}(x,t)>0} + \cdots \\ & + \lambda_{N-1} \, |I(x) - c_{N-1}|^2 \chi_{u_{i+1}(x,t)<0} \cdots \chi_{u_{N-2}(x,t)<0}\chi_{u_{N-1}(x,t)>0} \\ & + \lambda_N \, |I(x) - c_N|^2 \chi_{u_{i+1}(x,t)<0} \cdots \chi_{u_{N-2}(x,t)<0}\chi_{u_{N-1}(x,t)<0}.\end{aligned} \tag{11.23}$$

With $\chi_{u_i(x,t)>0} = H(\vec{\gamma}_i)$ if $u_i(x,t) > 0$ and $\chi_{u_i(x,t)\leq 0} = 1 - H(\vec{\gamma}_i)$ if $u_i(x,t) \leq 0$; k_{u_i} is the curvature of the level set of u_i and is given as a function as follows:

$$\mathrm{k} = \vec{\nabla} \cdot \frac{\vec{\nabla} u_i}{\|\vec{\nabla} u_i\|} = \frac{u_{xx}u_y^2 - 2u_x u_y u_{xy} + u_{yy}u_x^2}{(u_x^2 + u_y^2)^{3/2}}. \tag{11.24}$$

To implement the evolution equation, the functions $\{c_i\}_{i=1}^N$ are given as follows:

$$c_i = \begin{cases} \dfrac{\displaystyle\int_{R_1} I(x)\chi_{u_1(x,t)>0}dx}{\displaystyle\int_{R_1} \chi_{u_1(x,t)>0}dx} & i = 1 \\[3ex] \dfrac{\displaystyle\int_{R_i} I(x)\chi_{u_1(x,t)<0} \cdots \chi_{u_{i-1}(x,t)<0}\chi_{u_i(x,t)>0}dx}{\displaystyle\int_{R_i} \chi_{u_1(x,t)<0} \cdots \chi_{u_{i-1}(x,t)<0}\chi_{u_i(x,t)>0}dx} & i \in [2, N-1] \\[3ex] \dfrac{\displaystyle\int_{R_N} I(x)\chi_{u_1(x,t)<0} \cdots \chi_{u_{N-2}(x,t)<0}\chi_{u_{N-1}(x,t)<0}dx}{\displaystyle\int_{R_N} \chi_{u_1(x,t)<0} \cdots \chi_{u_{N-2}(x,t)<0}\chi_{u_{N-1}(x,t)<0}dx} & i = N \end{cases}. \tag{11.25}$$

Here, the segmentation procedure of the multiregion level set algorithm (MRLS) is summarized as follows:

Algorithm 1 MRLS Algorithm

---

1) For a given fixed region number N, set $k = 0, m = N-1$ and initialize the curves $\{\vec{\gamma}_i\}_{i=1}^{m}$, with $\{\vec{\gamma}_i^k\}_{i=1}^{N-1}$ defined as the distance function from initial curves.

2) For each $\vec{\gamma}_i$, compute the corresponding $c_i, i = 1, \cdots N$ as the averages for each region.

3) For each $\vec{\gamma}_i$, compute $\vec{\gamma}_i^{k+1}$ by solving the following:

$$\vec{\gamma}_i^{k+1} = \vec{\gamma}_i^{k} - \Delta t \frac{\partial E}{\partial t}\left(\{\vec{\gamma}_i\}_{i=1}^{N-1}, \{c_i\}_{i=1}^{N}\right) \tag{11.26}$$

Where Δt is the time step

4) Reinitialize $\vec{\gamma}_i^k$ locally from the queue $\{\vec{\gamma}_i\}_{i=1}^{m}$ to the signed distance function to the curve.

5) Run the following process until m =0:

For each curve $\vec{\gamma}_i^k$
  If the curve $\vec{\gamma}_i$ reaches convergence
    Delete the curve $\vec{\gamma}_i^k$ from the curves $\{\vec{\gamma}_i\}_{i=1}^{m}$
    m = m − 1
  Else
    Go to Step 2
  End if
End for

11.2.2.5 Multiresolution Analysis Level Set Method

For a given initialization of the level set function, the energy functional may be trapped in a local minimum solution and affect the quality of the segmentation result. This risk is especially increased when the image maintains much noise. To deal with these questions, we use a multiresolution approach [17] [18] which can analyze the image at different resolutions from coarse to fine by successively downsampling the image with a factor of two. First, the curve is evolved in the coarse resolution image up to convergence. Second, the resulting curve is interpolated and upsampled by a factor of two to create an initial curve for the next resolution, which, in turn, is updated with the same procedure until convergence. This iterative process is repeated over all the different considered resolutions until reaching the original image resolution stage. The solution not only improves the robustness of the segmentation procedure, but also decreases the computational cost by giving a good approximation to the original problem at a lower spatial resolution for each level. For this, we derived an important theoretical result relating solutions at different spatial resolutions. The proposed multiresolution MRLS (MR-MRLS) algorithm is shown as follows:

Algorithm 2 Proposed MR-MRLS Algorithm

1) Set a given integer L and the number of segmented regions N.

2) Generate the different spatial resolution of the original image by a factor of 2^L in each dimension.

3) Set initial resolution $i = L$, apply the MRLS algorithm on the downsampled image obtained at the current level i.

4) Upsample the MRLS algorithm by a factor of two and use it as the initial condition for the mask image obtained at the level $i - 1$ by bilinear interpolation. Repeat the following until the original spatial resolution is reached.

5) Repeat Steps 3 and 4 until the original spatial resolution is reached.

6) Generate the segmented map.

11.3 Statistical Formulation of Level Set Segmentation Method

11.3.1 Image Segmentation as Bayesian Inference

Let $\Omega \subset R^d$ be a given vector valued image, and $I : \Omega \rightarrow R^n$ be the image domain, and d the dimension of the vector $\boldsymbol{I}$. The image is being partitioned into N regions to find a partition $\{R_i\}_{i=1}^N$ from the image domain Ω so that each region is homogeneous with respect to some image characteristics in terms of region parametric models. That is to say, a family subset of Ω is pairwise disjoint such that it can cover Ω. In this case, it is convenient to cast segmentation in a Bayesian framework [23–26] by maximizing a posteriori (MAP) estimation. The problem would consist of finding an optimal partition $\{R_i\}_{i=1}^N$ which maximizes the a posteriori probability $p(\{R_i\}_{i=1}^N|I)$ over all possible $\boldsymbol{N}$-region partitions of the image plane Ω.

$$\begin{aligned}\{R_i\}_{i=1}^N &= \arg\max_{R_i \subset \Omega} p(\{R_i\}_{i=1}^N|I) \\ &= \arg\max_{R_i \subset \Omega} p(I|\{R_i\}_{i=1}^N)p(\{R_i\}_{i=1}^N)\end{aligned} \tag{11.27}$$

Maximization of the a posteriori probability (11.27) is equivalent to minimizing its negative logarithm. Here, we assume that $I(x)$ is independent o

$I(y)$ for $x \neq y$, the expression is given as follows:

$$\{R_i\}_{i=1}^N = \arg\min_{R_i \subset \Omega} E[\{R_i\}_{i=1}^N] \tag{11.28}$$

where the function $E[\{R_i\}_{i=1}^N]$ is defined as:

$$E[\{R_i\}_{i=1}^N] = -\sum_{i=1}^N \int_{x \in R_i} \log p\big(I(x)|\{R_i\}_{i=1}^N\big)dx - \log p\big(\{R_i\}_{i=1}^N\big) \tag{11.29}$$

where $p(I(x)|R_i)$ denotes the probability of observing an image ***I***. The first term, also called the Bayesian term, computers the conformity of image data within each region $R_i, i = 1, \cdots, N$, to a parametric distribution $p(I(x)|R_i)$. The Gaussian distribution has been considered in most studies because it can reduce the computational cost and be simply used [12]. In this case, the Gaussian distribution reads:

$$p(I(x)|R_i) = \frac{1}{\sqrt{2\pi\sigma_i^2}} e^{-\frac{(I(x)-u_i)^2}{2\sigma_i^2}} \tag{11.30}$$

where u_i and σ_i denote the mean value and variance within the region R_i. The Bayesian term are expressed as follows:

$$\begin{aligned} E^B[\{R_i\}_{i=1}^N] &= -\sum_{i=1}^N \int_{x \in R_i} \log p\big(I(x)|\{R_i\}_{i=1}^N\big)dx \\ &= \sum_{i=1}^N \left(\frac{(I(x)-u_i)^2}{2\sigma_i^2} + \log\left(\sqrt{2\pi\sigma_i^2}\right)\right) \end{aligned} \tag{11.31}$$

The second term, also called regularization term, embeds the length prior [12] on the segmentation and is commonly used for smooth segmentation boundaries.

$$E^R\big[\{R_i\}_{i=1}^N\big] = -\text{In}\,\big(p(\{R_i\}_{i=1}^N)\big) = \lambda \sum_{i=1}^{N-1} \int_{\gamma_i} ds \tag{11.32}$$

where ∂R_i is the boundary of the region R_i and λ is a positive factor.

11.3.2 Two-Region Level Set Formulation

Here, the Bayesian model will be used to deduce the level set evolution functional for two-region image segmentation. Let the image $I(x)$ be formed by two regions which may consist of several disconnected parts, we want to find a contour C which is the boundary of an open set and segments the image into non-overlapping regions. Assuming a given curve C is represented by a Lipschitz function $\phi(x, y)$, called level set function, such that:

$$\begin{cases} \phi(x,y) > 0 & (x,y) \in R_1 \\ \phi(x,y) = 0 & (x,y) \in C \\ \phi(x,y) < 0 & (x,y) \in R_2 \end{cases} \tag{11.33}$$

The evolving curve as C is completely determined by level set function $\phi(x, y)$. The Heaviside function is used to describe a region in which $\phi(x, y)$ is greater than zero or not. $H_\varepsilon(x)$ and $\delta_\varepsilon(x)$ are the regularized approximation of Heaviside function $H(x)$ and the derivative of $H_\varepsilon(x)$ called Dirac delta function $\delta_\varepsilon(x)$ as follows:

$$H(x) = \begin{cases} 1 & if\, x \geq 0 \\ 0 & if\, x < 0 \end{cases} \quad \delta(x) = \frac{d}{dx} H(x). \tag{11.34}$$

In practice, the Heaviside function $\boldsymbol{H}$ is approximated by a smooth function H_ε defined as:

$$H_\varepsilon(x) = \frac{1}{2}\left[1 + \frac{2}{\pi}\arctan\left(\frac{x}{\varepsilon}\right)\right], \quad \delta_\varepsilon(x) = H_\varepsilon'(x) = \frac{1}{\pi}\frac{\varepsilon}{\varepsilon^2 + x^2}. \tag{11.35}$$

Extending the approach of Chan and Vese [13], one can implement the functional (11.29) by:

$$\begin{aligned} E(\phi) = & \int_\Omega H(\phi)\left(\frac{(I(x) - u_1)^2}{2\sigma_1^2} + \log\left(\sqrt{2\pi\sigma_1^2}\right)\right) \\ & + \int_\Omega (1 - H(\phi))\left(\frac{(I(x) - u_2)^2}{2\sigma_2^2} + \log\left(\sqrt{2\pi\sigma_2^2}\right)\right) + \lambda \int_C ds \end{aligned} \tag{11.36}$$

The first two terms in Eq. (11.36) represent inside and outside the contour C while the last term represents the length of the separating interface. Minimizing Eq. (11.36), one can drive the Euler-Lagrange equations and update the level set function $\phi(x, y)$ by the gradient descent method:

$$\frac{\partial \phi}{\partial t} = \delta_\varepsilon(\phi)\left[\lambda \cdot div\left(\frac{\nabla\phi}{|\nabla\phi|}\right) + \left(\log\sigma_2 + \frac{(I - u_2)^2}{2\sigma_2^2}\right) - \left(\log\sigma_1 + \frac{(I(x) - u_1)^2}{2\sigma_1^2}\right)\right] \tag{11.37}$$

With initial condition $\phi(x, y, 0) = \phi_0(x, y)$ in Ω and boundary condition $(\delta_0(\phi)/|\nabla\phi|)(\partial\phi/\partial\vec{n}) = 0$ on $\partial\Omega$, where $\vec{n}$ is the unit normal at the boundary $\partial\Omega$ and $\partial\phi/\partial\vec{n}$ is the normal derivative of ϕ at the boundary.

Here, the optimal estimates for the mean u_i and the variance σ_i can be computed:

$$\begin{cases} u_1 = \dfrac{\displaystyle\int H(\phi)I(x)dx}{\displaystyle\int H(\phi)dx}, & \sigma_1^2 = \dfrac{\displaystyle\int H(\phi)(I(x)-u_1)^2dx}{\displaystyle\int H(\phi)dx} \\ u_2 = \dfrac{\displaystyle\int (1-H(\phi))I(x)dx}{\displaystyle\int (1-H(\phi))dx}, & \sigma_2^2 = \dfrac{\displaystyle\int (1-H(\phi))(I(x)-u_2)^2dx}{\displaystyle\int (1-H(\phi))\backslash dx} \end{cases} \tag{11.38}$$

11.3.3 Multiregion Level Set Segmentation

11.3.3.1 Representation of a Partition

Here, we first think that a fixed number of regions is considered for segmentation into multiple regions. We consider a family $\{\vec{\gamma}_i\}_{i=1}^{N}: [0,1] \to \Omega$ of plane curves parametrized by the arc parameter $s \in [0,1]$. To guarantee an unambiguous segmentation, we use a representation of a partition of the image domain by the following explicit correspondence between the family of regions $\{R_{\vec{\gamma}_i}\}$enclosed by the curves $\{\vec{\gamma}_i\}_{i=1}^{N-1}$. The regions of partition $\{R_i\}_{i=1}^{N}$ of the image domain Ω denotes similar to [1] as follows:

$$\begin{aligned} R_1 &= R_{\vec{\gamma}_1} \\ R_2 &= R_{\vec{\gamma}_1}^c \bigcap R_{\vec{\gamma}_2} \\ &\cdots\cdots \\ R_k &= R_{\vec{\gamma}_1}^c \bigcap R_{\vec{\gamma}_2}^c \bigcap \cdots \bigcap R_{\vec{\gamma}_k} \\ &\cdots\cdots \\ R_N &= R_{\vec{\gamma}_1}^c \bigcap R_{\vec{\gamma}_2}^c \bigcap \cdots \bigcap R_{\vec{\gamma}_{N-1}} \end{aligned} \; . \tag{11.39}$$

The family obtained by $\{\vec{\gamma}_i\}_{i=1}^{N-1}$ is a partition of the image domain. The partition representation is shown in Figure 11.1 with five regions divided by four curves.

11.3.3.2 Multiregion Segmentation Functional

With representation of a partition of the image domain into N regions, $N-1$ contours $\{\vec{\gamma}_i\}_{i=1}^{N-1}$ are represented by the zero level set of $N-1$ Lipschitz function. We define the energy functional with extension to two-region active contour models:

$$E\left[\{\vec{\gamma}_i\}_{i=1}^{N-1}\right] = \int_{R_1} \omega_1(x)dx + \int_{R_2} \omega_2(x)dx + \cdots + \int_{R_k} \omega_k(x)dx + \cdots$$
$$+ \int_{R_N} \omega_N(x)dx + \lambda \sum_{i=1}^{N-1} \int_{\gamma_i} ds \tag{11.40}$$
$$= \sum_{i=1}^{N} \int_{R_i} \omega_i(x)dx + \lambda \sum_{i=1}^{N-1} \int_{\gamma_i} ds$$

where

$$\omega_i(x) = \frac{(I(x) - u_i)^2}{2\sigma_i^2} + \log\left(\sqrt{2\pi\sigma_i^2}\right) \approx \frac{(I(x) - u_i)^2}{2\sigma_i^2} + \log \sigma_i \tag{11.41}$$

In most work, the number of regions for image segmentation is fixed in advance. In fact, the true number of regions is unknown. Here, the method of a region merging prior in [26] is used to allow the number of regions to vary automatically for image segmentation. The energy functional can be written as follows ($a_i \log a_i$ is replaced by $\int_{R_i} \log a_i$):

$$E[\{\vec{\gamma}_i\}_{i=1}^{N-1}] = \sum_{i=1}^{N} \int_{R_i} \omega_i(x)dx - \beta \sum_{i=1}^{N} a_i \log a_i + \lambda \sum_{i=1}^{N-1} \int_{\gamma_i} ds$$
$$= \sum_{i=1}^{N} \int_{R_i} \omega_i(x)dx - \beta \sum_{i=1}^{N} \int_{R_i} \log a_i dx + \lambda \sum_{i=1}^{N-1} \int_{\gamma_i} ds$$
$$= \sum_{i=1}^{N} \int_{R_i} (\omega_i(x) - \beta \log a_i)dx + \lambda \sum_{i=1}^{N-1} \int_{\gamma_i} ds \tag{11.42}$$

where a_i is the area of region R_i and β is a positive real constant to weigh the relative contribution of the region merging term in the segmentation functional. In [27], Ayed et al. interpret how to fix the weighting parameter β. The parameters are defined as:

$$a_i = \int_{R_i} dx \quad \text{and} \quad \beta = \alpha \frac{\int_\Omega \left(\frac{(I(x) - u)^2}{2\sigma^2} + \log \sigma\right)}{A \log A} \quad \forall A > 1 \tag{11.43}$$

where u and σ are the mean intensity and variance over the whole image; A is the image domain area; α is a constant and is close to 1.

The weighting parameter β is the ratio of the data term to the region merging term in the case of a partition for each region. Using expression (11.43), the sum of the data term and the term based on the region merging prior can be rewritten as follows:

$$\sum_{i=1}^{N} \int_{R_i} (\omega_i(x))dx - \alpha \frac{\sum_{i=1}^{N} a_i \log a_i}{A \log A} \int_\Omega \left(\frac{(I(x) - u)^2}{2\sigma^2} + \log \sigma\right) \tag{11.44}$$

From (A.1), we can note that the denominator in Eq. (11.43) can be viewed as a normalizing factor for the prior and the integral in the numerator as a normalizing factor for the data term because minimizing Eq. (11.44) is equivalent to minimizing:

$$\underbrace{\frac{\sum_{i=1}^{N}\int_{R_i}(\omega_i(x))dx}{\int_{\Omega}\left(\frac{(I(x)-u)^2}{2\sigma^2}+\log\sigma\right)}}_{\in[0,1]} - \alpha\underbrace{\frac{\sum_{i=1}^{N}a_i\log a_i}{A\log A}}_{\in[0,1]} \tag{11.45}$$

Thus, the parameter α should be a value of close to 1. The following important inequalities for any partition $R = \{R_i\}_{i=1}^{N}$ of Ω satisfies

$$1-\frac{\log N}{\log A}\leq\frac{\sum_{i=1}^{N}a_i\log a_i}{A\log A}\leq 1\ \forall A>1 \tag{11.46}$$

The process of proof in Eq. (11.46) is shown in Section 11.4 referred to [27]. In fact, the number of region N is generally much smaller than A and $\sum_{i=1}^{N}a_i\log a_i/A\log A$ is close to 1. The small interval of variation of the normalized prior in Eq. (11.46) suggests that will vary in a small interval centered close to 1, which makes the sum of the data and the region merging terms close to the in-between cluster distance.

11.3.3.3 Curve Evolution Equations

To minimize the functional E in Eq. (11.42) with respect to the curves $\{\vec{\gamma}_i\}_{i=1}^{N-1}$, we considered it is performed by embedding by the family $\vec{\gamma}_i : [0,1] \to \Omega, i = 1,2,\cdots,N-1$ of plane curves parameterized by arc parameter $s \in [0,1]$. The Euler-Lagrange descent equation corresponding to $\vec{\gamma}_i$ is obtained by embedding the curve into a family of one-parameter curves $\vec{\gamma}_i : [0,1] \times R^+ \to \Omega, i = 1,2,\cdots,N-1$ by solving the evolution equations:

$$\frac{d\vec{\gamma}_i}{dt}=-\frac{\delta E}{\delta\vec{\gamma}_i},\quad i=1,2,\cdots,N-1 \tag{11.47}$$

The functional derivatives $\delta E/\delta\vec{\gamma}_i$ can be easily computed by suitably rewriting the area integrals appearing in the energy functional. Beginning with $\vec{\gamma}_1$, we can rewrite region-based energy functional Eq. (11.42) as follows:

$$E\left[\{\vec{\gamma}_i\}_{i=1}^{N-1}\right]=\int_{R_1}(\omega_1(x)-\beta\log a_1)dx+\int_{R_1^c}(\Phi_1(x)-\theta_1(x))dx+\lambda\sum_{i=1}^{N-1}\int_{\gamma_i}ds \tag{11.48}$$

where $\Phi_1(x)$ is defined as

$$\begin{aligned}\Phi_1(x)=&\chi_{R_{\vec{\gamma}_2}}\omega_2(x)+\chi_{R_{\vec{\gamma}_2}^c}\chi_{R_{\vec{\gamma}_3}}\omega_3(x)+\cdots+\chi_{R_{\vec{\gamma}_2}^c}\cdots\chi_{R_{\vec{\gamma}_{N-2}}^c}\chi_{R_{\vec{\gamma}_{N-1}}}\omega_{N-1}(x)\\&+\chi_{R_{\vec{\gamma}_2}^c}\cdots\chi_{R_{\vec{\gamma}_{N-2}}^c}\chi_{R_{\vec{\gamma}_{N-1}}^c}\omega_N(x).\end{aligned} \tag{11.49}$$

$$\begin{aligned} \theta_1(x) &= \log a_2 \cdot \chi_{R_{\vec{\gamma}_2}}(x) + \log a_3 \cdot \chi_{R_{\vec{\gamma}_2^c}}(x)\chi_{R_{\vec{\gamma}_3}}(x) + \cdots \\ &\quad + \log a_{N-1} \cdot \chi_{R_{\vec{\gamma}_2^c}}(x) \cdots \chi_{R_{\vec{\gamma}_{N-2}^c}}(x)\chi_{R_{\vec{\gamma}_{N-1}}}(x) \\ &\quad + \log a_N \cdot \chi_{R_{\vec{\gamma}_2^c}}(x) \cdots \chi_{R_{\vec{\gamma}_{N-2}^c}}(x)\chi_{R_{\vec{\gamma}_{N-1}^c}}(x) \end{aligned} \tag{11.50}$$

where the parameter $\chi_{R_i}(x)$, $i = 1, \cdots, N$ is the characteristic function of the *i-th* region and makes $\sum_{i=1}^{N} \chi_{R_i}(x) = 1$, i.e. $\chi_{R_i}(x) = 1$ if $x \in R_i$ and $\chi_{R_i}(x) = 0$ if $x \in R_i^c$; λ_i is positive constants. Here, let H be the Heaviside function, χ_{R_i} is represented as follows:

$$\begin{cases} \chi_{R_i}(\vec{\gamma}_i) = \chi_{R_{\vec{\gamma}_1^c}}(\vec{\gamma}_k)\chi_{R_{\vec{\gamma}_2^c}}(\vec{\gamma}_k) \cdots \chi_{R_{\vec{\gamma}_{i-1}^c}}(\vec{\gamma}_i)\chi_{R_{\vec{\gamma}_i}}(\vec{\gamma}_i) \\ \qquad = \prod_{i=1}^{k-1} [1 - H(\vec{\gamma}_i)] \cdot H(\vec{\gamma}_i) \quad i = 1, \cdots, N-2 \\ \chi_{R_{N-1}}(\vec{\gamma}_{N-1}) = \chi_{R_{\vec{\gamma}_1^c}}(\vec{\gamma}_{N-1})\chi_{R_{\vec{\gamma}_2^c}}(\vec{\gamma}_{N-1}) \cdots \chi_{R_{\vec{\gamma}_{N-2}^c}}(\vec{\gamma}_{N-1})\chi_{R_{\vec{\gamma}_{N-1}^c}}(\vec{\gamma}_{N-1}) \\ \qquad = \prod_{i=1}^{N-1} [1 - H(\vec{\gamma}_i)] \quad k = N-1 \end{cases} \tag{11.51}$$

From (11.47), it is clear

$$\begin{aligned} \sum_{i=1}^{N} \chi_{R_i}(\vec{\gamma}_i) &= \chi_{R_{\vec{\gamma}_1}}(\vec{\gamma}_1) + \cdots + \chi_{R_{\vec{\gamma}_1^c}}(\vec{\gamma}_k)\chi_{R_{\vec{\gamma}_2^c}}(\vec{\gamma}_k) \cdots \chi_{R_{\vec{\gamma}_{i-1}^c}}(\vec{\gamma}_i)\chi_{R_{\vec{\gamma}_i}}(\vec{\gamma}_i) + \cdots \\ &\quad + \chi_{R_{\vec{\gamma}_1^c}}(\vec{\gamma}_{N-2})\chi_{R_{\vec{\gamma}_2^c}}(\vec{\gamma}_{N-2}) \cdots \chi_{R_{\vec{\gamma}_{N-2}^c}}(\vec{\gamma}_{N-2})\chi_{R_{\vec{\gamma}_{N-1}}}(\vec{\gamma}_{N-2}) \\ &\quad + \chi_{R_{\vec{\gamma}_1^c}}(\vec{\gamma}_{N-1})\chi_{R_{\vec{\gamma}_2^c}}(\vec{\gamma}_{N-1}) \cdots \chi_{R_{\vec{\gamma}_{N-2}^c}}(\vec{\gamma}_{N-1})\chi_{R_{\vec{\gamma}_{N-1}^c}}(\vec{\gamma}_{N-1}) = 1. \end{aligned} \tag{11.52}$$

The functional derivative $\delta E / \delta \vec{\gamma}_1$ is computed and given the following evolution equation:

$$\begin{aligned} \frac{d\vec{\gamma}_1}{dt} &= -\frac{\delta E}{\delta \vec{\gamma}_1} = -[(\omega_1(\vec{\gamma}_1) - \beta \log a_1) - (\Phi_1(\vec{\gamma}_1) - \beta\theta_1(\vec{\gamma}_1))) + \lambda k_1]\vec{n}_1 \\ &= -[(\omega_1(\vec{\gamma}_1) - \Phi_1(\vec{\gamma}_1)) - \beta(\log a_1 - \theta_1(\vec{\gamma}_1)) + \lambda k_1]\vec{n}_1 \end{aligned} \tag{11.53}$$

where $\vec{n}_1$ is the external unit normal of $\vec{\gamma}_1$. Proceeding similarly to compute the functional derivatives $\delta E^R / \delta \vec{\gamma}_i$ for all i, the minimization of the multiregion energy functional is obtained and given the following evolution equations:

$$\begin{cases} \dfrac{d\vec{\gamma}_1}{dt} = -[(\omega_1(\vec{\gamma}_1) - \Phi_1(\vec{\gamma}_1)) - \beta(\log a_1 - \theta_1(\vec{\gamma}_1)) + \lambda k_1]\vec{n}_1 \\ \qquad \vdots \\ \dfrac{d\vec{\gamma}_i}{dt} = -\left[\chi_{R_{\vec{\gamma}_1^c}}(\vec{\gamma}_i) \cdots \chi_{R_{\vec{\gamma}_{i-1}^c}}(\vec{\gamma}_i)((\omega_i(\vec{\gamma}_i) - \Phi_i(\vec{\gamma}_i)) - \beta(\log a_i - \theta_i(\vec{\gamma}_i))) + \lambda k_i\right]\vec{n}_i \\ \qquad \vdots \\ \dfrac{d\vec{\gamma}_{N-1}}{dt} = -\left[\chi_{R_{\vec{\gamma}_1^c}}(\vec{\gamma}_{N-1}) \cdots \chi_{R_{\vec{\gamma}_{N-1}^c}}(\vec{\gamma}_{N-1})((\omega_{N-1}(\vec{\gamma}_{N-1}) - \Phi_{N-1}(\vec{\gamma}_{N-1})) \right. \\ \qquad \left. - \beta(\log a_{N-1} - \theta_{N-1}(\vec{\gamma}_{N-1}))) + \lambda k_{N-1}\right]\vec{n}_{N-1} \end{cases} \tag{11.54}$$

where $\Phi_i(\vec{\gamma}_i)$ and θ_i are defined as follows, respectively:

$$\begin{aligned}\Phi_i(x) &= \omega_{i+1}(x)\chi_{R_{\vec{\gamma}_{i+1}}}(x) + \omega_{i+2}(x)\chi_{R_{\vec{\gamma}^c_{i+1}}}(x)\chi_{R_{\vec{\gamma}_{i+2}}}(x) + \cdots \\ &+ \omega_{N-1}(x)\chi_{R_{\vec{\gamma}^c_{i+1}}}(x)\cdots\chi_{R_{\vec{\gamma}^c_{N-2}}}(x)\chi_{R_{\vec{\gamma}_{N-1}}}(x) \\ &+ \omega_N(x)\chi_{R_{\vec{\gamma}^c_{i+1}}}(x)\cdots\chi_{R_{\vec{\gamma}^c_{N-2}}}(x)\chi_{R_{\vec{\gamma}^c_{N-1}}}(x)\end{aligned} \tag{11.55}$$

$$\begin{aligned}\theta_i(x) &= \log a_{i+1}\cdot\chi_{R_{\vec{\gamma}_{i+1}}}(x) + \log a_{i+2}\cdot\chi_{R_{\vec{\gamma}^c_{i+1}}}(x)\chi_{R_{\vec{\gamma}_{i+2}}}(x) + \cdots \\ &+ \log a_{N-1}\cdot\chi_{R_{\vec{\gamma}^c_{i+1}}}(x)\cdots\chi_{R_{\vec{\gamma}^c_{N-2}}}(x)\chi_{R_{\vec{\gamma}_{N-1}}}(x) \\ &+ \log a_N\cdot\chi_{R_{\vec{\gamma}^c_{i+1}}}(x)\cdots\chi_{R_{\vec{\gamma}^c_{N-2}}}(x)\chi_{R_{\vec{\gamma}^c_{N-1}}}(x)\end{aligned} \tag{11.56}$$

The derivative of the length prior E^R with respect to $\vec{\gamma}_i$ is:

$$\frac{\partial E^R\left(\{\vec{\gamma}_i\}_{i=1}^{N-1}\right)}{\partial\vec{\gamma}_i} = -\lambda k_i\vec{n}_i \tag{11.57}$$

where k_i is the mean curvature function of $\vec{\gamma}_i$. The level set equations in Eq. (11.54) show how region merging occurs intrinsically in multiple curve evolution. Ayed [27] et al. pointed out evolution of two curves, in which one curve encloses both regions and the other curve disappears, result in one region expanding and the other shrinking.

11.3.3.4 Level Set Implementation

The system of curves evolution equations (11.53) can be implemented by discretizing the interval $[0, 1]$ on which the curves $\{\vec{\gamma}_i\}_{i=1}^{N-1}$ are defined. This leads to an explicit representation of each curve $\vec{\gamma}_i$. A better alternative is to represent the curve $\vec{\gamma}_i$ implicitly by the zero level set function. It is well-known that the level set method has advantages over an implicit representation and topology independence. The level sets representation allows topological changes in a natural way and can be implemented by stable numerical schemes. With level sets, the curve $\vec{\gamma}_i$ is represented implicitly by the zero level set function $u_i : R^2 \to R$, i.e., we define $\vec{\gamma}_i$ as the set:

$$\begin{cases} u_i(x,t) > 0 & x \in Inside(\vec{\gamma}_i) \\ u_i(x,t) = 0 & x \in \vec{\gamma}_i \\ u_i(x,t) < 0 & x \in Outside(\vec{\gamma}_i)\end{cases} \quad \text{And } \vec{n}_i = \frac{\vec{\nabla}u_i}{\|\vec{\nabla}u_i\|}. \tag{11.58}$$

For zero level set function, we have: $u_i(x,t) = 0$. This implies that:

$$\frac{du_i(x,t)}{dt} = \frac{\partial u_i}{\partial t}(x,t) + \vec{\nabla}u_i\cdot\frac{d\vec{\gamma}_i}{dt} = 0. \tag{11.59}$$

The level set evolution equation minimizing the functional is therefore given by the following system of coupled partial deferential equations:

$$\begin{cases} \dfrac{du_1(x,t)}{dt} = -\left[(\omega_1(x) - \Phi_1(x)) - \beta(\log a_1 - \theta_1(x)) + \lambda k_{u_1}\right] \|\vec{\nabla} u_1(x,t)\| \\ \vdots \\ \dfrac{du_i(x,t)}{dt} = -\left[\chi_{u_1(x,t)<0}(x) \cdots \chi_{u_{i-1}(x,t)<0}(x)((\omega_i(x) - \Phi_i(x)) \right. \\ \quad \left. -\beta(\log a_i - \theta_i(\vec{\gamma}_i))) + \lambda k_{u_i}\right] \|\nabla u_i(x,t)\| \\ \vdots \\ \dfrac{du_{N-1}(x,t)}{dt} = -\left[\chi_{u_1(x,t)<0}(x) \cdots \chi_{u_{N-1}(x,t)<0}(x)((\omega_{N-1}(x) - \Phi_{N-1}(x)) \right. \\ \quad \left. -\beta(\log a_{N-1} - \theta_{N-1}(x))) + \lambda k_{u_{N-1}}\right] \|\nabla u_{N-1}(x,t)\| \end{cases} \tag{11.60}$$

where $\Phi_k(\vec{\gamma}_k)$ and θ_k are defined as follows, respectively:

$$\begin{aligned} \Phi_i(x) = {} & \omega_{i+1}(x)\chi_{u_{i+1}(x,t)>0} + \omega_{i+2}(x)\chi_{u_{j+1}(x,t)<0}\chi_{u_{i+2}(x,t)>0} + \cdots \\ & + \omega_{N-1}(x)\chi_{u_{i+1}(x,t)<0} \cdots \chi_{u_{N-2}(x,t)<0}\chi_{u_{N-1}(x,t)>0} \\ & + \omega_N(x)\chi_{u_{i+1}(x,t)<0} \cdots \chi_{u_{N-2}(x,t)<0}\chi_{u_{N-1}(x,t)<0} \end{aligned} \tag{11.61}$$

$$\begin{aligned} \theta_i(x) = {} & \log a_{i+1} \cdot \chi_{u_{i+1}(x,t)>0} + \log a_{i+2} \cdot \chi_{u_{j+1}(x,t)<0}\chi_{u_{i+2}(x,t)>0} + \cdots \\ & + \log a_{N-1} \cdot \chi_{u_{i+1}(x,t)<0} \cdots \chi_{u_{N-2}(x,t)<0}\chi_{u_{N-1}(x,t)>0} \\ & + \log a_N \cdot \chi_{u_{i+1}(x,t)<0} \cdots \chi_{u_{N-2}(x,t)<0}\chi_{u_{N-1}(x,t)<0} \end{aligned} \tag{11.62}$$

With $\chi_{u_i(x,t)>0} = H(\vec{\gamma}_i)$ if $u_i(x,t) > 0$ and $\chi_{u_i(x,t)\le 0} = 1 - H(\vec{\gamma}_i)$ if $u_i(x,t) \le 0$; k_{u_i} is the curvature of the level set of u_i and is given as a function as follows:

$$\mathrm{k} = \vec{\nabla} \cdot \frac{\vec{\nabla} u_i}{\|\vec{\nabla} u_i\|} = \frac{u_{xx}u_y^2 - 2u_x u_y u_{xy} + u_{yy}u_x^2}{(u_x^2 + u_y^2)^{3/2}}. \tag{11.63}$$

where u_x, u_y, u_{xx}, u_{yy} and u_{xy} are computed as follows:

$$\begin{aligned} & u_x = \frac{1}{2h}(u_{i+1,j} - u_{i-1,j}), u_y = \frac{1}{2h}(u_{i,j+1} - u_{i,j-1}), \\ & u_{xx} = \frac{1}{h^2}(u_{i+1,j} + u_{i-1,j} - 2u_{i,j}), u_{yy} = \frac{1}{h^2}(u_{i,j+1} + u_{i,j-1} - 2u_{i,j}), \\ & u_{xy} = \frac{1}{h^2}(u_{i+1,j+1} - u_{i-1,j+1} - u_{i+1,j-1} + u_{i-1,j-1}) \end{aligned} \tag{11.64}$$

where h is the grid spacing. And the optimal estimates for the mean u_i and the variance σ_i can be computed:

$$.u_i = \frac{\int \chi_{R_i}(\vec{\gamma}_i)I(x)dx}{\int \chi_{R_i}(\vec{\gamma}_i)dx}, \sigma_i^2 = \frac{\int \chi_{R_i}(\vec{\gamma}_i)(I(x) - u_i)^2 dx}{\int \chi_{R_i}(\vec{\gamma}_i)dx} \tag{11.65}$$

11.3.3.5 Description of our Proposed Method

Here, the segmentation procedure of our proposed method is summarized as follows:

Step 1: Set initial parameters: set a given fixed region number N, the number of iterations *Max_iter*, and the weighted factor α.

Step 2: Initialize the curves $\{\vec{\gamma}_i\}_{i=1}^m$, with $\{\vec{\gamma}_i^k\}_{i=1}^{N-1}$ defined as the distance function from initial curves, and computer the factor β to weigh the relative contribution of the region merging term based on the mean intensity and variance over the whole image.

Step 3: For each $\vec{\gamma}_i$, compute the corresponding u_i and $\sigma_i, i = 1, \cdots N$ as the averages for each region.

Step 4: For each $\vec{\gamma}_i$, compute $\vec{\gamma}_i^{k+1}$ by solving the following:

$$\vec{\gamma}_i^{k+1} = \vec{\gamma}_i^k - \Delta t \frac{\partial E}{\partial t}\left(\{\vec{\gamma}_i\}_{i=1}^{N-1}\right) \tag{11.66}$$

where Δt is the time step.

Step 5: Reinitialize each curve $\vec{\gamma}_i^k$ locally from the queue $\{\vec{\gamma}_i\}_{i=1}^m$ to the signed distance function to the curve.

Step 6: Run the process until the curves $\{\vec{\gamma}_i\}_{i=1}^m$ reaches convergence.

11.4 Results

To demonstrate the effectiveness of our proposed method, a large number of tests with different image types have been carried out. First, we analyze the feasibility of the MR-MRLS method through examples and experimental results are shown on medical imaging. Then, we do a large number of experiments on synthetic images, some of which have various noise models. To illustrate the flexibility of the method, we also show a representative sample of the tests with a real medical image. These methods are implemented using the Matlab and C programming language and experimented on a Pentium IV 2 × 2.2 GHZ computer with Memory 3G. In our experiments, we fixed to the parameter of the model $\lambda = 0.1$ and the time step $\Delta t = 0.2$.

11.4.1 Multiresolution Level Set Method with Multiple Regions to Implement

In the last experiment, Figure 11.1 shows different segmentation results for two medical images with noise and inhomogeneity levels using different schemes. The typical schemes include the clustering-based method (***Clust***) [27], the multiphase Chan-Vese (***Mean***) [9], and the method with a

TABLE 11.1

Average DC Values for Different Schemes on Two Different Medical Images

	Regions	Mean	Ker	Clust	Our
First image (192×220)	D1	0.470278	0.334662	0.714674	**0.947548**
	D2	0.410583	0.204184	0.610954	**0.894213**
	D3	0.680684	0.378026	0.758349	**0.918747**
Second image (154×169)	D1	0.613491	0.334662	0.737412	**0.937621**
	D2	0.513734	0.379843	0.546438	**0.876933**
	D3	0.640673	0.510972	0.720219	**0.908747**

kernel induced data term (***Ker***) [26]. In these models, the number of iterations and regions, and the step time is all 300, 3 and 0.01s, respectively. And they have the same initial curves. The results indicate that the ***Ker*** and ***Mean*** methods can lead to poor separation of different regions whereas noise can affect the result of ***Clust*** schemes. Since the size of the segmented image is not large, the SR-MGC model is used to partition the same medical images. From the segmentation results, the proposed model handles higher non-uniformity without degrading the final segmentation results. We further use the average DC values to show a comparison result with other related multiphase active contour methods as shown in Table 11.1. As can be seen, our proposed model performs better in terms of the DC compared with other related approaches in all of the three regions.

11.4.2 Image Segmentation using Statistical Approaches with Multiple Regions

The piecewise constant segmentation method based on Gaussian kernel has been the focus of most studies and applications [12] [26] because of its tractability. In the following, we use the synthetic images to illustrate the effectiveness of our proposed method. In the experiment, the parameter α for region merging prior is set at 1.

Figure 11.2 shows the segmentation process of our proposed method. The image is partitioned into four regions. The initial positions of the curves are shown in Figure 11.2 (b); After 30 iterations, the final position of the curves at convergence with multiple regions is shown Figure 11.2 (c); three segmented regions surrounding by three curves in Figure 11.2 (b) are shown in Figure 11.2 (d-f).

Next, the influence of the region merging prior is represented, which can make some curves disappear at convergence, and the segmentation result is shown in Figure 11.3. The initial number of regions for the synthetic image varies from four to seven regions. The first line of Figure 11.3 depicts the curve initializations corresponding to the different values of N. To illustrate the influence of the region merging prior, we show the results obtained with the

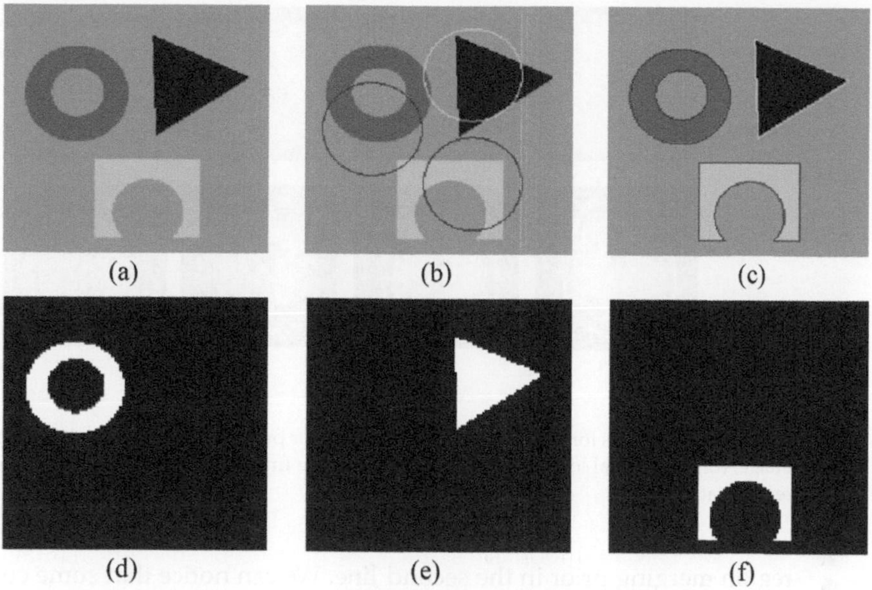

FIGURE 11.2
The synthetic image segmentation using our proposed level set method. (a) The input image; (b) The initial curves in the input image; (c) shows the final segmentation result of contour images; (d) Final segmentation result of the first region; (e) Final segmentation result of the second region; (f) Final segmentation result of the third region.

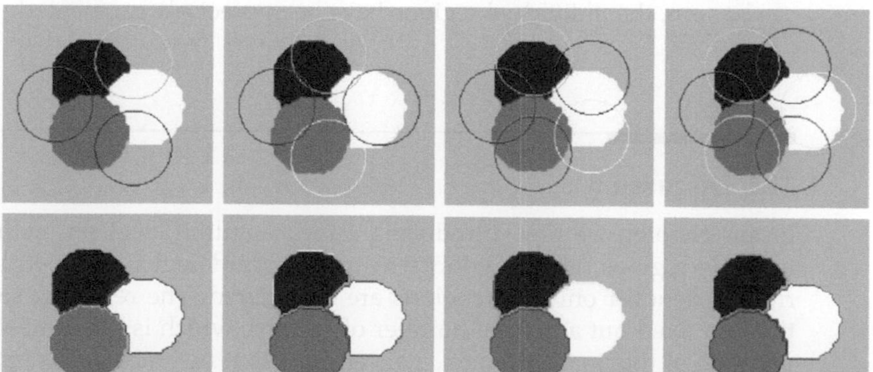

FIGURE 11.3
Segmentation of the synthetic image using our proposed level set method. Line 1: Different number of regions at the initialization; line 2: final curves which remained at convergence with the region segmentation.

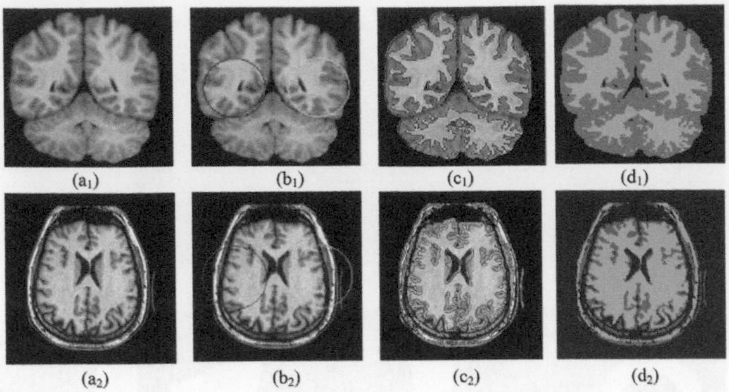

FIGURE 11.4
Segmentation results for the medical images using our proposed level set method: (ai) The input image; (bi) The initial location of the curves; (ci) The final location of the curves; (di) The final segmentation result.

region merging prior in the second line. We can notice that some curves disappear at convergence (Line 2), leading to the same correct segmentation into four regions. The term of the region merging prior balances the effect of the data term.

The results of the medical images using our proposed level set method are shown in Figure 11.4. In this experiment, the number of iterations for each image was set at 30 and 50, respectively. The first column of Figure 11.4 shows the input original image; the second column shows initial contour image with two circles for each image; the third column shows the final curves remaining at convergence; the forth column shows the result of image segmentation. As can be seen, the individual regions have been precisely segmented.

11.5 Discussion

In this chapter, we first introduce a multiresolution level set method with multiple regions, which reduces to the standard region competition algorithm whenever only two regions are considered. The resulting segmentation is a fixed but arbitrary number of regions, which is guaranteed to be a partition of the image domain. This ensures that no ambiguities arise when assigning points to the various segmented regions. The solution with multiresolution level set method not only improve the robustness of the segmentation procedure but also decreases the computational cost. The experimental results show that the final segmentation remains a partition of the image domain and that the method is efficient.

Next, we introduce an efficient level set method on statistical approach with multiple regions, which reduces to the standard region competition algorithm whenever only two regions are considered. The resulting segmentation is a number of regions, which is guaranteed to be a partition of the image domain. This ensures that no ambiguities arise when assigning points to the various segmented regions. The experimental results show that the final segmentation remains a partition of the image domain and that the method is efficient.

References

1. Ayed B., Mitchie A., and Belhadj Z. Multiregion level-set partitioning of synthetic aperture radar images. *IEEE Trans Pattern Anal Mach Intell.* 2005; 27: 793–800; doi: 10.1109/TPAMI.2005.106.
2. Pham D. L., Xu C., and Prince J. Current methods in medical image segmentation. *Ann Rev Biomed Eng.* 2000; 2: 315–338.
3. Cai Q., Aggarwal J. Human motion analysis: A review. *Comput Vis Image Underst.* 1999; 73: 428–440; doi: 10.1109/NAMW.1997.609859.
4. Zhao T., Nevatia R., Wu B. Segmentation and tracking of multiple humans in crowded environments. *IEEE Trans Pattern Anal Mach Intell.* 2008; 30: 1198–1211; doi: 10.1109/TPAMI.2007.70770.
5. Caselles V., Kimmel R., and Sapiro G. Geodesic active contours. *Int J Comput Vis.* 1997; 22: 61–79; doi: 10.1023/A:10079798.
6. Chan T. and Vese L. Active contours without edges. *IEEE Trans on Image Proc.* 2001; 10: 266–277; doi: 10.1016/S1470-2045(12)70388-1.
7. Li C., Kao C. Y., Gore J. C., Ding Z. Minimization of region-scalable fitting energy for image segmentation. *IEEE Trans on Image Proc.* 2008; 17: 1940–1949; doi: 10.1007/978-3-642-17274-8_12.
8. Mansouri A.-R., Mitiche A., Vazquez C. Multiregion competition: A level set extension of region competition to multiple region image partitioning. *Comput Vis Image Underst.* 2006;101:137–150; doi: 10.1200/JCO.2012.44.0586.
9. Vese L., Chan T. A multiphase level set framework for image segmentation using the Mumford and Shah model. *Int J Comput Vis.* 2002; 50: 271–293; doi: 10.1023/A:1020874308076.
10. Lankton S., Tannenbaum A. Localizing region-based active contours. *IEEE Trans on Image Proc.* 2008; 17 (11): 2029–2039; doi: 10.1109/TIP.2008.2004611.
11. Brox T., Weickert J. Level set segmentation with multiple regions. *IEEE Trans on Image Proc.* 2006; 15(10): 3213–3218; doi: 10.1109/TIP.2006.877481.
12. Cremers D., Rousson M., Deriche R. A review of statistical approaches to level set segmentation: Integrating color, texture, motion and shape. *Int J Comput Vis.* 2007; 72(2): 195–215; doi: 10.1007/s11263-006-8711-1A.
13. Bertelli L., Sumengen B., Manjunath B., Gibou F. A variational framework for multi-region pairwise similarity-based image segmentation. *IEEE Trans Pattern Anal Mach Intell.* 2008; 30(8): 1400–1414; doi: 10.1109/TPAMI.2007.70785.

14. Li C. M., Kao C. Y., Gore J. C., Ding Z. Implicit active contours driven by local binary fitting energy. *Proc of IEEE Conf Comput Vis and Pattern Recog* 2007;1–7; doi: 10.1109/CVPR.2007.383014.
15. Brox T. and Cremers D. On local region models and a statistical interpretation of the piecewise smooth Mumford-Shah functional. *Int J Comput Vis.* 2009; 84(2): 184–193; doi: 10.1007/s11263-008-0153-5.
16. Mumford D., and Shah J. Optimal approximations by piecewise smooth functions and associated variational problems. *Commun Pure Appl Math.* 1989; 42(5): 577–685.
17. Li C. M., Xu C., Gui C., Fox M. D. Level set evolution without re-initialization: A new variational formulation. *Proc of IEEE Conf Comput Vis and Pattern Recog.* 2005; 430–436; doi: 10.1109/CVPR.2005.213.
18. Law Y. N., Lee H. K., Yip A. M. A multiresolution stochastic level set method for Mumford-Shah image segmentation. *IEEE Trans on Image Proc.* 2008; 17(12): 2289–2300; doi: 10.1109/TIP.2008.2005823.
19. Bazi Y., Melgani F., Al-Sharari H. D. Unsupervised change detection in multispectral remotely sensed imagery with level set methods. *IEEE Trans. on Geoscience & Remote Sensing.* 2010; 48(8): 3178–3187; doi: 10.1109/TGRS.2010.2045506.
20. Zhu G. P., Zhang S. Q., Zeng Q. S., Wang C. H. Boundary-based image segmentation using binary level set method. *Opt. Eng.* 2007; 46: 050501; doi: 10.1117/1.2740762.
21. Zhu G. P., Zeng Q. S., Wang C. H. Dual geometric active contour for image segmentation. *Opt. Eng.* 2006; 45: 080505; doi: 10.1117/1.2333566.
22. Liu F., Luo Y. Q., Hu D. C. Adaptive level set image segmentation using the Mumford and Shah functional. *Opt. Eng.* 2002; 41: 3002–3003; doi: 10.1117/1.1519542.
23. Zhu S. C., Yuille A. Region competition: unifying snakes, region growing, and Bayes/MDL for multiband image segmentation. *IEEE Trans Pattern Anal Mach Intell.* 1996; 18(9): 884–900; doi: 10.1109/34.537343.
24. Martin P., Refregier P., Goudail F., Guerault F. Influence of the noise model on level set active contour segmentation. *IEEE Trans Pattern Anal Mach Intell.* 2004; 26(6): 799–803; doi: 10.1109/TPAMI.2004.11.
25. Kim J., Fisher J. W., Yezzi A., Cetin M. Nonparametric methods for image segmentation using information theory and curve evolution. In *Int. Conf. on Image Processing.* 2002; 3: 797–800; doi: 10.1109/ICIP.2002.1039092.
26. Ayed I. B., Mitiche A. A region merging prior for variational level set image segmentation. *IEEE Trans on Image Proc.* 2008; 17(12): 2301–2311; doi: 10.1109/TIP.2008.2006425.
27. Salah M. Ben, Mitiche A., Ayed I. B. Effective level set image segmentation with a kernel induced data term. *IEEE Trans on Image Proc.* 2010; 19(1): 220-232; doi: 10.1109/TIP.2009.2032940.

12

Image Segmentation With B-Spline Level Set

Shenhai Zheng, Bin Fang, and Laquan Li

CONTENTS

12.1 Introduction

Finding a general mechanism for switching between the continuous and discrete signal domains is one of the fundamental issues in signal processing [1]. During processing, an analog signal or image is represented in a discrete form using a sequence of numbers (discrete representation). Conversely, the need for a continuous signal representation comes up when one wishes to implement numerically an operator that is initially defined in the continuous domain [2]. An obvious approach is to fit a parametrized continuous image model to the observed data points and to derive algorithms that operate on the model's parameter values, such as edge detection and geometric transformations. Piecewise two-dimensional polynomial functions are frequently used in this context [3, 4]. For the few degrees of freedom and some built-in smoothness constraints, one usually chooses to use an approximate representation in which the function parameters are determined by minimizing some measure of the discrepancy between pixel values and real-valued image function at the grid points [5].

For image edge detection, early techniques relied on finite differences to estimate the spatial gradients or Laplacians [6]. However, these simple operators perform poorly for the noisy images. Some recent approaches were studied depending on the concept of fitting a continuous surface locally to the image data [4, 7]. Contrasted to the polynomial fits, the use of B-spline functions seems to have a number of advantages [5]. First, higher order polynomials tend to oscillate while spline functions are usually smooth and well behaved. Second, B-spline surfaces are continuous everywhere, especially in the connection regions where the juxtaposition of local polynomials tent to oscillate. Third, there is exactly one B-spline coefficient associated with each grid point, and the range of these coefficients is of the same order of magnitude as that of the initial gray level values [8]. Finally, either exact or approximate B-spline signal representations can be evaluated quite efficiently.

In the past two decades, active contour models (ACM), based on the principle of smoothness and continuity, have been proposed. They are successful deformable models and have been extensively studied in image segmentation because of the sub-pixel accuracy and closed object boundary. The level set based methods corresponding to the ACM capture the shape of the object by propagating an interface which is represented by the zero level set of a smooth implicit function (usually called the level-set function). Level sets are widely used for 2D image segmentation [9, 10] and 2D or 3D medical image segmentation [11–14] among other areas.

As an alternative to this well-known implicit scheme, there is a continuous approach where the level-set function is expressed as a continuous parametric function. In [15] and [16], the continuous representation is based on radial-basis functions (RBFs), which are then used to solve the level-set PDE. In [17, 18], the level-set function is expressed as a continuous parametric function using B-splines. In contrast with the RBFs-based approaches, the B-spline method is to fit the level-set function to the B-spline coefficients which allows one to formulate the B-spline level set from the initial level-set energy functional and compute the solution as a restriction of the variational problem onto the space spanned by the B-splines. As a consequence, the minimization of the functional is directly obtained in terms of the B-spline coefficients [18]. Before that, B-splines have already been used in the context of deformable models. Realization of Snakes using B-splines was developed in [19], [20] and [21]. In [22], the shape contour is modelled as quadratic B-spline curves in order to introduce statistical shape priori into the MS [23] model. In [24], in order to constrain the domain transformations to a linear combination of a set of predefined transformations, B-splines are used for shape gradient-based level-set evolution for image segmentation.

In this chapter, the use of B-spline level-set segmentation model in medical image segmentation is presented. Compared to the traditional implicit presentation, the use of B-splines as a basis for the level-set representation provides some specific additional benefits, such as fast convergence and the intrinsic smoothing contour to the segmentation solution.

12.2 Spline Interpolation

12.2.1 Polynomial Splines

A function $s(x)$ is a polynomial spline of degree n with knots $(\cdots < x_k < x_{k+1} < \cdots)$ if it satisfies the following two properties:

1. Piecewise polynomial: $s(x)$ is a polynomial of degree n with each interval $[x_k, x_{k+1})$;
2. Higher-order continuity: $s(x), s^{(1)}(x), \ldots, s^{(n-1)}(x)$ are continuous at the knots x_k.

Splines are piecewise polynomials with pieces that are smoothly connected together. The joining points of the polynomials are called knots. For a spline of degree n, each segment is a polynomial of degree n. In this case, one needs $n+1$ coefficients to describe each segment. However, there is an additional smoothness constraint that imposes the continuity of the spline and its derivatives up to order $(n-1)$ at the knots, so that, effectively, there is only one degree of freedom per segment. Here, we will only consider splines with uniform knots and unit spacing. Consider splines with uniform knots and unit spacing one analog signal $s(x)$ has a unique and stable representation of B-spline expansion:

$$s(x) = \sum_{k \in Z} c(k)\beta^n(x - k) \tag{12.1}$$

This B-spline model is linear, which involves the integer shifts of the central B-spline of degree n denoted by β^n; the parameters of the model are the B-spline coefficients $c(k)$ (discrete signal).

Firstly, the definition of a rectangular function $\beta^0(x)$ is given as:

$$\beta^0(x) = \begin{cases} 1, & |x| < \dfrac{1}{2} \\ 0, & otherwise \\ \dfrac{1}{2}, & |x| = \dfrac{1}{2} \end{cases} \tag{12.2}$$

Then the symmetrical, bell-shaped functions β^n is constructed from the $(n+1)$-fold convolution of a rectangular pulse $\beta^0(x)$, i.e., the central B-spline of degree n is given as:

$$\beta^n(x) = \underbrace{\beta^0 * \beta^0 * \cdots * \beta^0(x)}_{(n+1)\ times} \tag{12.3}$$

With the Fourier transform and Euler formula, Eq. (12.3) can be written as:

$$\beta^n(x) = \frac{1}{n!}\sum_{k=0}^{n+1} \binom{n+1}{k} (-1)^k \left(x - k + \frac{n+1}{2}\right)_+^n \tag{12.4}$$

The $(x)_+^n = \{\begin{smallmatrix} x^n, & x \geq 0 \\ 0, & x < 0 \end{smallmatrix}$ is the one-side power function. The B-splines of degrees 0 to 3 are shown in Figure 12.1.

Thanks to the representation of (12.1), each spline is unambiguously characterized by its sequence of B-spline coefficients $c(k)$, which has the convenient structure of a discrete signal, even though the underlying model is continuous (discrete/continuous representation).

Within the family of polynomial splines, cubic splines tend to be the most popular in applications-perhaps due to their minimum curvature property.

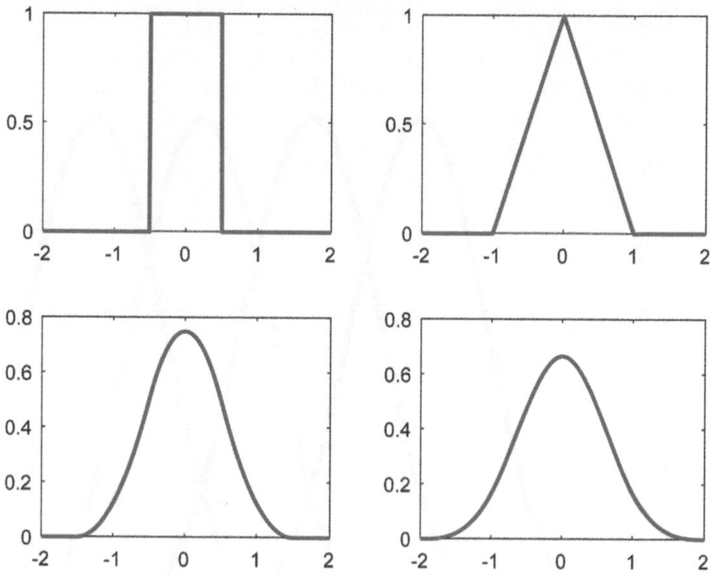

FIGURE 12.1
The centered B-splines of degree 0 to 3.

The closed-form representation of the cubic B-spline is given as:

$$
\begin{aligned}
\beta^3(x) &= \frac{1}{6}(x+2)_+^3 - \frac{4}{6}(x+1)_+^3 + (x)_+^3 - \frac{4}{6}(x-1)_+^3 + \frac{1}{6}(x-2)_+^3 \\
&= \begin{cases} \dfrac{(2-|x|)^3}{6}, & 1 \le |x| < 2 \\ 0, & 2 \le |x| \\ \dfrac{2}{3} - |x|^2 + \dfrac{|x|^3}{2}, & 0 \le |x| < 1 \end{cases}
\end{aligned}
\tag{12.5}
$$

which is often used for performing high-quality interpolation.

Let $\beta_k^n = \beta^n(x-k)$ is the transformed B-splines, then the B-splines of β_{-1}^3, β_0^3, β_1^3 and β_2^3, which are shown in Figure 12.2, have the property of $\sum_{i=-1}^{3} \beta_i^3(x) = 1$.

Use these transformed B-splines functions, many image geometric transformation (scaling, rotation and translation) can be performed efficiently. Let (x, y) and (x_0, y_0) are the pixel coordinates of output and input image, respectively. The relationship between them is shown in Figure 12.3. With the same size of output and input image, generally, image geometric transformation

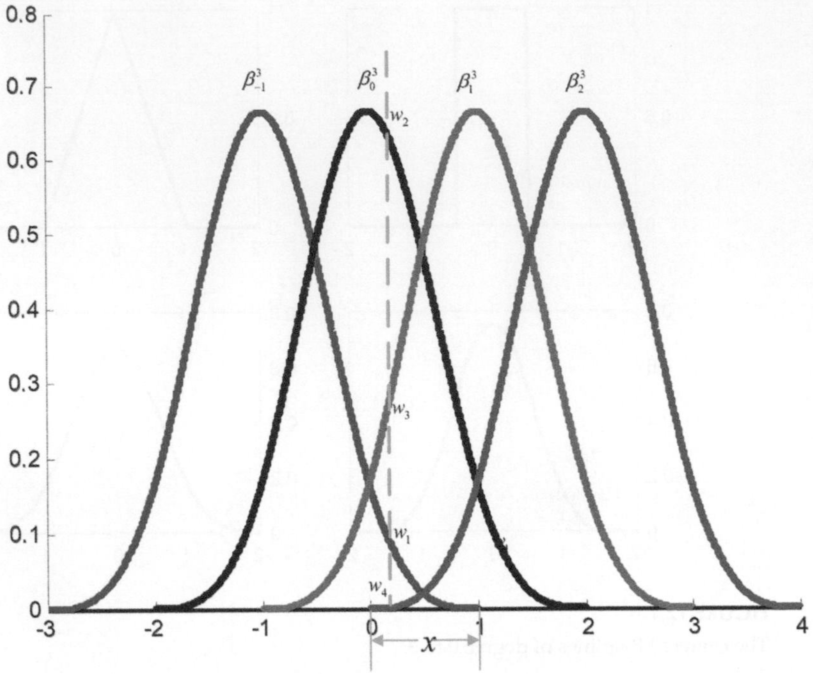

FIGURE 12.2
Four transformed B-splines functions.

can be written as:

$$\begin{cases} x_0 = \dfrac{(x - x_c - a)\cos\theta + (y - y_c - b)\sin\theta}{r} + x_c \\ y_0 = \dfrac{-(x - x_c - a)\sin\theta + (y - y_c - b)\cos\theta}{r} + y_c \end{cases} \tag{12.6}$$

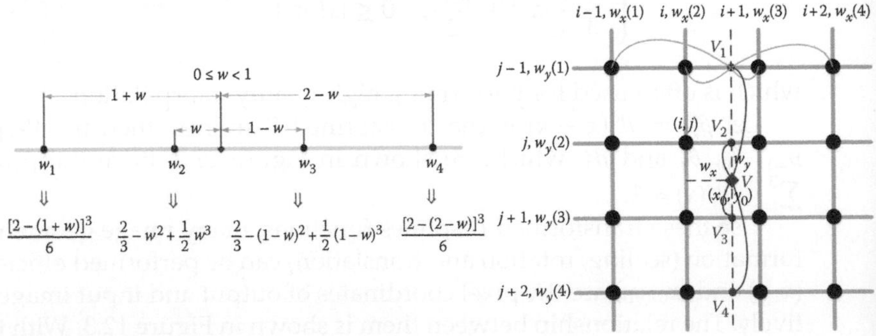

FIGURE 12.3
Bi-linear cubic B-spline interpolation model.

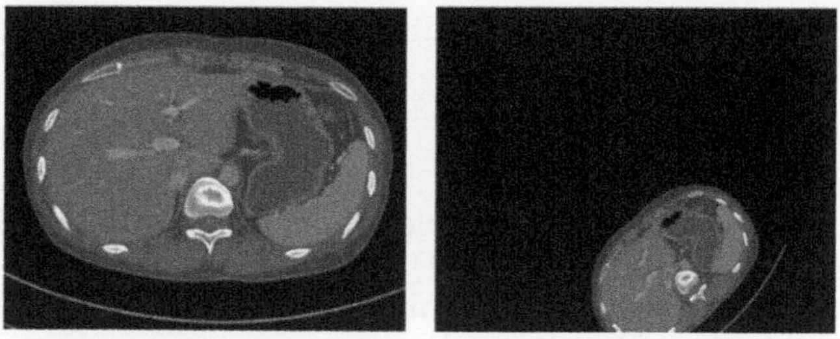

(a) (b)

FIGURE 12.4
The image geometric transformation results. (a) is the original image. (b) is the geometric transformation result with $a = 30$, $b = 80$, $r = 0.5$ and $\theta = \frac{\pi}{4}$.

where $(x_c, y_c) = (0.5W, 0.5H)$ (W and H are the width and height of image), θ is the rotation angle, r is the scaling parameter and (a, b) is the transformation.

Let $w_1(x) = \beta^3_{-1}(x)$, $w_2(x) = \beta^3_0(x)$, $w_3(x) = \beta^3_2(x)$ and $w_4(x) = \beta^3_3(x)$ as the interpolation weights (as show in Figure 12.2 and left of Figure 12.3.). So the bi-linear cubic B-spline image interpolation model is shown right of Figure 12.3. That is to say, the gray scale at point (x_0, y_0) is interpolated by:

$$V = V_1 w_y(1) + V_2 w_y(2) + V_3 w_y(3) + V_4 w_y(4) \tag{12.7}$$

where $V_k = \sum_{m=1}^{4} I(i-2+m, j-2+k) w_x(m), k \in \{1, 2, 3, 4\}$ and $w_x(m) = w_m(x)$.

Figure 12.4 shows some image geometric transformation results.

12.2.2 B-Spline Interpolation via Digital Filtering

Now considering to determine a B-spline interpolation model of a given input signal $s(k)$ such that the B-spline function goes through the data points exactly. This is a trivial matter for splines of degree 0 (piece wise constant) and splines of degree 1 (piecewise linear) because the B-spline coefficients are identical to the signal samples: $c(k) = s(k)$. For higher-degree splines the situation is more complex. Traditionally, the B-spline interpolation problem has been approached by setting up and solving a band-diagonal system of equations [8, 25]. An alternative to this problem could also be approached using simpler digital filtering techniques [1, 26, 27].

To derive this type of signal processing algorithm, one needs to introduce the discrete B-spline kernel b^n_m, which is obtained by sampling the B-spline of degree n expanded by a factor of 2^m.

$$b^n_m(k) = \beta^n\left(\frac{x}{2^m}\right)\bigg|_{x=k} \quad (m = 0, 1, 2, \cdots\cdots) \tag{12.8}$$

For example, $b^3_0(-2) = \beta^3(-2) = 0$ and $b^3_0(-1) = b^3_0(1) = \frac{1}{6}$.

Introduce the Z-transformation of b_m^n, one have:

$$b_m^n(k) \overset{Z}{\longleftrightarrow} B_m^n(z) = \sum_{k \in Z} b_m^n(k) z^{-k} \tag{12.9}$$

Now, given the signal samples $s(k)$, one wants to determine the coefficients $c(k)$ of the B-spline model (12.1) such that $\sum_{l \in Z} c(l)\beta^n(x-l)\big|_{x=k} = s(k), \forall k \in Z$. Using the discrete B-splines, this formulation can be rewritten in the form of a convolution: $s(k) = (b_l^n * c)(k)$.

Defining the inverse convolution operator:

$$\left(b_l^n\right)^{-1}(k) \overset{Z}{\longleftrightarrow} 1/B_l^n(z) \tag{12.10}$$

Then the solution is found by inverse filtering, i.e., $c(k) = (b_l^n)^{-1} * s(k)$.

Since b_l^n is symmetric finite impulse response, the so-called direct B-spline filter $(b_l^n)^{-1}$ is an all-pole system that can be implemented very efficiently using a cascade of first-order causal and anti-causal recursive filters [27, 28]. This algorithm is stable numerically and is faster and easier to implement than any other numerical technique. The explicit procedure for the cubic spline case is described in [1].

Example of B-spline interpolation via digital filtering is shown in Figure 12.5. The original signal is sampled from an image. With the computed B-spline coefficient $c(k)$, one can get the interpolation signal using $(b_l^n * c)(k)$.

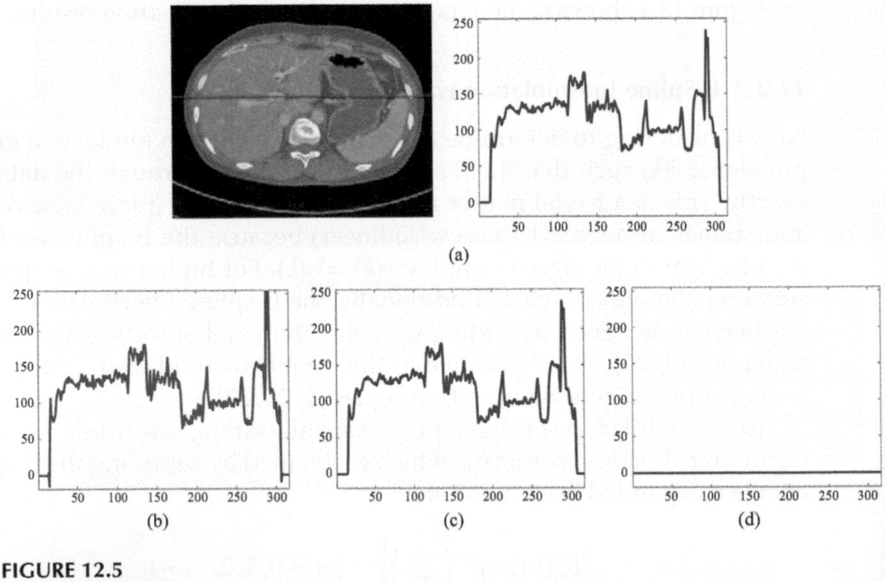

FIGURE 12.5
B-spline interpolation via digital filtering. (a) is the original signal which sampled from an image. (b) is the B-spline coefficient $c(k)$. (c) is the interpolation signal using B-spline coefficient and (d) is the absolute difference between the sampled signal and interpolation signal, respectively.

Results shown in Figure 12.5 demonstrate the efficiency of the numerical technique.

12.3 Variational B-Spline Level Set

12.3.1 Variational Level Set

Let $\Omega \in \mathbb{R}^d (d = 2, 3)$ is an image domain, and $I : \Omega \to \mathbb{R}$ is a given d-dimensional image. Chan and Vese (CV) [29] formulated a simplified global binary fitting image segmentation model based on the homogeneous of object and background regions:

$$F^{CV}\left(c_1, c_2, C\right) = \int_{inside(C)} |I(x) - c_1|^2 \, dx + \int_{outside(C)} |I(x) - c_2|^2 \, dx + v\,|C| \quad (12.11)$$

where *inside*(C) and *outside*(C) represent the object and background regions, $|C|$ is the length of contour, v are positive weight parameters. Intensity of each region is approximated by c_1 and c_2 respectively. The first two terms in Eq. (12.11) are global binary fitting energy which drive contours toward the true boundaries of objects. In the level-set framework, the evolving interface $C \subset \mathbb{R}^d$ is represented as the zero level set of a Lipschitz-continuous function ϕ of dimension $d + 1$ that satisfies:

$$\begin{cases} \phi(x) = 0, & x \in C \\ \phi(x) > 0, & x \in inside(C) \\ \phi(x) = 0, & x \in outside(C) \end{cases} \quad (12.12)$$

By using the Heaviside function H and Dirac function δ, the variational level-set formalism of CV model can be formulated as:

$$E\left(\phi, c_1, c_2\right) = \int_{\Omega} (I - c_1)^2 H(\phi) dx + \int_{\Omega} (I - c_2)^2 \left[1 - H(\phi)\right] dx + v \int_{\Omega} \delta(\phi)\, |\nabla \phi|\, dx \quad (12.13)$$

12.3.2 B-Spline Level-Set Model

The B-spline level-set model is obtained by expressing the level-set function ϕ as the linear combination of B-spline basis functions [18]:

$$\phi(x) = \sum_{k \in \mathbb{Z}^d} c[k] \beta^n \left(\frac{x}{h} - k\right) \quad (12.14)$$

$\beta^n(\bullet)$ is the uniform symmetric d-dimensional B-spline of degree n. This function is separable and is built as the product of d 1-Dimensional B-splines, so that $\beta^n(\mathbf{x}) = \prod_{j=1}^{d} \beta^n(x_j)$. The knots of the B-splines are located on a grid spanning Ω, with a regular spacing given by h. The coefficients of the B-spline representation are gathered in $c[\mathbf{k}]$.

12.3.3 B-Spline Level-Set Model Minimization

In contrast with the classical variational approaches, the minimization of this model is respect to the B-spline coefficients. Such minimization implies computing the derivatives of (12.13) with respect to each B-spline coefficient $c[\mathbf{k}_0]$.

Using differentiation with respect to parameter $c[\mathbf{k}_0]$, one has:

$$\frac{\partial E}{\partial c[\mathbf{k}_0]} = \int_\Omega \delta(\phi)\left[(I-c_1)^2-(I-c_2)^2 - v div\left(\frac{\nabla\phi}{|\nabla\phi|}\right)\right]\frac{\partial\phi}{\partial c[\mathbf{k}_0]}dx \qquad (12.15)$$

where $\frac{\partial\phi}{\partial c[\mathbf{k}_0]} = \beta^n(\frac{x}{h} - \mathbf{k}_0)$.

For the sake of simplicity, Eq. (12.15) is rewritten as:

$$\frac{\partial E}{\partial c[\mathbf{k}_0]} = \int_\Omega w(\mathbf{x})\beta^n\left(\frac{\mathbf{x}}{h} - \mathbf{k}_0\right)d\mathbf{x} \qquad (12.16)$$

where $w(\mathbf{x}) = \delta(\phi)[(I-c_1)^2-(I-c_2)^2 - v div(\frac{\nabla\phi}{|\nabla\phi|})]$ reflects the features of image and will be called the feature function in the sequel.

The minimization of the energy criterion (12.13) with respect to the B-spline coefficients generally does not lead to a closed-form solution. In order to obtain a local minimum, we then perform a gradient-descent method which yields:

$$c^{(i+1)} = c^{(i)} - \lambda\nabla_c E(c^{(i)}) \qquad (12.17)$$

where λ is the iteration step length and ∇_c corresponds to the gradient of the energy relative to the B-spline coefficients, the components of which being given by (12.16).

Equation (12.16) yields an interesting interpretation of the minimization process. Let $\beta_h^n(x) = \beta_h^n\left(x/h\right)$, which is the B-spline of degree n up scaled by a factor h. The expression of the energy gradient is then given by:

$$\nabla_c E = \frac{\partial E}{\partial c[\mathbf{k}]} = \int_\Omega w(\mathbf{x})\beta_h^n(\mathbf{x} - h\mathbf{k})d\mathbf{x} \qquad (12.18)$$

Let $w(\mathbf{u})$ is the corresponding discrete feature function, with $\mathbf{u} \in \mathbb{Z}^d$. One immediately obtains the discrete version of the gradient (12.18) by applying the discrete B-spline formulation of [5]. The centered d-dimensional discrete B-spline of degree n is noted $b^n(\mathbf{u})$ which is obtained by sampling its continuous version $\beta^n(\mathbf{x})$ at integer values. Similar to its continuous counterpart the sequence $b^n[\bullet]$ is separable and is built as the product of d 1-dimentional B-splines, so that $b^n[\mathbf{u}] = \prod_{j=1}^{d} b^n[u_j]$. By using an integer spacing of the knots (i.e., $h \in \mathbb{N} \setminus \{0\}$), one may define the discrete B-spline of degree scaled by a factor h as $b^n[u] = \beta^n(u/h)$.

Then, the discrete version of the formulation is then obtained from (12.18) as:

$$\langle \nabla_c E \rangle [k] = \left\langle \frac{\partial E}{\partial c[k]} \right\rangle = \sum_{u \in \mathbb{Z}^d} w[u] b_h^n[u - hk] \tag{12.19}$$

Thus, the energy gradient corresponds to the convolution of the feature image and the B-spline, down-sampled by a factor h; put differently: $\langle \nabla_c E \rangle [k] = (w * b_h^n)_{\downarrow h}[k]$. This expression provides an efficient way of calculating the gradient and, thus, the evolution of the level set through (12.17). Since the B-spline kernel $b_h^n[u]$ is separable, the gradient may indeed be computed as a simple series of d convolutions of the feature image with a 1-dimentional B-spline kernel.

In effect, each step of the level-set evolution corresponds to filtering the feature image with a B-spline kernel—that is, performing a low-pass filtering operation. This induces an intrinsic smoothing in the algorithm. For a fixed B-spline degree n, the amount of smoothing can be controlled by choosing the scale of the filter $b_h^n[u]$ (i.e., by choosing the knot spacing h). This provides a way to efficiently deal with noisy images. In the implementation of this model, the flow chart of the B-spline level-set model is shown in Figure 12.6.

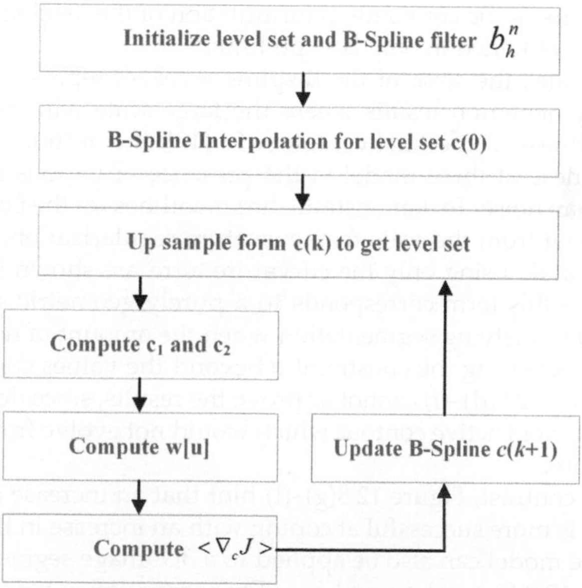

FIGURE 12.6
The flow chart of the B-spline level-set model.

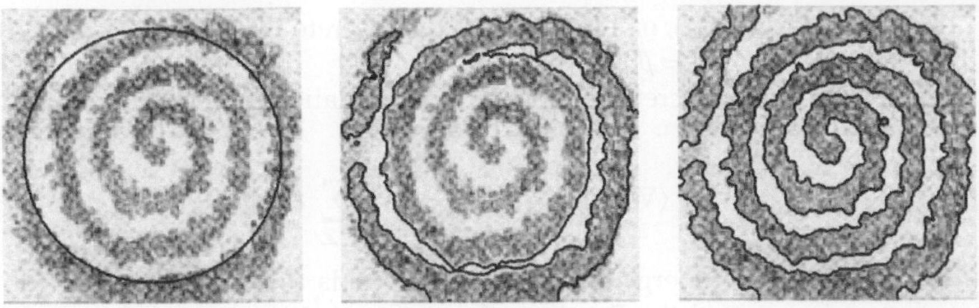

(a) (b) (c)

FIGURE 12.7
Segmentation of a textured spiral image. Full-scale model ($h = 1$) with curvature weight $v = 0.08 \times 255^2$. (a) Initialization; (b) level set after 11 iterations; (c) segmentation result obtained after 46 iterations, the cpu time is 20s.

12.3.4 B-Spline Level-Set Model Experiment

Figure 12.7 gives the segmentation results obtained on an image containing a textured spiral. From the initial solution, the zero-level interface propagates into the spiral and converges to the final curve after 46 iterations. In this case, the B-spline representation is applied at full scale ($h = 1$), which corresponds to a knot placed at every pixel of the image of size 256 × 256. In this example, the curvature regularization is set as $v = 0.08 \times 255^2$. Thanks to the separable nature of the convolution formulation of the level-set evolution, the final result is obtained in only 20s cpu time.

Usually, the scale of the B-spline level-set representation will influence the segmentation results where the large scale will increase the degree of smoothness of the final contours. In [18], the author also demonstrate the robustness of these model in the presence of various amounts of additive Gaussian noise. To demonstrate the smoothness of the final contours are more beneficial from the scale than curvature regularization, the results obtained at full scale using only the curvature term are shown in Figure 12.8(d)–(f). Because this term corresponds to a purely geometric smoothing, it cannot provide satisfying segmentation when the amount of noise is important. Indeed, increasing the constraint v beyond the values corresponding to those of Figure 12.8(d)–(f) cannot improve the results, since doing this would yield a quasi-rigid active contour which would not evolve from the initial solution anymore.

By contrast, Figure 12.8(g)–(l) hint that an increase of the scale of the B-spline is more successful at coping with an increase in the amount of noise.

The model can also be applied to a 3D image segmentation, as shown in Figure 12.9 for a calcaneus bone. The segmentation was obtained at full scale without curvature term. Results of three image slices and 3D visualization of the resulting segmentation are shown in Figure 12.9. These results show the ability of the model to handle complex topology.

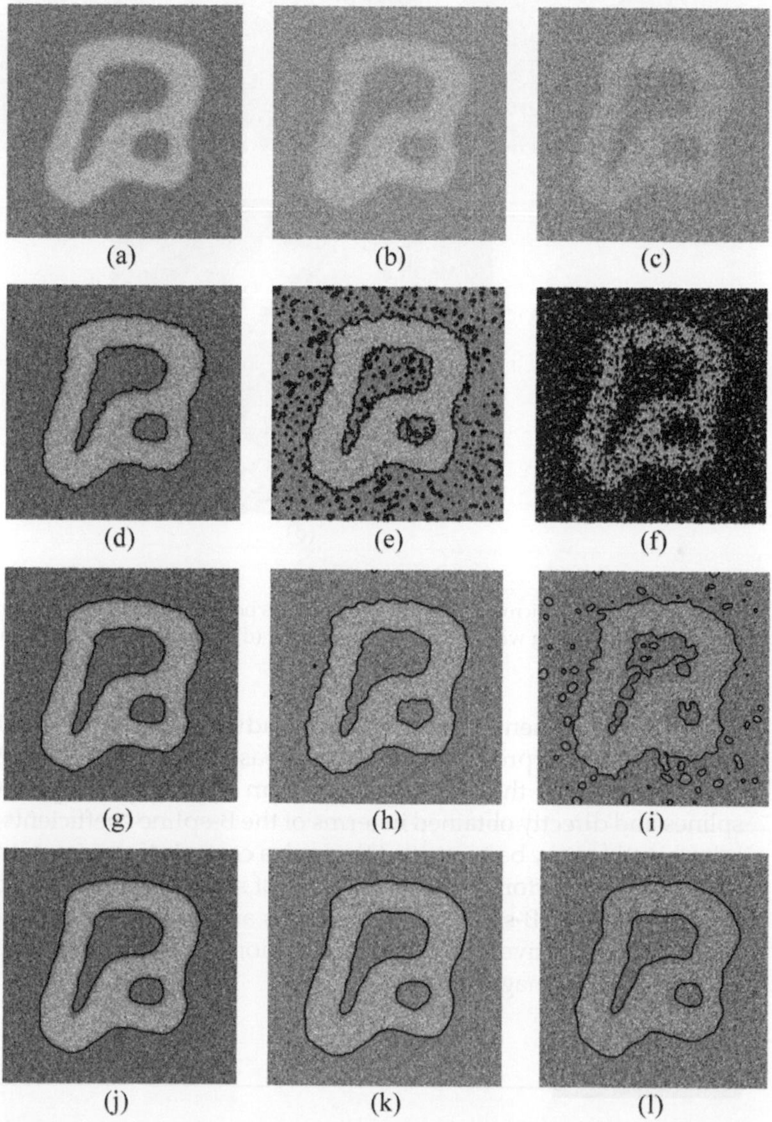

FIGURE 12.8
Segmentation of images with different SNR values. Each column corresponds to a given noise level (left: 25 dB, middle: 20 dB, right: 15 dB); each row corresponds to a given scale. Top row: original images. Second row: $h = 1$ with curvature term. Third row: $h = 4$ without curvature term. Bottom row: $h = 8$ without curvature term.

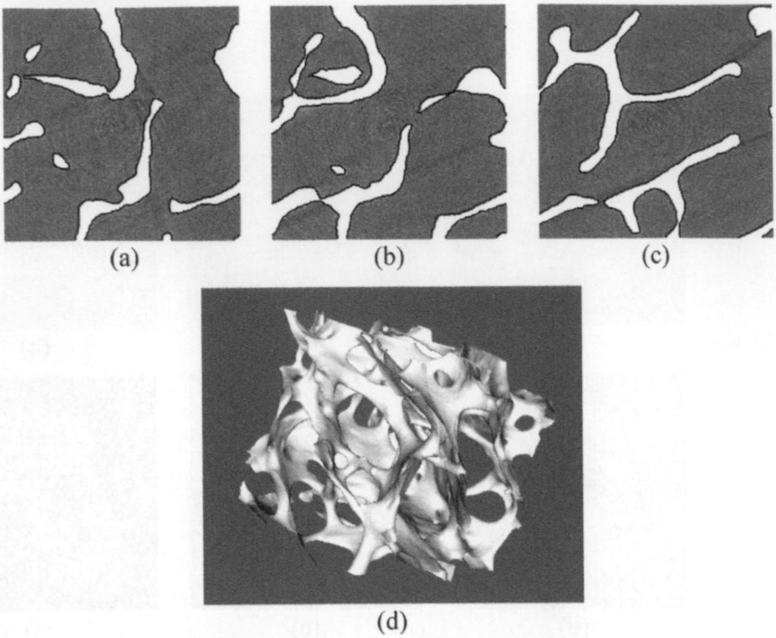

FIGURE 12.9
Segmentation of 3D micro-CT images of a calcaneus bone. (a)–(c) Three slices through the original data volume, along with the obtained contours; (d) 3D rendering of the resulting segmentation.

These experiments demonstrate the advantages of the continuous parametric function expressed on a B-spline basis: The solution can be computed as a restriction of the variational problem on the space spanned by the B-splines and directly obtained in terms of the B-spline coefficients; Each step of minimization may be expressed through a convolution operation, this convolution may be performed as a sequence of simple 1D convolutions; Filtering operation with a B-spline kernel induces an intrinsic smoothing of the contour. This alternative level-set segmentation method show more advantages in handling the image noise.

12.4 Variational B-Spline Level Set with Moment-Based Shape Prior

This section presents a new shape prior-based implicit level-set model for image segmentation based on linear combination of B-spline basic functions. In [30], they proposed an energy functional including a data term and a shape prior term. The data term comes from the region information of the image to segment. The shape prior term constraints the evolution of the contour with respect to the reference shape.

12.4.1 Moment-Based Shape Description

In most shape prior-based approaches, a fundamental step is to align the shapes such as the training shape and the shape to be segmented, to account for possible pose variations. The pose parameters are associated with rotation, scaling, and translation. Different from the general partial differential equations based alignment, one can takes into account the affine transformation to compute the pose transformation utilizing the theory of moment invariants and shape normalization [31–33]. Moments naturally provide region-based shape descriptors.

The set of geometric moments [34] of function $f(x, y)$ is commonly defined as:

$$m_{pq} = \int_{-\infty}^{\infty} \int_{-\infty}^{\infty} x^p y^q f(x, y) dx dy \tag{12.20}$$

where p and q are nonnegative integers, $(p + q)$ is the order of the moment. The zero order moment is the area of an object and the first order moments are used to locate the image centroids or center of mass which computed by $(\bar{x}, \bar{y}) = (m_{10}/m_{00}, m_{01}/m_{00})$.

Then, the central moments can be defined as:

$$\mu_{pq} = \int_{-\infty}^{\infty} \int_{-\infty}^{\infty} (x - \bar{x})^p (y - \bar{y})^q f(x, y) dx dy \tag{12.21}$$

To make the shape invariant to translation, scaling, and rotation, the shape normalization procedure must be considered and the procedure can be summarized as for steps (please refer [31] to learn the details of these procedure):

Step 1: Compute covariance matrix M of the original shape.

Step 2: Align the coordinates with the eigenvectors of M.

Step 3: Rescale the coordinates according to the eigenvalues of M to get the compact shape.

Step 4: Rotate the compact shape with respect to the ellipse tilt angle to get the normalized shape, which is invariant under translation, scaling, and rotation.

After the above processes, the transformation equation from the original to the normalized shape is achieved as:

$$\begin{bmatrix} \tilde{x} \\ \tilde{y} \end{bmatrix} = RWE \begin{bmatrix} x - \bar{x} \\ y - \bar{y} \end{bmatrix} \tag{12.22}$$

where R, W and E are three transformation matrixes. As mentioned in [31], the shape normalization procedure presented above is applicable for non-symmetric shapes while results in unsatisfactory results for symmetric shapes. So the called normalization to second rotation is utilize to address this problem.

12.4.2 B-Spline Level-Set Model with Moment-Based Shape Prior

Simply, the energy functional of the shape prior model is given as the following equation:

$$E = E_{image} + \alpha E_{shape} \tag{12.23}$$

Where E_{image} is the term respected to the image region and edge, E_{shape} is the shape energy measuring the distance between the evolving shape and a reference shape and $\alpha \geq 0$ is a weighting factor. Without loss of generality, one can consider the E_{image} is the data fitting term of the CV model [29].

The term E_{image} is defined as:

$$\begin{aligned} E_{image}(\phi, c_1, c_2) = & \int_\Omega (I - c_1)^2 H(\phi(x,y))dxdy \\ & + \int_\Omega (I - c_2)^2 \left[1 - H(\phi(x,y))\right] dxdy \end{aligned} \tag{12.24}$$

The term E_{shape} is given as follows:

$$E_{shape}(\phi, \tilde{\phi}) = \int_\Omega \left[H(\phi(x,y)) - H(\tilde{\phi}(x,y))\right]^2 dxdy \tag{12.25}$$

ϕ and $\tilde{\phi}$ are the signed distance function for the evolving shape and reference shape, respectively. As used in Section 12.3, the function ϕ is expressed as Eq. (12.14), where $\boldsymbol{x} = (x, y)$. One can see that, in the image term, the length term of CV model is omitted because the shape prior term is capable of controlling the smoothness of the segmentation.

In numerical approximation, the Heaviside function H is approximated by a smooth function H_ε as defined in [35]. Thus, the energy functional in (12.23) is approximated by:

$$\begin{aligned} E_\varepsilon(\phi, c_1, c_2, \tilde{\phi}) = & \int_\Omega (I - c_1)^2 H_\varepsilon(\phi(x,y))dxdy \\ & + \int_\Omega (I - c_2)^2[1 - H_\varepsilon(\phi(x,y))]dxdy \\ & + \alpha \int_\Omega [H_\varepsilon(\phi(x,y)) - H_\varepsilon(\tilde{\phi}(x,y))]^2 dxdy \end{aligned} \tag{12.26}$$

For the minimization of energy functional (12.26), one can use the standard gradient descent method.

Firstly, keeping ϕ fixed, the energy functional with respect to c_1 and c_2 is minimized by:

$$c_1 = \frac{\int_\Omega IH_\varepsilon(\phi(x,y))dxdy}{\int_\Omega H_\varepsilon(\phi(x,y))dxdy}, \quad c_2 = \frac{\int_\Omega I[1 - H_\varepsilon(\phi(x,y))]dxdy}{\int_\Omega 1 - H_\varepsilon(\phi(x,y))dxdy} \tag{12.27}$$

Then, keeping c_1 and c_2 fixed, the energy functional with respect to ϕ is approached by computing the derivatives of (12.26) with respect to each B-spline coefficient $c[k]$:

$$\frac{\partial E}{\partial c[k]} = \int_\Omega w_\varepsilon(x)\beta^n\left(\frac{x}{h} - k\right)dx \tag{12.28}$$

where $w_\varepsilon(x) = \delta_\varepsilon(\phi)[(I - c_1)^2 - (I - c_2)^2 + 2\alpha(H_\varepsilon(\phi) - H_\varepsilon(\tilde{\phi}))]$.

In implementation, the segmentation algorithm with shape prior can be outlined in following steps:

Step 1: Choose an initial level-set function and B-spline coefficients.

Step 2: Calculate the two intensity means inside and outside the evolving contour according to Eq. (12.27).

Step 3: Normalize the reference shape and evolving shape using the normalization procedure in Section 12.4.1. Then, align the reference shape with the evolving shape.

Step 4: Evolve the level-set function φ to obtain B-spline coefficients and the level-set function for the next iteration.

Step 5: Check whether the evolution of the level-set function has converged, or a specified maximum iteration number is reached. If not, return to Step 2.

12.4.3 Prior Shape from a Set of Training Samples

There are many limitations for the one shape template to capture the object in an image. An intuitive approach is to reconstruct a prior shape from a set of training samples, i.e., at each iteration during the segmentation, a prior shape is reconstructed according to the evolving curve [31].

Let $\{\tilde{\phi}_j\}_{j=1}^N$ and ϕ_s are the set of aligned training samples and an evolving level-set function, respectively. The kernel density estimation of the ϕ_s is given as [36]:

$$P(\phi_s) \propto \frac{1}{N}\sum_{j=1}^{N}\exp\left(-\frac{1}{2\sigma^2}d^2(H(\phi_s), H(\tilde{\phi}_j))\right) \tag{12.29}$$

where $\sigma^2 = \frac{1}{N}\sum_{j=1}^{N}\min_{i \neq j} d^2(H(\tilde{\phi}_i), H(\tilde{\phi}_j))$ and $d^2(H(\phi_s), H(\tilde{\phi}_j)) = \int_\Omega [H(\phi_s(x)) - H(\tilde{\phi}(x))]^2 dx$.

So, the shape reconstruction energy using a set of training samples is given as:

$$E_R(\phi_s) = -\log(P(\phi_s)) \tag{12.30}$$

To solve this energy, the level-set function ϕ_s is firstly express as in (12.14), and then perform the gradient descent with respect to these B-spline coefficients. Similar to the minimization step in Section 12.4.2, one obtain:

$$\frac{\partial E_R}{\partial c[\boldsymbol{k}]} = \frac{\sum_{j=1}^{N} w_j \left(\frac{\partial}{\partial \phi_s} d_2(H(\phi_s), H(\tilde{\phi}_j)) \right)}{2\sigma^2 \sum_{j=1}^{N} w_j} \beta^n \left(\frac{\boldsymbol{x}}{h} - \boldsymbol{k} \right) \tag{12.31}$$

where $w_j = \exp(-\frac{1}{2\sigma^2} d_2(H(\phi_s), H(\tilde{\phi}_j)))$.

The reconstructed level-set function is obtained when the final B-spline coefficients $c[\boldsymbol{k}]$ converged:

$$\tilde{\phi}(\boldsymbol{x}) = \sum_{\boldsymbol{k} \in \mathbb{Z}^d} c[\boldsymbol{k}] \beta^n \left(\frac{\boldsymbol{x}}{h} - \boldsymbol{k} \right) \tag{12.32}$$

This reconstructed function $\tilde{\phi}$ will be used as the prior shape template in the energy functional (12.26). So, the final segmentation method with a set of training samples is then back to the case of a reference shape in Section 12.4.2.

12.4.4 Experiment Results

Usually, segmentation incorporating shape prior is effective when segmenting images even in the presence of clutter and occlusion. In this section, experimental results are provided to validate the effectiveness of the variational B-spline level set with moment-based shape prior.

In the experiments, the following parameters are set: $\varepsilon = 1, h = 1, n = 3$ and $\lambda = 0.1$. The value of the weighing coefficient α should be chosen depending on specific applications.

The first experiment in this section is shown in Figure 12.10. It is clearly seen that the desired object ellipse is partially occluded by two other objects, which is prone to fail when using intensity image information alone. This is illustrated in Figure 12.10(b), when using the model in [18], the contour stops at the boundary of the occluded object and could not encompass the real shape of the ellipse. On the contrary, by utilizing both region information and shape information (Figure 12.10(c)), the model in this section successfully segments the object of interest, as shown in Figure 12.10(d).

To validate the ability of the shape prior shape model in the case that a set of training shapes are given, an experiment on some images having different poses, noise and occlusion is conducted. The training set in this experiment includes 46 shapes, extracted from 2D views of a 3D terracotta warrior. Each shape in such training set is in different modes. Some samples of the training data set with different modes are provided in Figure 12.11.

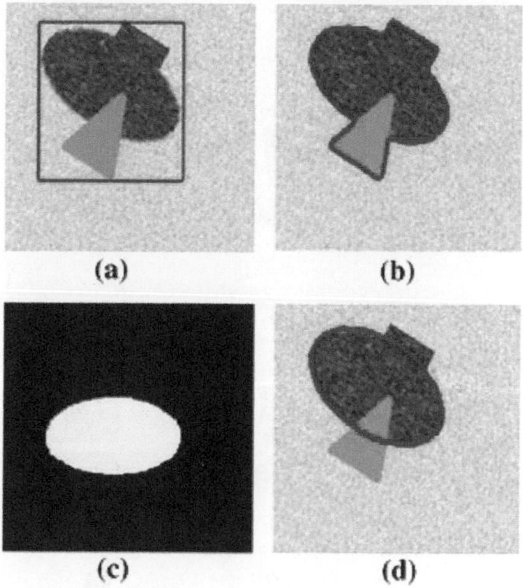

FIGURE 12.10
Segmentation results on the ellipse image with occlusion. (a) Original image and initial contour; (b) segmentation result without shape prior; (c) reference shape; (d) segmentation result using the shape prior model.

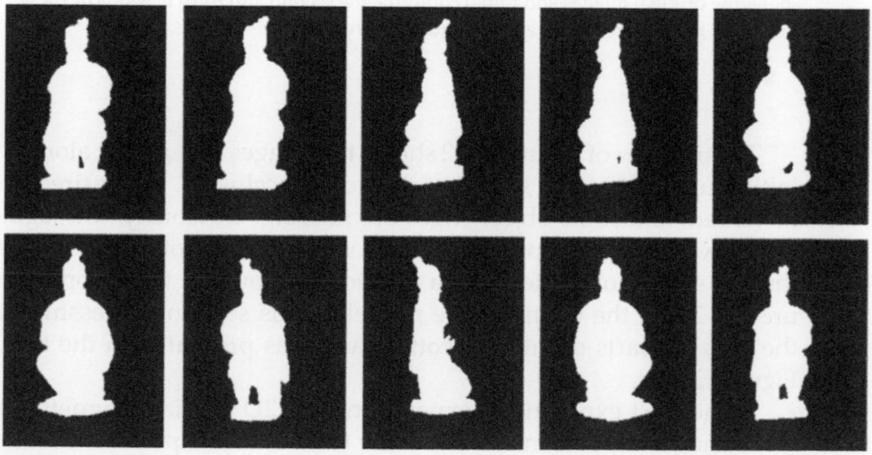

FIGURE 12.11
Some selected sample shapes from a set of terracotta warrior training data.

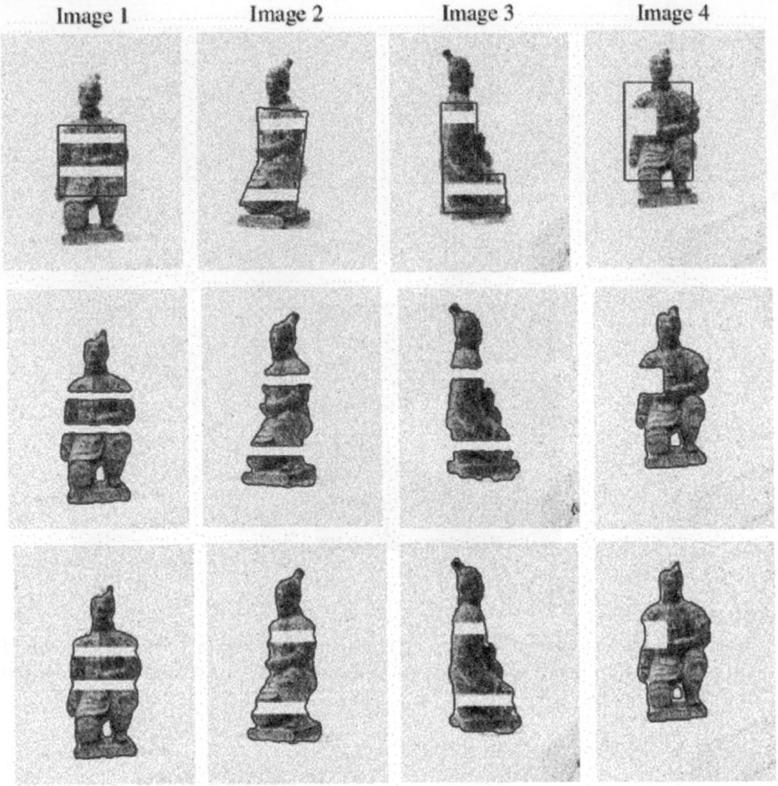

FIGURE 12.12
Segmentation results on the terracotta warrior images with a set of training shapes. The first row shows the original images and initial contours, the second and third rows show the segmentation results by Bernard et al. [18] and the model of this section.

The first row of Figure 12.12 shows the images to segment along with their initial curves. It can be seen that due to the occlusion, the desired objects are disturbed, and some object edges are missing. Obviously, the segmentation model without shape prior information [18] could not successfully segment the real shapes of the terracotta warrior as shown in the second row of Figure 12.12. On the contrary, the model of this section successfully recovers the missing parts of the terracotta warrior as presented in the third row of Figure 12.12.

In the next experiment, experiments on 2D cardiac magnetic resonance (MR) images are presented. The other two tested shape prior-based level-set models are Tsai et al. [37] and Liu et al. [38]. The purpose of this experiment is to extract the endocardium boundaries of the Left Ventricle. Figure 12.13 shows some sample segmentation results on the Left Ventricle in 2D cardiac

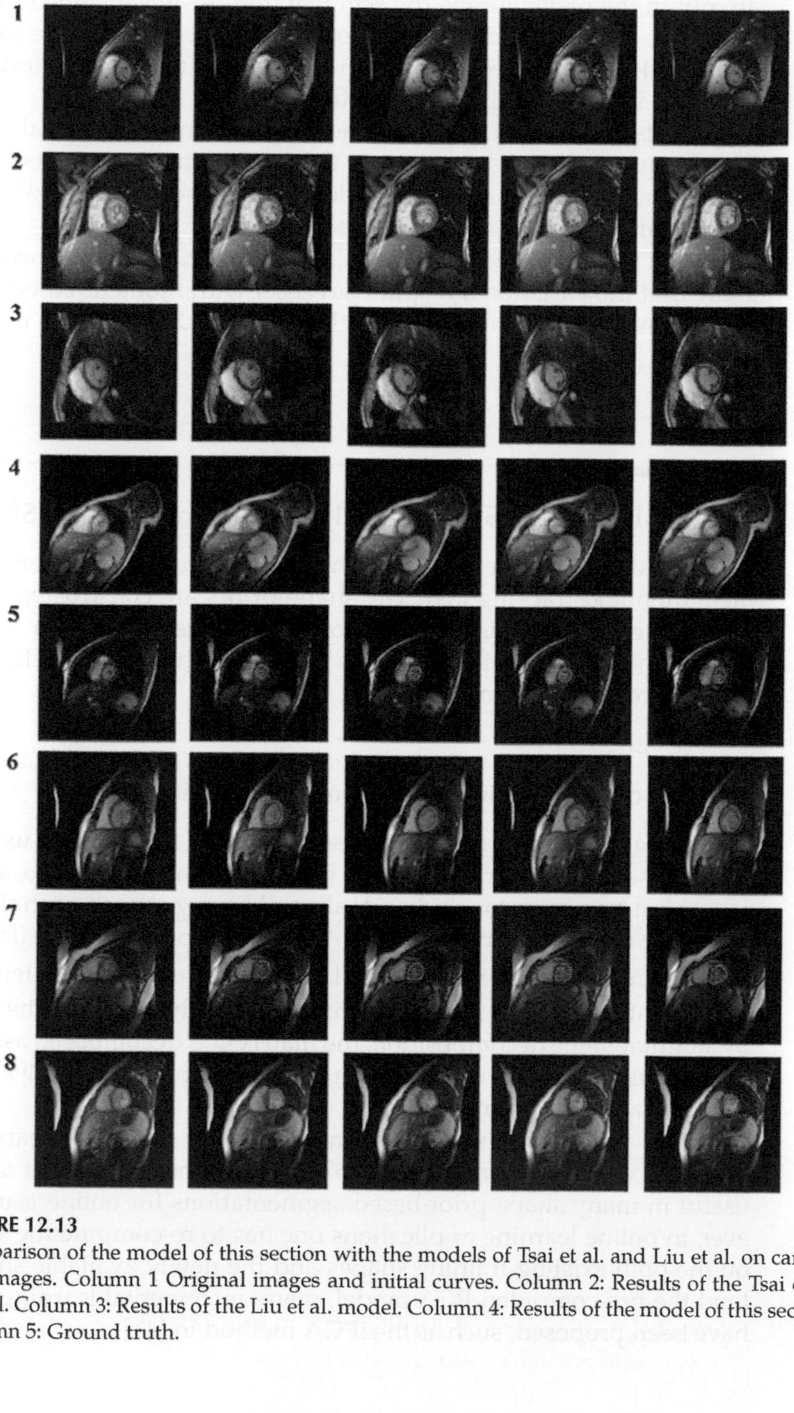

FIGURE 12.13
Comparison of the model of this section with the models of Tsai et al. and Liu et al. on cardiac MR images. Column 1 Original images and initial curves. Column 2: Results of the Tsai et al. model. Column 3: Results of the Liu et al. model. Column 4: Results of the model of this section. Column 5: Ground truth.

MR images. In this figure, the original images together with the initial curves are put in the first column. The segmentation results obtained by Tsai et al., Liu et al., and the models of this section are presented in the second, third and fourth columns, respectively. The ground truths of these test images are provided in the last column of this figure.

Results shown that the three models are similar by visual comparison. But the quantitative assessment of these segmentation results demonstrate that the matching errors of the model in of this section are lower than those in the Tsai et al., and Liu et al. models.

All in all, experimental results on synthetic, real, and medical images show that the variational B-spline level set with moment-based shape prior model have more advantages than the traditional shape prior model [30].

12.5 Multiphase B-Spline Level Set with Incremental Shape Priors

This section presents a new multiphase active contour model for object segmentation and tracking [39]. The shape priors are constructed by performing the incremental principal component analysis (iPCA) on a set of training shapes and newly available shapes which are the resulting shapes derived from preceding segmented images.

12.5.1 Incremental Principal Component Analysis

Traditionally, the methods for constructing the shape prior use PCA on a training set of familiar shapes can be outlined as follows [36, 40]: Let $A = \{S_i\}_{i=1}^{N}$ is a training set including N aligned binary shapes, each shape has the same size $m \times n$. To perform the PCA on the shapes set A, one first computes the mean shape as $m_A = \frac{1}{N}\sum_{i=1}^{N} S_i$. Let $\bar{S}_i = S_i - m_A$ is the centered map and Φ is a centered $(mn) \times N$ data matrix whose each column is the vector of $\bar{S}_i$. By singular value decomposition, the matrix Φ is decomposed as: $\Phi = U\Sigma V^T$, where U is a matrix whose each column is an eigenvector of Φ and Σ is a diagonal matrix of the corresponding eigenvalues.

Many prior-based segmentations are based on offline learning from a given set of reference shapes [30, 37, 38, 40]. The PCA-based approach are useful in many shape prior-based segmentations for online learning. However, in online learning applications one has to re-compute the shape model on the both existing training shapes and the newly available shapes. To extend the pre-computed PCA model, many incremental learning approaches have been proposed, such as the iPCA method in [41].

Suppose that one has already performed PCA on existing training shapes and would like to use the newly available shapes to update the previous results. Let $B = \{\tilde{S}_j\}_{i=1}^{M}$ is the newly aligned binary shape set. The mean shape for the newly available shapes is $m_B = \frac{1}{M}\sum_{j=1}^{M}\tilde{S}_j$. Similar to the stated above, let Ψ is a centered the centered data matrix of the newly available shape set. Supposing C is the concatenation of the shape set A and B, the mean shape of all the shape set is given as [41]:

$$m_C = \frac{fN}{fN+M}m_A + \frac{M}{fN+M}m_B \tag{12.33}$$

where $0 \leq f \leq 1$ is a forgetting factor.

Let $\tilde{\Psi}$ be the component of Ψ orthogonal to U, and $\hat{\Psi} = [\Psi_1, \cdots, \Psi_M\sqrt{\frac{NM}{N+M}}(m_A - m_B)]$. The concatenated matrix Θ can be expressed as $\Theta = [\Phi\Psi] = [U\tilde{\Psi}]R[\begin{smallmatrix} V^T & 0 \\ 0 & I \end{smallmatrix}]$ and the matrix of R is $[\begin{smallmatrix} f\Sigma & U^T\hat{\Psi} \\ 0 & \tilde{\Psi}(\hat{\Psi} - UU^T\hat{\Psi}) \end{smallmatrix}]$.

Finally, the incrementally updated shape statistics of C: $C = U'\Sigma'V'^T$ where $U' = [U\tilde{\Psi}]\tilde{U}$, $\Sigma' = \tilde{\Sigma}$, and $\tilde{U}\tilde{\Sigma}\tilde{V}^T$ is the singular value decomposition of R [39, 41].

Let $\hat{u}$ denotes the aligned evolving shape during the segmentation, the coordinates b^k of the projection of $\hat{u}$ onto the first k components is $b^k = U_k'^T(\hat{u} - m_C)$, where U_k' is a matrix consisting of the first k columns of U'. Given the coefficients b^k, an estimate of the prior shape can be reconstructed as:

$$\tilde{\psi} = m_C + U_k'^T b^k \tag{12.34}$$

It is noted that the number of components k should be chosen such that the accuracy of the fitting is 98%.

12.5.2 Endocardium and Epicardium B-Spline Segmentation Model

In the left ventricle MR images, the endocardium shape is located inside the epicardium shape which is illustrated in Figure 12.14. The segmentation model considers three disjoint regions: endocardium, myocardium, and the background.

Using two level-set function ϕ_1 and ϕ_2, the regions of Endocardium, Myocardium and background can be represented as $\Omega_1 \triangleq \{x \in \Omega : \phi_1(x) > 0\}$, $\Omega_2 \triangleq \{x \in \Omega : \phi_1(x) < 0, \phi_2(x) > 0\}$ and $\Omega_3 \triangleq \{x \in \Omega : \phi_2(x) > 0\}$, respectively.

Using the general segmentation model (12.23), B-spline level set based image data fitting term for left ventricle MR images segmentation model is

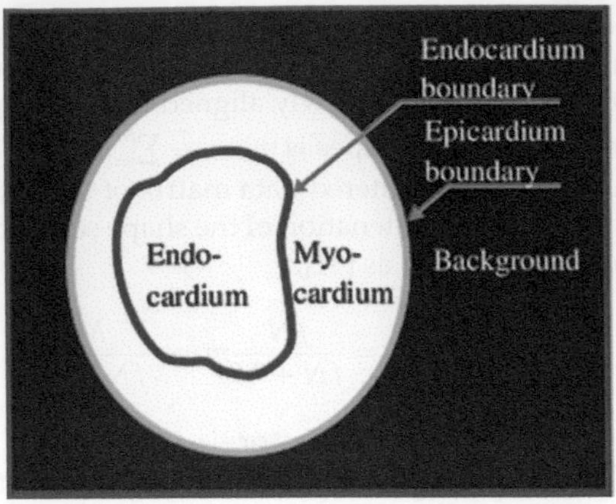

FIGURE 12.14
Relationship of the three regions in a left ventricle image.

given as:

$$\begin{aligned} E_{image}(\phi_1, \phi_2, \mu_1, \mu_2, \mu_3) &= \int_\Omega (I - \mu_1)^2 H_\varepsilon(\phi_1(x))dx \\ &+ \int_\Omega (I - \mu_3)^2 [1 - H_\varepsilon(\phi_2(x))]dx \\ &+ \int_\Omega (I - \mu_2)^2 [1 - H_\varepsilon(\phi_1(x))] H_\varepsilon(\phi_2(x))dx \end{aligned} \tag{12.35}$$

and the definition of the shape term which measure the distance or dissimilarity between shapes is presented as follows:

$$E_{shape}(\phi_1, \tilde{\phi}_1, \phi_2, \tilde{\phi}_2) = \sum_{i=1}^{2} \int_\Omega [H_\varepsilon(\phi_i(x)) - H_\varepsilon(\tilde{\phi}_i(x))]dx \tag{12.36}$$

where $\phi_1(x) = \sum_{k \in \mathbb{Z}^d} c_1[k]\beta^n(\frac{x}{h_1} - k)$ and $\phi_2(x) = \sum_{k \in \mathbb{Z}^d} c_2[k]\beta^n(\frac{x}{h_2} - k)$ are two evolving level-set function representing evolving shapes. $\tilde{\phi}_i (i = 1, 2)$ is signed distance functions representing the reference shapes.

During implementation, one may exploit the shape normalization procedure to align the evolving shape and each reference shape. Note that the binarization shapes can be reprented by $H(\phi_i)$ and $H(\tilde{\phi}_i)$, respectively. Let $\hat{u}_i = H(\phi_i)$ denote the aligned evolving shape of the current segmentation and $b^k = U_k^T(\hat{u}_i - m_C)$, an estimate of the prior shape $\tilde{\psi}_i$ can be reconstructed as Eq. (12.34). Finally, by normalizing $\tilde{\psi}_i$ to the range $[0, 1]$, one obtains a binary map representation $H(\tilde{\phi}_i)$.

By take into account the lengths of contours and an edge detecting function as a regularization term, the final energy functional is expressed as [39]:

$$E_\varepsilon(\phi_1, \phi_2, \tilde{\phi}_1, \tilde{\phi}_2, \mu_1, \mu_2, \mu_3) = E_{image} + \alpha E_{shape} + v \sum_{i=1}^{2} \int_\Omega g(x) \, |\nabla H(\phi_i(x))| \, dx \tag{12.37}$$

12.5.3 Energy Minimization and Implementation

The standard gradient descent method is used to minimize the energy functional (12.37).

Firstly, keeping level-set functions ϕ_1 and ϕ_2 fixed, the energy functional with respect to μ_1, μ_2 and μ_3 is minimized by:

$$\mu_1 = \frac{\int_\Omega I H_\varepsilon(\phi_1(x))dx}{\int_\Omega H_\varepsilon(\phi_1(x))dx}, \quad \mu_2 = \frac{\int_\Omega I[1 - H_\varepsilon(\phi_1(x))]H_\varepsilon(\phi_2(x))dx}{\int_\Omega 1 - H_\varepsilon(\phi_1(x))H_\varepsilon(\phi_2(x))dx},$$

$$\mu_3 = \frac{\int_\Omega I[1 - H_\varepsilon(\phi_2(x))]dx}{\int_\Omega 1 - H_\varepsilon(\phi_2(x))dx} \tag{12.38}$$

Then, keeping μ_1, μ_2 and μ_3 fixed, the energy functional with respect to ϕ_1 and ϕ_2 is approached by computing the derivatives of (12.37) with respect to each B-spline coefficient $c_1[k]$ and $c_2[k]$:

$$\frac{\partial E_\varepsilon}{\partial c_1[k]} = \int_\Omega V_1(x) \beta_1^n \left(\frac{x}{h_1} - k \right) dx \tag{12.39}$$

and

$$\frac{\partial E_\varepsilon}{\partial c_2[k]} = \int_\Omega V_2(x) \beta_2^n \left(\frac{x}{h_2} - k \right) dx \tag{12.40}$$

where

$$V_1(x) = \Bigg[(I - \mu_1)^2 - (I - \mu_2)^2 H_\varepsilon(\phi_2) - v\,div\left(g \frac{\nabla \phi_1}{|\nabla \phi_1|} \right) + 2\alpha (H_\varepsilon(\phi_1) - H_\varepsilon(\tilde{\phi}_1)) \Bigg] \delta_\varepsilon(\phi_1),$$

and

$$V_1(x) = \Bigg[(I - \mu_2)^2 (1 - H_\varepsilon(\phi_1)) - (I - \mu_3)^2 - v\,div\left(g \frac{\nabla \phi_2}{|\nabla \phi_2|} \right) + 2\alpha (H_\varepsilon(\phi_2) - H_\varepsilon(\tilde{\phi}_2)) \Bigg] \delta_\varepsilon(\phi_2).$$

Finally, with a iteration step λ, the B-spline coefficients are updated by:

$$c_1[\mathbf{k}]^{(t+1)} = c_1[\mathbf{k}]^{(t)} - \lambda \frac{\partial E_\varepsilon}{\partial c_1[\mathbf{k}]} \tag{12.41}$$

and

$$c_2[\mathbf{k}]^{(t+1)} = c_2[\mathbf{k}]^{(t)} - \lambda \frac{\partial E_\varepsilon}{\partial c_2[\mathbf{k}]} \tag{12.42}$$

In summary, the segmentation algorithm can be outlined in following steps:

Step 1: Choose initial level-set functions and B-spline coefficients.

Step 2: Calculate intensity means of each region according to Eq. (12.38).

Step 3: Reconstruct the prior shapes templates as Eq. (12.34). Normalize and alignment the prior shape templates and evolving shapes.

Step 4: Evolve the level-set functions ϕ_1 and ϕ_2 to obtain B-spline coefficients and the level-set functions for the next iteration.

Step 5: If the level-set functions are not converged or a specified maximum iteration number is not reached, return to Step 2. Otherwise, output the segmentation results.

12.5.4 Experiment Results

To build the training data in [39], they chosen 100 images in which both endocardium and epicardium have been manually delineated. Figure 12.15 show some representative shapes in the training sets before and after alignment.

Firstly, an experiment is conducted to show the advantages of utilizing shape prior information for segmentation. It can be seen from Figure 12.16(a), the results without shape prior ($\alpha = 0$) are not satisfactory since the inner curve that segments the endocardium is spilling into the background region, meanwhile the outer curve expected to segment the epicardium seems to be trapped due to the cluttered background. On the contrary, with the same initial curves, the satisfying results are obtained when using the shape priors, as shown in Figure 12.16(b).

To validate the effectiveness of the segmentation method of this section three recent multiphase model with shape prior, proposed in [42], [43], and [44], are compared in [39]. To this end, In [42], the multiphase model of Vese and Chan is extended by encoding the shape prior into the energy functional. Four models including the multiphase level-set model [42] with shape prior the Woo et al. [44], the multiphase graph cut-based model with shape prior [43] in which the shape energy is incorporated via the weights of the edges connected with the terminals [54], and the models of this section to segment a test subject. Some representative segmentation results on the test subject by the above models are depicted in Figure 12.17. From these results, one can

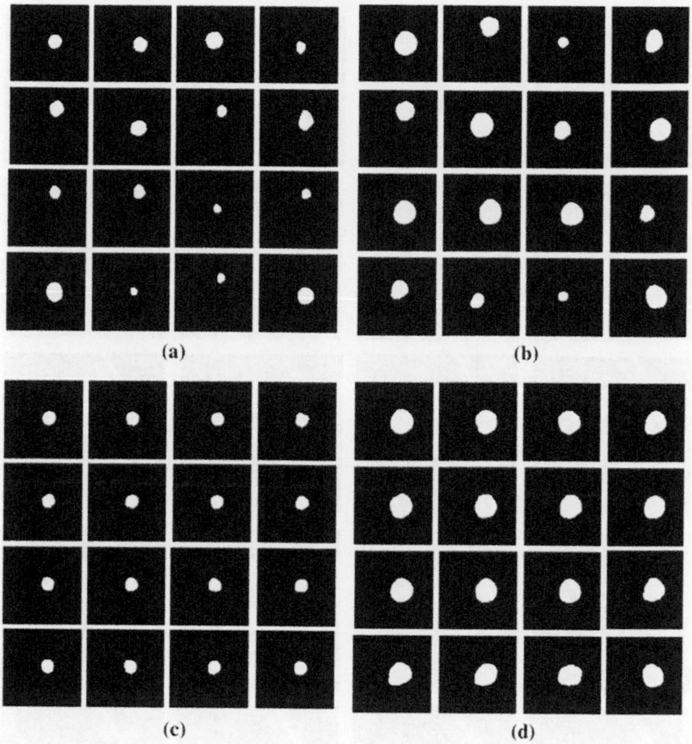

FIGURE 12.15
Representative training shapes used in experiments. (a) Training shapes for endocardium before alignment; (b) training shapes for epicardium before alignment; (c) aligned shapes of (a); and (d) aligned shapes of (b).

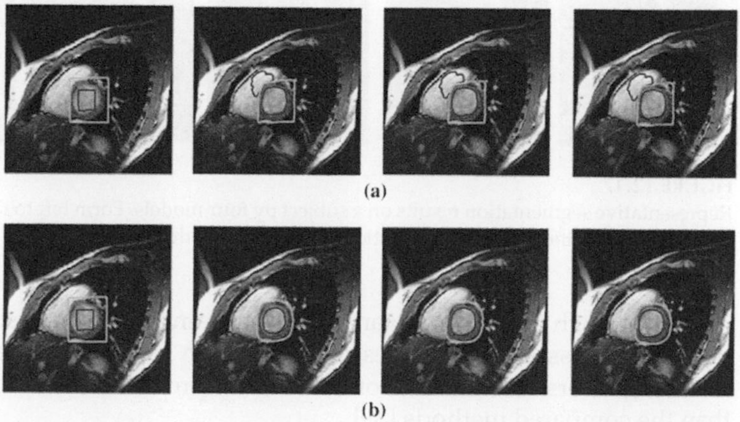

FIGURE 12.16
Curve evolution in segmentation of the LV image by the multiphase B-spline model (a) without shape prior, and (b) with shape prior. From left to right: initial curve, and the curve evolution at iteration 2, 4, and 30.

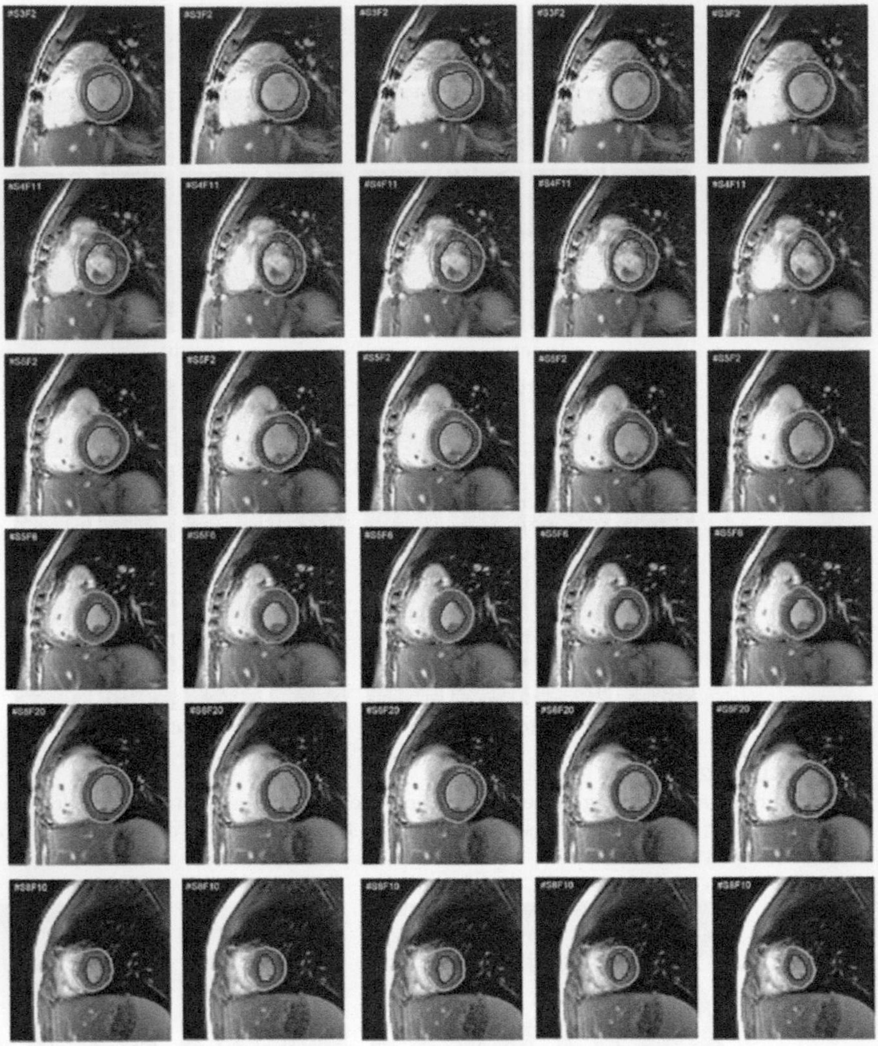

FIGURE 12.17
Representative segmentation results on a subject by four models. Form left to right are the reults of [42], [43], [44], the model of this section and ground truth, respectively.

see that though four models can deal with frames in the test subject. But the quantitative assessment of these segmentation results demonstrate that the matching errors of the model of this section produces more accurate results than the compared methods [39].

All in all, the multiphase B-spline level set with shape priors for segmentation and tracking the left ventricle in MR images have more advantages than traditional shape prior model. Additionally, using the iPCA to incrementally updating the resulted shape information without repeatedly performing PCA on the entire training set including the existing shapes and the newly available shapes is excellent in shape prior segmentation model.

12.6 B-Spline Based Globally Optimal Segmentation Combining Low-Level and High-Level Information

Variational-based segmentation methods are widely studied due to their good performance, but they still suffer from incapability to deal with images bearing weak contrast, overlapped noise and cluttered texture. To tackle this problem, we propose a new statistical information analysis based multi-scale and global optimization method for image segmentation. The multi-scale segmentation methods can be summarized in Figure 12.18. Firstly, Gaussian pyramid of original image is constructed and the proposed Gaussian statistical model is employed to each scale of the pyramid. Secondly, we use multiple Gaussian kernel gray equalization to get the rough contours of interest object. Third, contours achieved at coarse scale are used as high-level information for both contours initialization and constraint of finer scale. Different above shape prior models, the high-level of this proposed method needn't any reference shapes.

12.6.1 Gaussian Statistical Segmentation Model

As Gaussian functions are widely used in statistics, in this section, we consider a general combining region- and edge-based segmentation problem based on Gaussian distribution:

$$E_{low} = E_{region} + vE_{boundary} \tag{12.43}$$

Let Ω_1 and Ω_2 are object and background region with region characteristic function $M_i(x) = 1_{\Omega_i}(i = 1, 2)$ i.e., $M_i(x)$ is 1 if $x \in \Omega_i$ or 0 otherwise. Then the general region- and edge-based functional is immediately rewritten as (dropping the constant terms):

$$E(M_1, M_2, \theta_1, \theta_2) = \sum_{i=1}^{2} \int_{\Omega} \left(log\sigma_i + \frac{(I(x) - \mu_i)^2}{2\sigma_i^2} \right) M_i(x)dx + v \sum_{i=1}^{2} \int_{\Omega} g|\nabla M_i(x)|dx \tag{12.44}$$

where $\theta_i = (\mu_i, \sigma_i^2)$ are parameters of mean and variance corresponding to region Ω_i. Using maximum likelihood estimation, these parameters can be

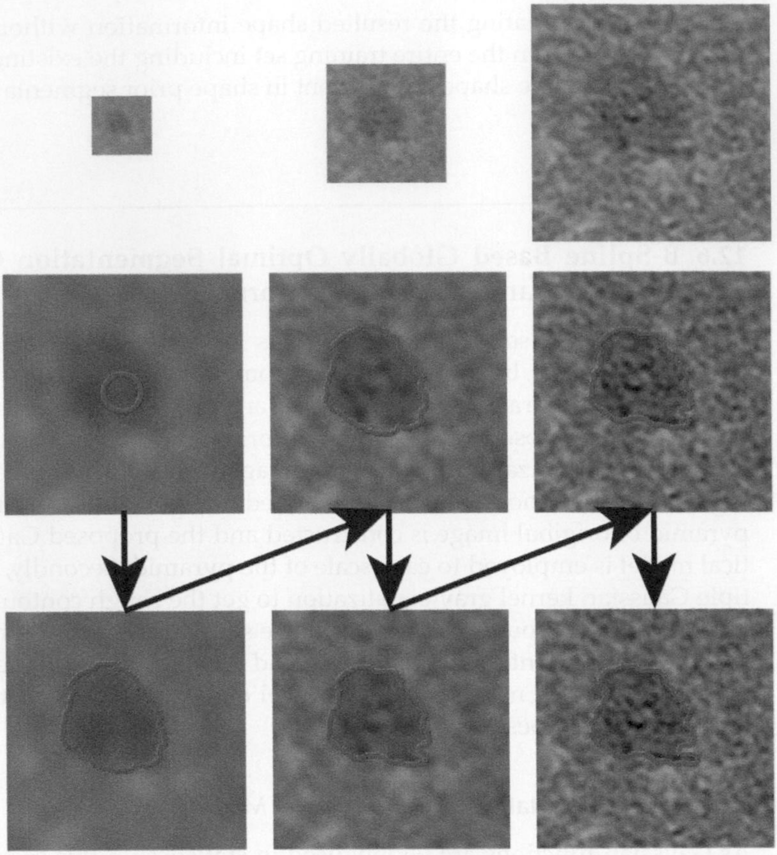

FIGURE 12.18
Diagram of the proposed method. First row are multi-scale image sequences. Second row are the initial contours at each scale, which are enlarged to the original image size for better view. With the exception of the red circle, this contours are also used as high-level information to constraint the evolution of contours. Third row are final contours at each scale.

expressed as:

$$\mu_i = \frac{\int_\Omega I(x)M_i(x)dx}{\int_\Omega M_i(x)dx} \quad (12.45)$$

$$\sigma_i^2 = \frac{\int_\Omega \left(I(x) - \mu_i\right)^2 M_i(x)dx}{\int_\Omega M_i(x)dx} \quad (12.46)$$

In the framework of level-set method, $M_1(x) = H(\phi(x))$ and $M_2(x) = 1 - H(\phi(x))$. g is a newly defined edge stopping function which is given by:

$$g = \min\left\{\frac{1}{1 + |\nabla G_\sigma * I|^2}, \exp\left(-\frac{|\nabla G_\sigma * I|^2}{\sigma^2}\right)\right\} \tag{12.47}$$

G_σ is a Gaussian kernel with standard deviation σ and $*$ is a convolution operator used to smooth the image and to reduce noise. This new stopping function can rapidly drive the contour and stop at the correct object boundaries [45]. Then the low-level based segmentation problem is to deduce the minimization of this functional respect to region characteristic function and Gaussian parameters.

12.6.2 Gaussian Gray Equalization and Multi-Scale Shape Evolution

This model works well for many scenarios. But there are some limitations for images with low contrast, noise or texture. Firstly, for noisy images, the edge stopping function will produce small values near noise and the contours may be attracted to these false edges. Secondly, at weak boundaries of low contrast image, because of the low response at weak boundaries, the contours may pass through these weak boundaries. Thirdly, lots of edges may arise from internal discontinuity and background clutter of texture images.

In this section, we tackle the above problems by combining low-level (gray scale intensity) and high-level (prior shape) information. Firstly, the Gaussian pyramid of the original image is constructed and the proposed model presented in Eq. (12.44) is employed to each scale of the pyramid. This strategy can solve the influence of noise and intensity inhomogeneity to some extent at coarse scale. Secondly, we use multiple Gaussian kernels at the coarsest scale: A large Gaussian kernel is used firstly, and decreased from coarse scale to fine scale. We name this multiple Gaussian kernel gray equalization. Contours achieved at coarse scale are used as high-level information for both contours initialization and constraints of finer scale. These prior shapes are continually updated at different scale by up-sampling. Third, to avoid weak boundary leakages in low contrast, noise and texture images, shape similarity between different scales is incorporated. This similarity constraint does not allow large deformation of the contours as the initialized contours are already close to the object boundaries.

The boundary similarity constraint function (high-level) can be defined as the symmetric difference between the two characteristic function which is given as:

$$E_{high}(M_1, M_2) = \sum_{i=1}^{n} \int_\Omega (M_i(x) - L_i(x))^2 dx \tag{12.48}$$

where $L_i(x)$ is the characteristic function with related to prior object region Ω_i. In this section, $L_i(x)$ was achieved by the coarser scale related to the current scale. That is to say, the object regions achieved in the coarse scale were up-sampled to finer scale as the constrained prior object region.

Finally, energy functional combining low-level and high-level using special Gaussian distribution can be rewritten as follows:

$$F = E_{low}(M_1, M_2, \mu_1, \mu_2, \sigma_1, \sigma_2) + \lambda E_{shape}(M_1, M_2) \tag{12.49}$$

where λ is a weight parameter related to the shape constraint term.

A diagram of these procedures and corresponding results are shown in Figure 12.18. As we can see, multiple Gaussian kernel gray equalization and image pyramids will weakly blur the object boundaries. But high-frequency noise is smoothed out at coarse scale of the pyramid, and neighboring pixels in these scales are more likely to be independent as sub-sampling reduces their correlation (as shown in the first column in Figure 12.18). At the coarse scale, we can get the prior shape of interested object. This prior is very useful for the boundary detection at finer scales. The effectiveness of boundary shape similarity constraint with the combining low-level and high-level information is proved in the bottom right in Figure 12.18. We can see that the proposed method precisely captures the object boundary at each scale by taking advantage of boundary shape similarity constraint in the multi-scale framework.

12.6.3 B-Spline Based Global Optimization Segmentation Model

The drawbacks of this proposed model are its non-convex property and local optimal minima as a traditional variational segmentation model. In this subsection, we propose to determine a global minimum of the proposed energy functional. The key idea is to reformulate this functional as the convex energy by introducing L^1-norm and B-spline functions.

Inspired by the work of [46], the convex segmentation model is given by [45]:

$$\begin{aligned} \arg\min_{0 \le u \le 1} F_G(u) = \arg\min_{0 \le u \le 1} \bigg| \int_\Omega r(x)u(x)dx + v \bigg| \int_\Omega g\,|\nabla u|\,dx \\ + \lambda \int_\Omega \|u(x) - \psi(x)\|^2\,dx \end{aligned} \tag{12.50}$$

where $r(x) = \log \sigma_1 + \frac{(I(x)-\mu_1)^2}{2\sigma_1^2} - \log \sigma_2 - \frac{(I(x)-\mu_2)^2}{2\sigma_2^2}$ is the global region statistic term, and $u(x)$ is called as convex relaxation function. ψ is the level-set representation of prior object region (normalized to [0, 1]).

12.6.4 Energy Minimization of the Convex Model

In this subsection, we will apply the Split Bregman method to minimize the proposed convex model of u. The split Bregman method is an efficient technique to L^1-regularized optimization problems, such as TV denoising and compressed sensing (CS) problems [47].

We introduce the auxiliary variable d such that $d = \nabla u$. This constrained problem can be reformulated to the unconstrained one by add the equality to the Eq. (12.50) as a quadratic penalty term:

$$(u^*, d^*) = \arg\min_{0 \le u \le 1} \int_\Omega r(x)u(x)dx + v\int_\Omega g|d|dx + \lambda\int_\Omega \|u(x) - \psi(x)\|^2 dx + \frac{\gamma}{2}\int_\Omega \|\nabla u(x) - d(x)\|^2 dx \tag{12.51}$$

where γ is the penalty coefficient. Using the Split Bregman method, we get the following elegant two-phase Split Bregman iteration:

$$(u^{k+1}, d^{k+1}) = \arg\min_{0 \le u \le 1, d} \int_\Omega r(x)u(x)dx + \lambda\int_\Omega \|u(x) - \psi(x)\|^2 dx + v\int_\Omega g|d(x)|dx + \frac{\gamma}{2}\int_\Omega \|d(x) - \nabla u(x) - b^k\|^2 dx \tag{12.52}$$

$$b^{k+1} = b^k + \nabla u^{k+1} - d^{k+1} \tag{12.53}$$

In order to implement the Bregman updates, we must be able to solve problem (24). By the split of the L^1 and L^2 components of this functional, we perform this minimization efficiently by iteratively minimizing with respect to u and d. The two steps we must perform are:

Step 1:

$$u^{k+1} = \arg\min_u \int_\Omega r(x)u(x)dx + \lambda\int_\Omega \|u(x) - \psi(x)\|^2 dx + \frac{\gamma}{2}\int_\Omega \|d(x) - \nabla u(x) - b^k\|^2 dx \tag{12.54}$$

Step 2:

$$d^{k+1} = \arg\min_d v\int_\Omega g|d(x)|dx + \frac{\gamma}{2}\int_\Omega \|d(x) - \nabla u(x) - b^k\|^2 dx \tag{12.55}$$

To solve Step 1, we propose to explicitly represent the function $u(x)$ by the cubic B-spline basis functions which allows fast convergence and intrinsic smooth segmentation model:

$$u(x) = \sum_{k \in \mathbb{Z}^d} c[k]\beta^n\left(\frac{x}{h} - k\right) \tag{12.56}$$

Different than in traditional Split Bregman updates, we give a smooth version of the unknown u by the intrinsic smooth B-spline function. Because u is differentiable in Eq. (12.54), the standard calculus of variation model can be used to find a minimum of the Eq. (12.54). The gradient flow is given by:

$$\frac{\partial c[k]}{\partial t} = -\int_{\Omega} w(x)\beta\left(\frac{x}{h} - k\right)dx \tag{12.57}$$

where $w(x) = r(x) + 2\lambda(u(x) - \psi(x)) + \gamma\nabla(d - b) + \gamma\Delta u$.

The discrete version of Eq. (12.57) to solve the B-spline coeffecients:

$$c[k]^{n+1} = c[k]^n - \Delta t\nabla_c F_G\left(c[k]^n\right) \tag{12.58}$$

where Δt is the time step and $\nabla_c F_G(c[k]^n) = (W * b_h)\ _h[k]$. This expression shows that each step of the coefficients computation corresponds to a low-pass filtering and a down-sampling operation. So these coefficients ensure the smoothness of the relaxation function.

To solve Step 2, since the function $f(x) = |x|$ is differentiable in $\mathbb{R}\backslash\{0\}$, we get the following equation minimizing with respected to d:

$$d^k = shink\left(\nabla u^{k+1} + b^k, \frac{vg}{\gamma}\right) \tag{12.59}$$

where $shrink\left(\alpha, \beta\right)$ is the shrinkage operator given by:

$$shrink\left(\alpha,\beta\right) = \begin{cases} \frac{\alpha}{|\alpha|}\max\left(|\alpha| - \beta, 0\right), & \alpha \neq 0 \\ 0, & \alpha = 0 \end{cases} \tag{12.60}$$

The brief implementation steps of the proposed combining low-level and high-level globally optimal segmentation model are given in Algorithm 1.

Note that we claim the proposed method in Eq. (12.50) is convex which means that it is convex respected to u for the fixed σ_i, μ_i and ψ. In Algorithm 1, each time when we update u, the value of others are fixed. σ_g is usually set large enough to equal the image gray intensity using Gaussian filtering and $s < 1$ is a scale parameter. Many advantages of this model can be founded in [45].

12.6.5 Experiment Results

To demonstrate the validity of the proposed method, we just apply the proposed method on synthetic image polluted by salt and pepper noise as shown in Figure 12.19. The salt and pepper noise with noise density 0.01, 0.1, 0.2, 0.3 and 0.4 are added from the first column to the fifth column. First row gives the original noise images and initial contours. The second row and third row show the results of the prior using multiple Gaussian kernel gray equalization (enlarged for better view) and final segmentation results respectively.

Algorithm 1

Get multi-scale image sequence, $\{LPIMG\}_{np=1}^{n}$, using Gaussian pyramid decomposition;
At the coarsest scale ($np = 1$)**:**
while $\sigma_g \geq 0.01$ **do:**
  Gaussian gray equalization: $I \leftarrow LPIMG_1 * G_{\sigma_g}$;
  while $\|u^{k+1} - u^k\| > \varepsilon$ **do:**
    Update μ_i and σ_i^2 as in Eq. (12.45) and (12.46);
    Update the B-spline coefficients $c[k]$ as Eq. (12.58);
    Update u^{k+1} as in Eq. (12.56) with $\lambda = 0$;
    Update d^{k+1} as in Eq. (12.59);
    Update b^{k+1} as in Eq. (12.53);
  end while
  $\sigma_g \leftarrow s\sigma_g$;
end while
Find and normalize the signed distance function ψ on the region $\Omega = \{x : u^{k+1}(x) > \mu\}$;
At finer scale ($np > 1$)**:**
for $np = 2 : n$ **do:**
  $I \leftarrow LPIMG_{np}$;
  Up-sample $\Omega' \leftarrow \Omega$ to the same size as I;
  Find and normalize the signed distance function ψ on the region Ω';
  while $\|u^{k+1} - u^k\| > \varepsilon$ **do:**
    Update μ_i and σ_i^2 as in Eq. (12.45) and (12.46);
    Update the B-spline coefficients $c[k]$ as Eq. (12.58);
    Update u^{k+1} as in Eq. (12.56);
    Update d^{k+1} as in Eq. (12.59);
    Update b^{k+1} as in Eq. (12.53);
  end while
  Find the segmentation region $\Omega = \{x : u^{k+1}(x) > \mu\}$
end for

From Figure 12.19, we can see that since even the noise density reaches 0.4, our proposed method can also success to segment the object.

We also referenced many famous and newly-published level-set methods on the medical image segmentation, such as, CV [29], DRLSE [48], LGD [49], BLS [18], NLAC [50], LSMPDF [51], PSM [52], InH_ACM [53] and LSAII [54].

In Figure 12.20, we perform different methods on micrograph (first and second row), X-ray (third and fourth row), MRI (fifth and sixth row) and CT (the last three rows) images. These images exhibit low contrast or intensity inhomogeneity. Most of the tested images in these experiments can be found at http://www.engr.uconn.edu/~cmli/. The visually compared segmentation results are shown in Figure 12.20 with the same initializations. It can be

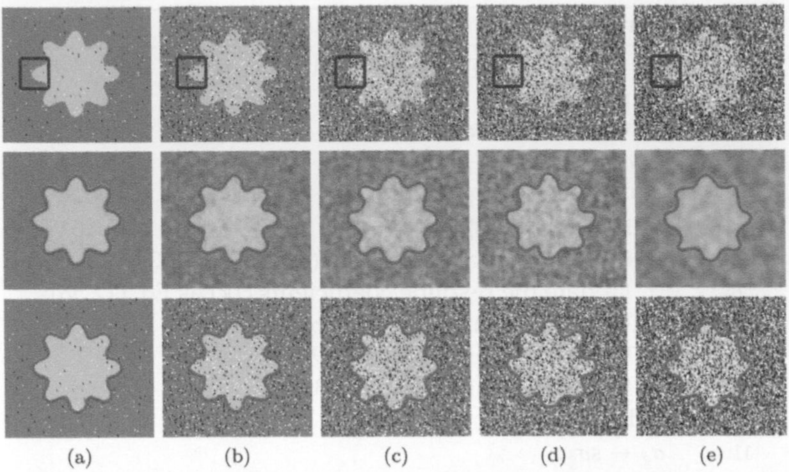

FIGURE 12.19
The evaluation for synthetic image polluted by salt and pepper noise. First to fifth columns show the images with noise density level 0.01, 0.1, 0.2, 0.3 and 0.4, respectively. The first row: noisy image with blue initial contours. The second row: results of the coarsest scale and multiple Gaussian kernel gray equalization which are enlarged for a better view. The third row: final results by the proposed model.

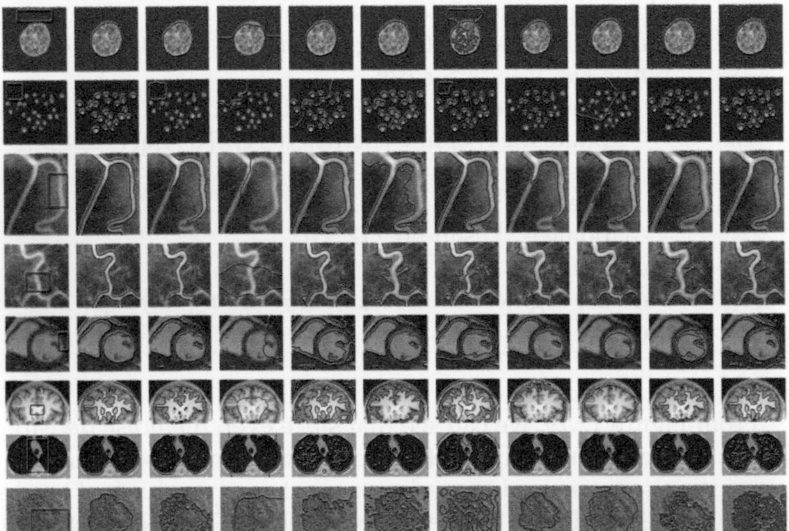

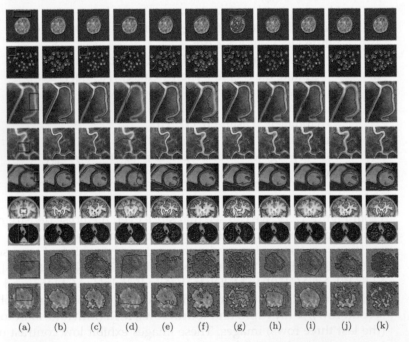

FIGURE 12.20
Segmentation results of natural images with different methods. (a) Initializations (blue solid contours); (b) The computed gray images; (c) Final contours (red solid lines) of the proposed method, (d) CV; (e) DRLSE; (f) LGD; (g) BLS; (h) NLAC; (i) LSMPDF; (j) PSM; (k) InH_ACM; (l) LSAII.

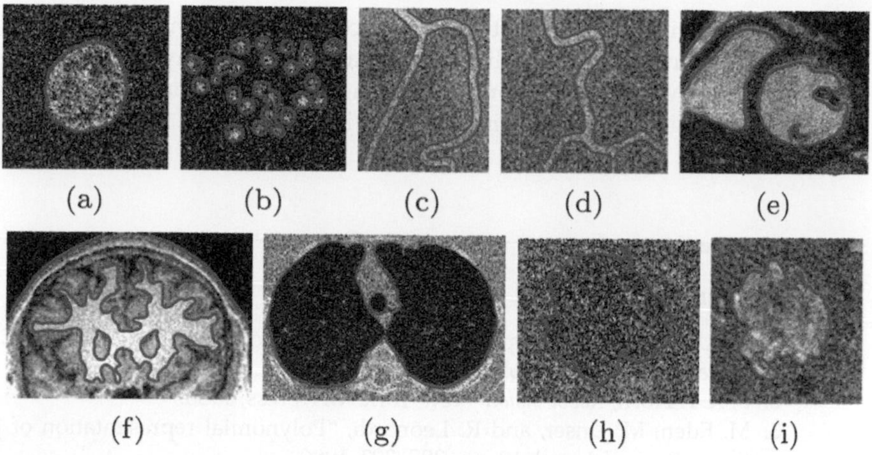

FIGURE 12.21
Segmentation results of medical images with Gaussian noise (variance is 0.02). Note that the initial contours are given as Figure 12.20.

seen that most of the referred methods miss the object contours, while the proposed method can segment most of the objects with low contrast and inhomogeneity.

The proposed method is also tested on these images (in Figure 12.20) with overlapped Gaussian noise (variance is 0.02) which are shown in Figure 12.21. However, despite the destroyed edge structure by noise, the results of these images show the ability of the proposed method to avoid interference. We mentioned that due to the multiple Gaussian kernel gray equalization, global Gaussian fitting energy and global optimization method, the proposed methods have exhibited a certain capability of handling intensity inhomogeneity and high noise robustness.

Experiments demonstrate that the proposed method yields efficient and robust image segmentation in low contrast, noisy, and texture images compared to many famous and newly published level-set methods. Numerical validation experiments on synthesized and medical images demonstrated the advantage of the proposed method.

12.7 Summary and Conclusion

In the field of deformable image segmentation models using B-spline based methods, the key strategy is to express the level-set function as a continuous parametric B-spline functions. This expression show many advantages in segmentation, such as fast convergence and the intrinsic smoothing contour. From the information outlined this chapter, we can say that the B-spline level set can be widely used in medical image segmentation, both in the low-level segmentation model and in models with shape prior.

References

1. M. Unser, "Splines: a perfect fit for signal and image processing," *IEEE Signal Processing Magazine*, vol. 16, pp. 22–38, 1999.
2. B. K. P. Horn, *Robot vision*. New York: MIT Press, 1986.
3. M. Eden, M. Unser, and R. Leonardi, "Polynomial representation of pictures," *Signal Processing*, vol. 10, pp. 385–393, 1986.
4. V. Torre and T. A. Poggio, "On edge detection," *IEEE Transactions on Pattern Analysis and Machine Intelligence*, vol. 8, pp. 147–163, 1986.
5. M. Unser, A. Aldroubi, and M. Eden, "B-spline signal processing: part I-Theory," *Signal Processing IEEE Transactions on*, vol. 41, pp. 821–833, 1993.
6. J. Kittler, "On the accuracy of the Sobel edge detector," *Image and Vision Computing*, vol. 1, pp. 37–42, 1983.
7. Hueckel and H. Manfred, "A Local Visual Operator Which Recognizes Edges and Lines," *Journal of the Association for Computing Machinery*, vol. 20, pp. 634–647, 1973.
8. C. De Boor, *A practical guide to splines*. New York: Springer Verlag, 1978.
9. V. Caselles, R. Kimmel, and G. Sapiro, "Geodesic active contours," *International Journal of Computer Vision*, vol. 22, pp. 61–79, 1997.
10. N. Paragios and R. Deriche, "Geodesic Active Contours and Level Sets for the Detection and Tracking of Moving Objects," *IEEE Transactions on Pattern Analysis and Machine Intelligence*, vol. 22, pp. 266–280, 2000.
11. D. Lingrand, A. Charnoz, P. M. Koulibaly, J. Darcourt, and J. Montagnat, "Toward Accurate Segmentation of the LV Myocardium and Chamber for Volumes Estimation in Gated SPECT Sequences," in *European Conference on Computer Vision*, 2004, pp. 267–278.
12. N. Paragios, M. Rousson, and V. Ramesh, "Knowledge-based Registration & Segmentation of the Left Ventricle: A Level Set Approach," in *IEEE Workshop on Applications of Computer Vision*, 2002, p. 37.
13. J. Park, S. Park, and W. Cho, "Medical Image Segmentation Using Level Set Method with a New Hybrid Speed Function Based on Boundary and Region Segmentation," *Ieice Transactions on Information and Systems*, vol. 95, pp. 2133–2141 2012.
14. T. Mcinerney and D. Terzopoulos, "Deformable models in medical image analysis a survey," in *Mathematical Methods in Biomedical Image Analysis, 1996., Proceedings of the Workshop on*, 2002, pp. 171–180.
15. B. S. Morse, W. Liu, T. S. Yoo, and K. Subramanian, "Active contours using a constraint-based implicit representation," in *ACM SIGGRAPH*, 2005, p. 252.
16. A. Gelas, O. Bernard, D. Friboulet, and R. Prost, "Compactly supported radial basis functions based collocation method for level-set evolution in image segmentation," *IEEE Transactions on Image Processing*, vol. 16, pp. 1873–1887, 2007.

17. O. Bernard, D. Friboulet, P. Thevenaz, and M. Unser, "Variational B-spline level-set method for fast image segmentation," in *IEEE International Symposium on Biomedical Imaging: From Nano To Macro*, 2008, pp. 177–180.
18. O. Bernard, D. Friboulet, P. Thevenaz, and M. Unser, "Variational B-Spline Level-Set: A Linear Filtering Approach for Fast Deformable Model Evolution," *IEEE Transactions on Image Processing A Publication of the IEEE Signal Processing Society*, vol. 18, pp. 1179–1191, 2009.
19. R. Cipolla and A. Blake, "The dynamic analysis of apparent contours," *Proceedings Third International Conference on Computer Vision*, 1990, pp. 616–623.
20. S. Menet, P. Saint-Marc, and G. Medioni,"B-snakes: implementation and application to stereo," *IEEE Transactions on Image Processing*, vol. 9, pp. 720–726, 1990.
21. G. E. Hinton, C. K. I. Williams, and M. D. Revow, "Adaptive elastic models for hand-printed character recognition," in *International Conference on Neural Information Processing Systems*, 1992, pp. 512–519.
22. D. Cremers, F. Tischhäuser, J. Weickert, and C. Schnörr, "Diffusion Snakes: Introducing Statistical Shape Knowledge into the Mumford-Shah Functional," *International Journal of Computer Vision*, vol. 50, pp. 295–313, 2002.
23. D. Mumford and J. Shah, "Optimal approximations by piecewise smooth functions and associated variational problems," *Communications on Pure and Applied Mathematics*, vol. 42, pp. 577–685, 1989.
24. É. Debreuve, M. Gastaud, M. Barlaud, and G. Aubert, "Using the Shape Gradient for Active Contour Segmentation: from the Continuous to the Discrete Formulation," *Journal of Mathematical Imaging and Vision*, vol. 28, pp. 47–66, 2007.
25. P. M. Prenter, *Splines and variational methods*. New York: Wiley, 1975.
26. A. Goshtasby, F. Cheng, and B. A. Barsky, "B -spline curves and surfaces viewed as digital filters," *Computer Vision Graphics & Image Processing*, vol. 52, pp. 264–275, 1990.
27. M. Unser, A. Aldroubi, and M. Eden, "Fast B-spline Transforms for Continuous Image Representation and Interpolation," *IEEE Trans. Pattern Anal. Mach. Intell.*, vol. 13, pp. 277–285, 1991.
28. M. Unser, A. Aldroubi, and M. Eden, "B-spline signal processing: part II-Efficiency design and applications," *IEEE Transactions on Signal Processing*, vol. 41, pp. 834–848, 2002.
29. T. F. Chan and L. A. Vese, "Active contours without edges," *IEEE Transactions on Image Processing*, vol. 10, pp. 266–277, 2001.
30. T.-T. Tran, V.-T. Pham, and K.-K. Shyu, "Moment-based alignment for shape prior with variational B-spline level set," *Machine Vision and Applications*, vol. 24, pp. 1075–1091, 2013.
31. T. T. Tran, V. T. Pham, and K. K. Shyu, *Moment-based alignment for shape prior with variational B-spline level set*: Springer-Verlag New York, Inc., 2013.
32. J. G. Leu, "Shape normalization through compacting," *Pattern Recognition Letters*, vol. 10, pp. 243–250, 1989.
33. S. C. Pei and C. N. Lin, "Image normalization for pattern recognition," *Image & Vision Computing*, vol. 13, pp. 711–723, 1995.
34. H. Ming-Kuei, "Visual pattern recognition by moment invariants," *IRE Transactions on Information Theory*, vol. 8, pp. 179–187, 1962.
35. L. Chunming, X. Chenyang, G. Changfeng, and M. D. Fox, "Level set evolution without re-initialization: a new variational formulation," in *2005 IEEE Computer*

Society Conference on Computer Vision and Pattern Recognition (CVPR'05), vol. 1, pp. 430–436, 2005.

36. D. Cremers, S. J. Osher, and S. Soatto, "Kernel Density Estimation and Intrinsic Alignment for Shape Priors in Level Set Segmentation," *International Journal of Computer Vision*, vol. 69, pp. 335–351, 2006.
37. A. Tsai, A. Yezzi, W. Wells, C. Tempany, D. Tucker, A. Fan, *et al.*, "A shape-based approach to the segmentation of medical imagery using level sets," *IEEE Transactions on Medical Imaging*, vol. 22, pp. 137–154, 2003.
38. W. Liu, Y. Shang, X. Yang, R. Deklerck, and J. Cornelis, "A shape prior constraint for implicit active contours," *Pattern Recognition Letters*, vol. 32, pp. 1937–1947, 2011.
39. V.-T. Pham, T.-T. Tran, K.-K. Shyu, L.-Y. Lin, Y.-H. Wang, and M.-T. Lo, "Multiphase B-spline level set and incremental shape priors with applications to segmentation and tracking of left ventricle in cardiac MR images," *Machine Vision and Applications*, vol. 25, pp. 1967–1987, November 01 2014.
40. M. E. Leventon, W. E. L. Grimson, and O. Faugeras, "Statistical shape influence in geodesic active contours," in *5th IEEE EMBS International Summer School on Biomedical Imaging, 2002*.
41. D. A. Ross, J. Lim, R. S. Lin, and M. H. Yang, "Incremental Learning for Robust Visual Tracking," *International Journal of Computer Vision*, vol. 77, pp. 125–141, 2008.
42. L. A. Vese and T. F. Chan, "A Multiphase Level Set Framework for Image Segmentation Using the Mumford and Shah Model," *International Journal of Computer Vision*, vol. 50, pp. 271–293, 2002.
43. N. Vu and B. S. Manjunath, "Shape prior segmentation of multiple objects with graph cuts," in *Computer Vision and Pattern Recognition, 2008. CVPR 2008. IEEE Conference on*, 2008, pp. 1–8.
44. J. Woo, P. J. Slomka, C. C. J. Kuo, and B. W. Hong, "Multiphase segmentation using an implicit dual shape prior: Application to detection of left ventricle in cardiac MRI," *Computer Vision & Image Understanding*, vol. 117, pp. 1084–1094, 2013.
45. S. Zheng, B. Fang, L. Li, M. Gao, R. Chen, and K. Peng, "B-Spline based globally optimal segmentation combining low-level and high-level information," *Pattern Recognition*, vol. 73, pp. 144–157, 2018.
46. T. F. Chan, S. Esedoglu, and M. Nikolova, "Algorithms for Finding Global Minimizers of Image Segmentation and Denoising Models," *SIAM Journal on Applied Mathematics*, vol. 66, pp. 1632–1648, 2006.
47. T. Goldstein and S. Osher, "The Split Bregman Method for L1-Regularized Problems," *SIAM Journal on Imaging Sciences*, vol. 2, pp. 323–343, 2009.
48. C. Li, C. Xu, C. Gui, and M. D. Fox, "Distance Regularized Level Set Evolution and Its Application to Image Segmentation," *IEEE Transactions on Image Processing*, vol. 19, pp. 3243–3254, 2010.
49. L. Wang, L. He, A. Mishra, and C. Li, "Active contours driven by local Gaussian distribution fitting energy," *Signal Processing*, vol. 89, pp. 2435–2447, 2009.
50. M. Jung, G. Peyré, and L. D. Cohen, "Nonlocal Active Contours," *SIAM Journal on Imaging Sciences*, vol. 5, pp. 1022–1054, 2012.
51. V. Estellers, D. Zosso, R. Lai, S. Osher, J. P. Thiran, and X. Bresson, "Efficient Algorithm for Level Set Method Preserving Distance Function," *IEEE Transactions on Image Processing*, vol. 21, pp. 4722–4734, 2012.

52. J. Wang and K. L. Chan, "Incorporating Patch Subspace Model in Mumford–Shah Type Active Contours," *IEEE Transactions on Image Processing*, vol. 22, pp. 4473–4485, 2013.
53. L. Dai, J. Ding, and J. Yang, "Inhomogeneity-embedded active contour for natural image segmentation," *Pattern Recognition*, vol. 48, pp. 2513–2529, 2015.
54. K. Zhang, L. Zhang, K. M. Lam, and D. Zhang, "A Level Set Approach to Image Segmentation With Intensity Inhomogeneity," *IEEE Transactions on Cybernetics*, vol. 46, pp. 546–557, 2016.

Index

Note: Page numbers in *italics* indicate figure and those in **bold** indicate table.

Printed and bound by CPI Group (UK) Ltd, Croydon, CR0 4YY
17/10/2024
01775660-0013